The Treatment of
Renal Failure

The Treatment of Renal Failure

Edited by
J. E. Castro

BSc, MRCS, LRCP, MB, BS, FRCSE, FRCS, MS, PhD
146 Harley Street, London

Springer-Science+Business Media, B.V.

British Library Cataloguing in Publication Data

Treatment of renal failure.
 1. Renal insufficiency
 I. Castro, J. E.
 616.6'14   RC918.R4

ISBN 978-94-011-7706-1   ISBN 978-94-011-7704-7 (eBook)
DOI 10.1007/978-94-011-7704-7

Copyright © 1982 Springer Science+Business Media Dordrecht
 Originally published by MTP Press Limited in 1982
 Softcover reprint of the hardcover 1st edition 1982

Mather Bros (Printers) Ltd Preston

Contents

List of Contributors

V. E. ANDREUCCI
Department of Nephrology, Second Faculty of Medicine, University of Naples, Via S. Pansini, 80131 Naples, Italy

F. H. BACH
Department of Laboratory Medicine and Pathology, University of Minnesota, Minnesota, USA

J. E. CASTRO
Consultant Urologist and Transplant Surgeon, 146 Harley Street, London W1N 1AH, England

D. N. S. KERR
Department of Medicine, Royal Victoria Infirmary, Newcastle upon Tyne, NE1 4LP, England

D. G. OREOPOULOS
Department of Medicine, University of Toronto: Peritoneal Dialysis Unit, Toronto Western Hospital, 399 Bathurst Street, Toronto, Ontario M5T 2S8, Canada

D. J. RAINFORD
Department of Renal Medicine, Princess Mary's Royal Air Force Hospital, Halton, Aylesbury, Bucks., HP22 5PS, England

B. H. B. ROBINSON
Consultant Physician, East Birmingham Hospital, Bordesley Green East, Birmingham B9 5ST, England

G. WILLIAMS
Department of Surgery, Royal Postgraduate Medical School, Hammersmith Hospital, Du Cane Road, London W12 0HS, England

1

Acute renal failure

D. J. Rainford

INTRODUCTION

The management of acute renal failure (ARF) is perhaps one of the most exciting and satisfying aspects of modern medicine. The fact that acute renal failure may follow vasomotor or nephrotoxic insults of such a wide variety means that the physician can expect to encounter patients from every department of the hospital. He can therefore also expect to learn a great deal about the practice of his colleagues' specialities.

The modern management of acute renal failure is an exercise in intensive care. It is important to be meticulous and to pay strict attention to detail if the desired result is to be achieved. As in all other aspects of intensive care, interdepartmental co-operation is essential. The presence of renal failure must never allow one to lose sight of the patient's underlying condition, as failure to appreciate this will reduce the chances of effective renal recovery. As will be seen, the mortality rate of patients with acute renal failure is very closely related to the antecedent underlying condition.

There has been a change in the pattern of acute renal failure over the years since treatment first became available. In the early years, many cases were of obstetric origin or due to early shock and poor initial resuscitation. The advent of intensive care, improved resuscitation and antenatal care has had a profound influence on the sort of cases with which we are now being presented. The importance of early and adequate resuscitation after trauma has been well demonstrated by the American Services in the South East Asian conflicts. Adherence to this principle with early evacuation of the injured reduced the incidence of acute renal failure in the seriously injured from 1:200 in Korea to 1:600 in Vietnam[1]. Today, many of our patients are severely ill, often with late-onset acute renal failure due to sepsis or nephrotoxic drug administration. Their survival to the stage of developing renal

1

failure is a tribute to modern nursing and medical care and their ultimate survival a tribute to the work of the pioneers of dialysis.

THE PATHOPHYSIOLOGY OF ACUTE RENAL FAILURE

The pathophysiology of acute renal failure has been the subject of several excellent reviews[2-4]. However, the precise mechanisms involved have still to be elucidated. Following the initial ischaemic or nephrotoxic insult, the questions arise as to why some people develop ARF, and, in those that do, what pathogenetic factors are involved. Various theories have been put forward over the years and each has been studied in depth. Each has its merits and its pitfalls and it is even possible that we should not be looking for a common answer to all forms of acute renal failure.

The four main theories which are commonly recognized are:

(1) Tubular obstruction.
(2) Interstitial oedema and passive backflow of glomerular filtrate at tubular level.
(3) Altered renal haemodynamics.
(4) Disseminated intravascular coagulation.

Tubular obstruction

The recognition by York and Nauss[5] in 1911 of tubular casts of haemoglobin in patients with acute renal failure and haemolytic disease suggested that tubular obstruction may be an important causative factor in acute renal failure. The presence of myoglobin casts in the tubules was highlighted again in the early papers on crush syndrome, but their inconstant presence as a histological feature led Bywaters and Dible[6] to reject the cast blockage theory. In patients with ARF consequent upon heat exhaustion, casts of myoglobin have been demonstrated in the distal tubules of those cases who have been biopsied[7]. Jaenike[8], using a rat model of acute renal failure induced by methaemoglobin, found, by micropuncture studies, that intratubular pressure was raised in some tubules, whilst others were collapsed. Cirksena[9] found a fall in intratubular pressure despite the presence of pigment casts. Oken and his colleagues[10] found no rise in intratubular pressure and were able to wash out early sludge using pressures below that of the presumed filtration pressure, although high pressures were required to dislodge fully formed casts. Their conclusion was that tubular obstruction did not cause oliguria but could have a role in maintaining it.

The literature is both contradictory and confusing, but it is certainly difficult to justify, on the evidence that we have, a primary role for tubular obstruction in the pathogenesis of acute renal failure.

Interstitial oedema and passive backflow of filtrate

The gross macrosopic finding of large swollen kidneys in acute renal failure, together with histological features of interstitial oedema, led to the belief that increased interstitial pressure may cause tubular collapse. Flanigan and Oken[11] found pressures in the tubules and the peritubular capillaries to be similar, and Munck[12] found 'wedged renal venous pressure' to be similar in normal patients and those with acute renal failure. The demonstration of breaks in the basement membrane of the tubules by Oliver and his colleagues[13] in their elegant microdissection studies suggested that back diffusion of filtrate may be the cause of oliguria. This theory was enhanced by Bank and his colleagues[14], who recorded excessive reabsorption of lissamine green from proximal tubules in acute renal failure. This work has never really been substantiated. Indeed, Flamembaum[15], using micropuncture techniques in rats with HgCl-induced ARF, found a constant single nephron glomerular filtration rate (SNGFR), measured by inulin clearance, whatever the site of tubular micropuncture. The latest evidence from extensive studies in several models of ARF by Mason and Thurau[16] puts yet another nail in the coffin of the theory that back diffusion of filtrate plays a primary role.

The author's feelings are that passive back diffusion, if it does occur to any extent, is an epiphenomenon that has little contribution to make in the pathogenesis of ARF, but again may contribute to the maintenance of oliguria.

Altered renal haemodynamics

Trueta[17] showed that stimulation of the splanchnic and sciatic nerves of rabbits caused a redistribution of blood flow away from the cortex to the medulla with relative cortical ischaemia. This same redistribution of blood flow has now been shown to occur in human acute renal failure, both in postsurgical and nephrotoxic cases. What causes this redistribution of blood flow, and what perpetuates it, are questions which are not as yet fully answered.

Goormaghtigh[18], as long ago as 1945, recognized that, in histological specimens of the kidney from patients with crush syndrome, there was increased granularity and hypertrophy of cells in the juxtaglomerular apparatus. His conclusions have stimulated considerable research into the role of the renin–angiotensin–aldosterone system in the pathogenesis of acute renal failure.

Plasma renin levels in acute renal failure are raised in some cases, but not in others[19]. Certainly, acute renal failure is more likely to occur in dehydrated, salt-depleted states when renin levels are often at their highest. Renin depletion of rats by chronic salt loading has been shown in several models to protect the animal from acute renal failure[20,21]. However, measures which reduce plasma renin without depleting intrarenal renin are not protective [21]. It is clear, therefore, that, if renin has a role to play, it is at a local level within the kidney. It has been shown[22,23] that there is a tubulo-glomerular feedback mechanism acting to control salt excretion by continuously adjusting the glomerular filtration rate to the reabsorptive capacity of the proximal tubule. The presentation of increasing amounts of sodium chloride acutely to the macula densa leads to an increase in local renin production. Angiotensin I is converted locally to angiotensin II which will cause afferent arteriolar constriction, thus lowering GFR. This could help to explain the oliguria of AFR, providing the tubuloglomerular feedback mechanisms are still active in the pathological state. Mason[24], in her beautiful micropipette studies, has shown that this mechanism is operative in her model of acute renal failure.

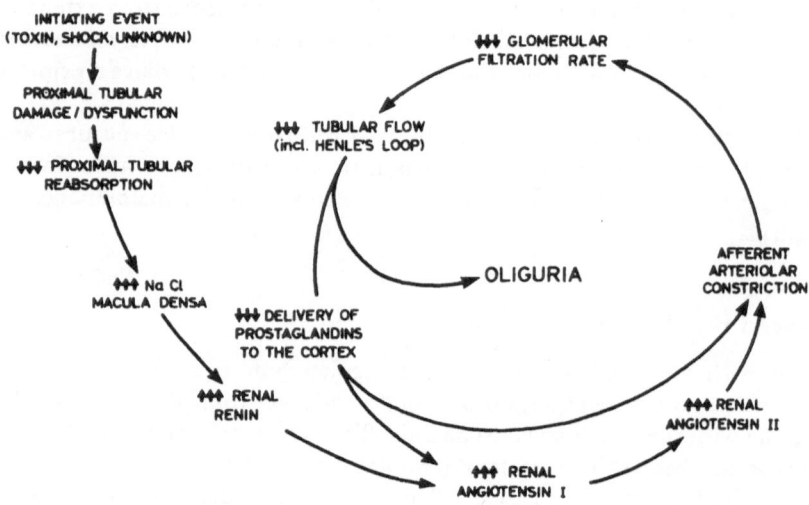

Figure 1 Pathogenesis of acute renal failure. From reference 4, by kind permission of Dr Andreucci

Prostaglandins, produced in the renal medulla, are powerful vasodilators, acting mainly at cortical level. Why are they not protective against the action of the angiotensin II? Torres[25] has produced evidence that prostaglandins will protect against circulatory but not nephrotoxic acute renal failure and administration of prostaglandin antagonists will predispose to acute renal failure in circulatory ARF. Oken[26] has been unable to substantiate this and could not produce an increased susceptibility to ARF in salt-loaded rats treated with very large doses of indomethacin.

Prostaglandins probably travel to the site of their action via the loop of Henle. As Oken[26] hypothesizes, initially the renin–angiotensin mechanism swamps the prostaglandin activity and the subsequent fall in GFR reduces effective delivery to their site of action. Therefore, less intense vasoconstrictor stimuli, unopposed by prostaglandins, might be enough to perpetuate acute renal failure. In terms of the protective effects of salt loading, he also points out that this will not only deplete renin, but also enhance prostaglandin synthesis and decrease vascular susceptibility to catecholamines.

Andreucci[4] has evaluated all the foregoing evidence and produced his theory as shown graphically in Figure 1. The author considers that this summarizes well the state of present knowledge and presents a workable hypothesis.

Disseminated intravascular coagulation

No section on the pathogenesis of acute renal failure can be considered complete without considering disseminated intravascular coagulation (DIC). Acute renal failure can be perhaps divided into two groups. Firstly, where DIC is primary and histologically demonstrable as important, and secondly, where the role of DIC is tenuous.

Histologically identifiable evidence of DIC in the pathogenesis of acute renal failure can be seen in the haemolytic uraemic syndrome[27], Robson's syndrome[28] and accelerated hypertension[29].

However, what part, if any, does it play in the pathogenesis of acute tubular necrosis? DIC is a common phenomenon in many situations where acute tubular necrosis is likely to develop, viz. septicaemia, shock, postpartum haemorrhage, pancreatitis and burns. In the author's experience, frank DIC is uncommon in uncomplicated acute tubular necrosis, but fibrin degradation products in the blood are often raised to around 40 µg/ml. It is not always possible to demonstrate the presence of fibrin in the kidneys of all patients with ARF, and it has been suggested by Menon[30] and his colleagues that this is due to rapid fibrinolysis in the kidney.

The importance of endotoxinaemia in stimulating DIC as a contribution to the pathogenesis of ARF has been well described by Wardle[31].

Spink[32] and his colleagues have shown that, during the generalized Schwartzmann reaction, there is excessive catecholamine release. This may be the instigator of initial renal vasoconstriction, thus stimulating the cycle shown in Figure 1. Even if DIC is a transient phenomenon in uncomplicated ARF, the possibility exists that it may be the arbiter of initial vasconstriction.

DIC may be more important in the pathogenesis of bilateral cortical necrosis, which, though uncommon, seems to occur more often in patients where frank DIC is evident and renal vasoconstriction is much more severe.

THE DIAGNOSIS OF ACUTE RENAL FAILURE

The diagnosis of established acute renal failure rarely presents a problem, except perhaps in the search for the aetiology. Many biochemical variables and ratios have been suggested, each of which will be discussed briefly, but there is no doubt in my mind that simple measurement of an incessant rise in serum creatinine is by far the most important marker.

There is no substitute for suspicion and clinical awareness in the early diagnosis. Patients who are particularly at risk, particularly post-aortic graft and bypass cases, severe trauma, septicaemias and obstetric accidents, should be carefully monitored with daily creatinine clearance measurements. Differentiation between pre-renal and intrinsic renal failure is important, because failure to treat the former may rapidly lead to the latter. All patients with oliguria should have a central venous pressure line inserted to assess hydration. If the central venous pressure is low, simple volume repletion may be all that is required to re-establish urine flow. It should be remembered that diuresis following rehydration may be delayed by several hours[33]. This delay in diuresis may well explain some of the recorded good responses to frusemide in 'averting' acute renal failure[34]. The author's experience is that if there is no response to volume repletion, then renal failure is established and frusemide has no place in management. The administration of mannitol may have a prophylactic place in high risk situations[35, 36]. Thurau[37] has suggested that it maintains the flow of urine in the region of the macula densa, preventing activation of vasoconstriction via the renin–angiotensin system. In the fully hydrated patient, its use to try to promote a diuresis must be cautious to prevent fluid overload. In keeping with Thurau's[37] theory the author has only found it useful in renal shutdown after uncomplicated haemorrhagic shock.

Urine volume

The measurement of urine volume to diagnose acute renal failure is notoriously unreliable. Non-oliguric renal failure is not uncommon in burns, and this was first highlighted by Graber and Sevitt[38]. It is also common in patients with renal failure due to acute interstitial nephritis[39]. In this situation, however, urine output rarely exceeds 2–2.5 l/day. A falling urinary output in a well-hydrated patient at risk for acute renal failure should nevertheless alert the physician to investigate the patient further.

Blood urea

Unlike creatinine, the blood urea level is dependent on too many other factors to be of use in isolation in the diagnosis of acute renal failure. For example, dehydration and the heavy protein meal of gastrointestinal haemorrhage will both cause a rise in blood urea in the presence of normal renal function. The author has seen several cases of severe acute renal failure with normal or low blood urea levels in the presence of severe hepatic failure. However, the rate of rise of blood urea in established ARF is the best indicator of the rate of catabolism and has a profound influence on further management.

The use of urine:plasma urea ratios as an indication of concentrating ability, and hence of tubular integrity, is only helpful if the ratio is > 10:1. Ratios below this do not necessarily imply that ARF is present.

Urinary sodium

Urinary sodium in established ARF is usually > 70 mmol/l. However, the levels are so variable that its diagnostic significance is of limited value[36].

Urine/plasma osmolality ratio

Eliahou and Bata[40] in 1965 described the use of urine:plasma osmolality ratios to distinguish reversible pre-renal from established ARF. A high ratio (> 1.8–2.0) will certainly distinguish those patients who are dehydrated, presuming they have antecedent normal renal function. Ratios of < 1.1:1, however, can be seen without ARF, especially if prior administration of a high dose of frusemide has occurred, and indeed in normal subjects[2].

Urinary sediment

Haematuria, proteinuria and increased cell excretion are common features of acute renal failure. However, the presence of casts may be useful in suggesting glomerulonephritis as the cause of the acute renal failure.

Serum creatinine

Serum creatinine is relatively independent of factors other than glomerular filtration rate, and, in the author's experience, creatinine clearance is the best indicator of declining renal function and a rising serum creatinine the best marker of acute renal failure. All the other variables are of little use in isolation, but, used together, will help to confirm a diagnostic suspicion.

Obstruction

In order to differentiate obstruction of the urinary tract from acute intrinsic renal failure, the use of high dose intravenous urography, isotope renography and grey-scale ultrasound are extremely useful and obviate the

necessity for retrograde pyelography in most cases. The high-dose intravenous urogram may also be of some assistance in the differential diagnosis
of the cause of acute renal failure[41].

Intravenous urography

High-dose intravenous urography is a safe procedure in patients with acute
renal failure[42]. The slow appearance of a nephrogram which becomes denser
over 24 hours is indicative of obstructive uropathy. Occasionally a pyelo-
gram will be seen which may even indicate the site of obstruction. Cattell
and his colleagues[41] showed the appearance of an early dense persisting
nephrogram in all patients with acute uncomplicated tubular necrosis and in
patients with acute oliguric pyelonephritis. It is, however, important that
their protocol is strictly adhered to in order to maintain reproducible and
valid results. We have not always found this particular pattern in uncomplicated acute tubular necrosis, even when confirmed by renal biopsy, but,
when it occurs, it is indeed additional confirmatory evidence of one's clinical
suspicion (Figure 2). The subject of renal radiology in acute renal failure has
been excellently reviewed recently[43].

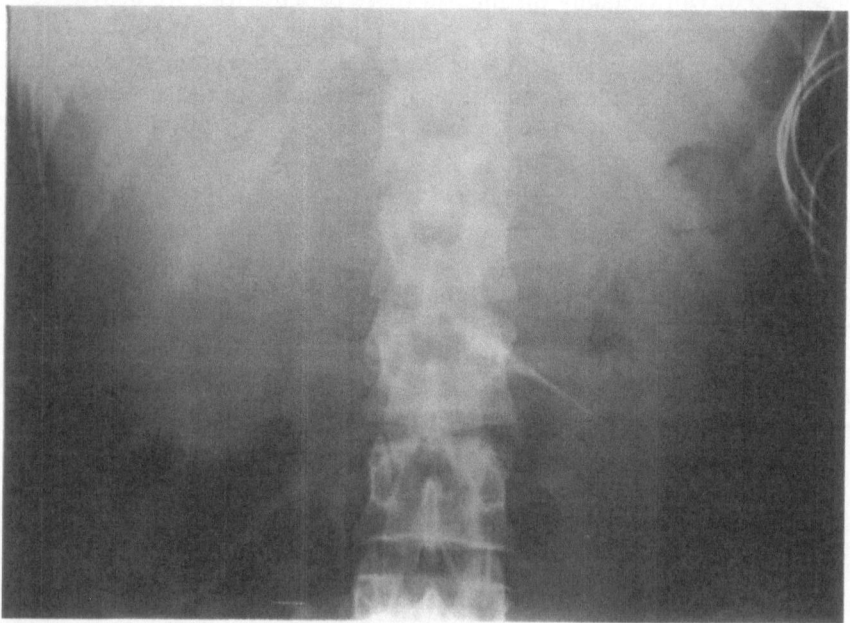

(a)

Figure 2   This patient was struck a glancing blow by a car and developed acute renal failure.
(a) Shows an instant dense persistent nephrogram on the right but just a renal outline on the
left. (b) Angiography shows suspected avulsion of left kidney. (c) Post-recovery IVU shows
normal right kidney. Diagnosis—avulsed left kidney, ATN on the right

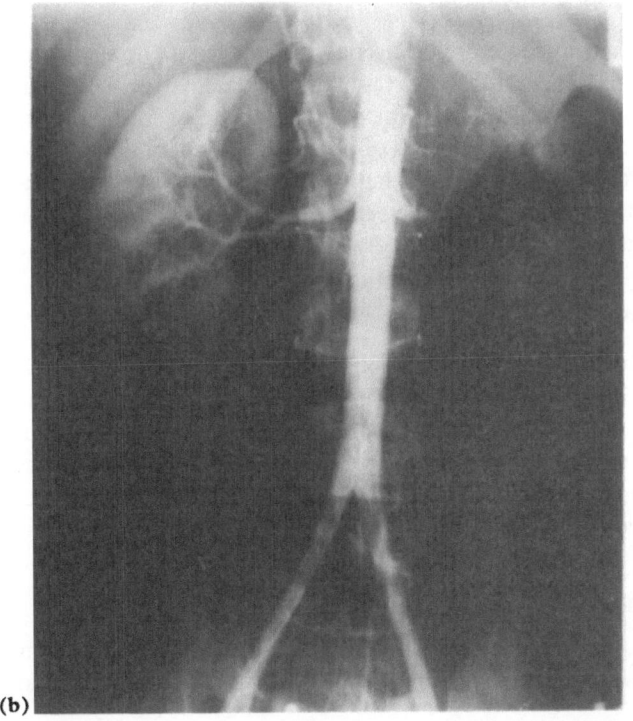

(b)

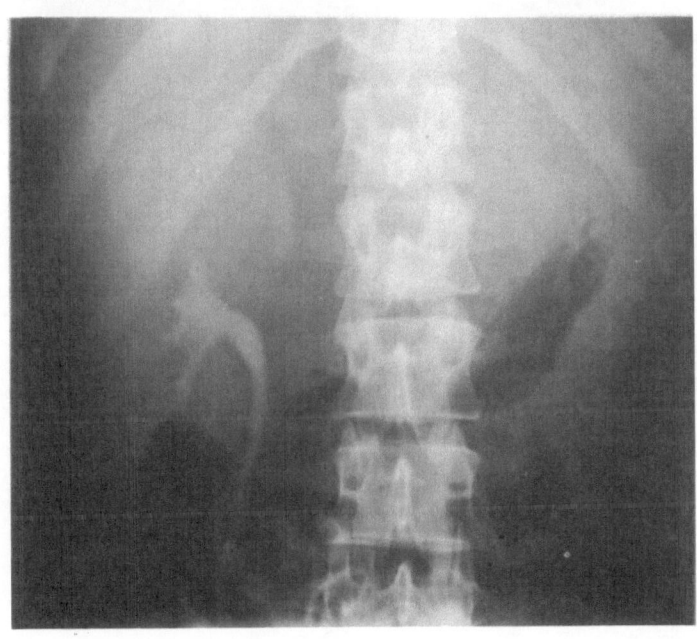

(c)

Isotope renography

The renogram in acute oliguric renal failure shows initially symmetrically slowly rising traces which progressively become flatter as tubular necrosis becomes more established[44]. The only real value of isotope renography in this situation is in the exclusion of obstruction, where the traces tend to be asymmetrical. After acute renal failure has been established for more than a few days, the results of isotope renography become confusing and should not be used in isolation to diagnose obstruction.

Ultrasound

The use of ultrasound to exclude obstruction of the urinary tract is now our first line of investigation. In experienced hands it takes only a few minutes to give an answer. It also has the advantage of being non-invasive and requires no preparation of the patient (Figure 3). It is also possible to assess renal size, which may be of assistance in the diagnosis, particularly when chronic renal failure is suspected.

Angiography

In patients who are anuric after aortic grafting or where renal artery occlusion is suspected, it is important to know if the renal arteries are patent.

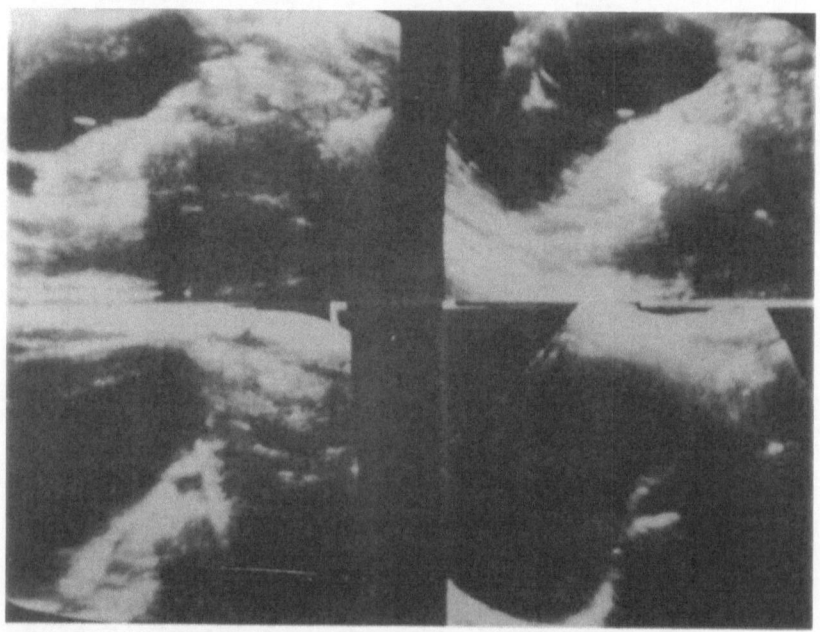

(a)

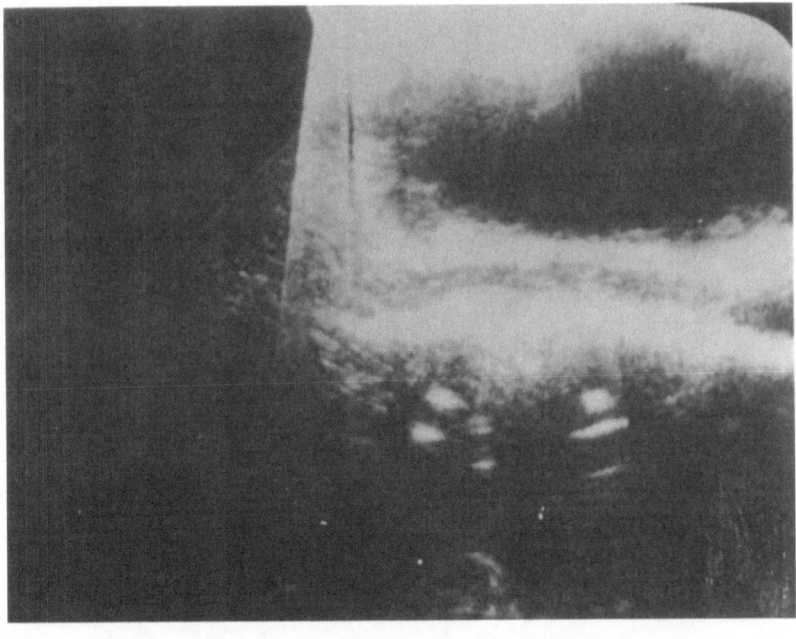

(b)

Figure 3 (a) Grey-scale ultrasound scan in the transverse plane shows large hydronephrosis. (b) Longitudinal scan to show extent of obstruction

If an aorto-iliac trouser graft has been inserted, transfemoral arteriography is not without hazard. Radiographs can, however, be taken using the brachial approach. We have found the technique of intravenous arteriography, as described by Joffre and his colleagues[45], particularly useful. In essence, a high dose of contrast is given rapidly intravenously and a previously determined level of tomogram cut taken at 15 seconds (see Figure 4).

Renal biopsy

The value of renal biopsy in the investigation and diagnosis of acute renal failure is undoubted but is not without hazard and should be reserved for those cases where:

    (1) There is reason to doubt a diagnosis of acute tubular necrosis.
    (2) Acute glomerular nephritis or a systemic disorder is suspected.
    (3) Historically acute interstitial nephritis is suspected.
    (4) Oliguria is prolonged beyond 6 weeks.

It is the author's practice to dialyse the patient adequately first to reduce bleeding tendencies and to perform a percutaneous renal biopsy 6 hours

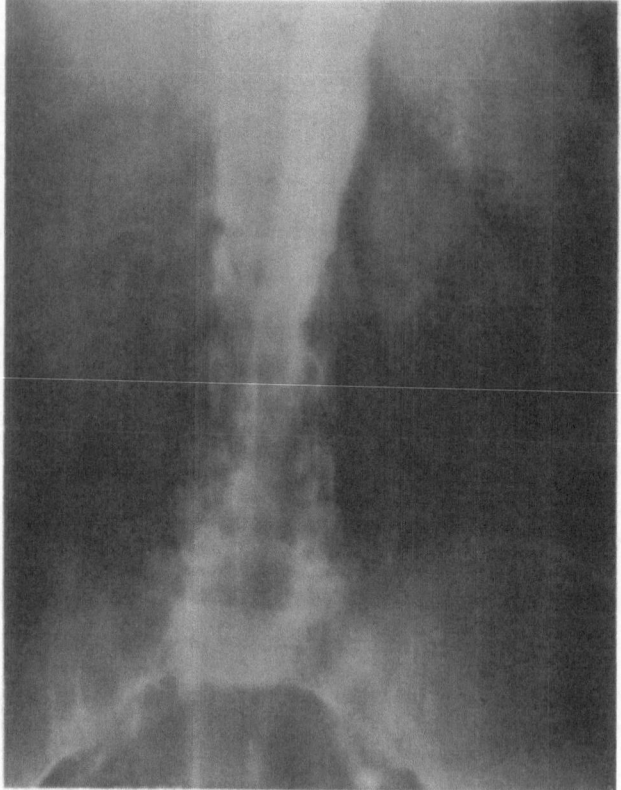

Figure 4 Shows patent renal vessels in a patient with acute anuria following aortic graft, using high-dose intravenous arteriography

later. If possible dialysis is deferred for 24 hours. To date, we have had no post-biopsy bleeding that has necessitated transfusion.

When the diagnosis is one of acute glomerular nephritis or a systemic disorder, such as lupus erythematosus, immunosuppression or plasma-phoresis may be indicated (see below).

If acute interstitial nephritis is present, the judicious administration of high-dose methyl prednisolone often reverses the acute renal failure within 48 hours[39].

The finding of cortical necrosis in a patient with prolonged oliguria should not deter one from continuing therapy. Cortical necrosis is often patchy, especially following the haemolytic uraemic syndrome or a severe disseminated intravascular coagulapathy. The author now has several patients who have ultimately diuresed and attained creatinine clearances of greater than 50 ml/min.

The diagnosis of acute renal failure is therefore not difficult. A good history, if obtainable, paying particular attention to exposure to toxins (including drug administration!), a thorough clinical examination and the use of some of the more specialized techniques described above will usually give some clues as to aetiology.

The majority of patients will have acute tubular necrosis and management should be directed along the lines described.

THE MANAGEMENT OF ACUTE RENAL FAILURE

The management of established acute renal failure is based on four main principles:

(a) Regulation of fluid and electrolyte balance.
(b) Control of nitrogen retention.
(c) Provision of adequate nutrition.
(d) Treatment of the underlying condition.

These principles are inseparable and therapy should be directed so that they can be strictly observed. Figure 5 outlines the initial management of a patient with oliguria and a rising blood urea.

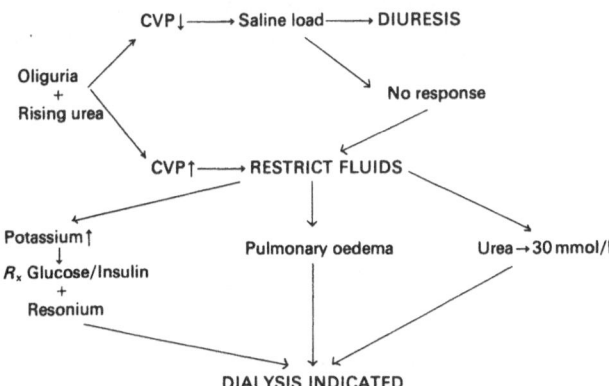

Figure 5   The initial management of suspected acute renal failure

The use of dialysis therapy allows easy regulation of fluid and electrolyte balance and control of nitrogen retention. It also provides intravascular 'space' for administration of adequate nutrition to prevent a negative nitrogen balance. In many cases, as will be seen, the provision of space for feeding is often the most cogent reason for dialysis[46]. There is virtually no place nowadays for conservative management of established oliguric acute renal failure as the fluid limitations preclude the administration of adequate nutrition, even in non-catabolic patients.

Haemodialysis or peritoneal dialysis?

Having decided that a patient must embark on a course of dialysis, a decision must be made as to whether haemodialysis or peritoneal dialysis is more appropriate.

Peritoneal dialysis has the advantage that it can be performed adequately without resort to expensive or sophisticated equipment. However, in patients who are severely catabolic (i.e. blood urea levels rising faster than 10 mmol/24 h), peritoneal dialysis is not efficient enough to cope[47]. The only exception is in the child, where peritoneal dialysis is more efficient than in the adult, as the peritoneal surface area is proportionately greater. Patients who have recently undergone abdominal surgery, particularly if there are drains *in situ*, are not suitable for peritoneal dialysis for obvious reasons.

Peritoneal dialysis should be reserved for the uncomplicated non-catabolic patient, children, and those where acute or chronic renal failure is suspected. In the latter situation, peritoneal dialysis is less likely to cause disequilibration and it buys time to assess suitability for long-term haemodialysis in the event of inadequate recovery. We have found no contra-indication to haemodialysis even in haemorrhagic states[46].

Occasionally, peritoneal dialysis and haemodialysis may be combined. In our practice, this has been used in patients with acute pancreatitis and renal failure. The series is too small to derive any definite conclusions, but, on theoretical grounds, washing the peritoneum clear of pancreatic enzymes should be of some help in preventing autodigestion.

Peritoneal dialysis will not be discussed here, as it will be dealt with in Chapter 3.

Haemodialysis

In order to practise good haemodialysis, it is important to establish efficient vascular access. The principles of vascular access surgery are discussed in Chapter 4. However, there are certain points about vascular access in acute renal failure which are worth noting.

It is the author's practice to insert arteriovenous shunts in these patients under local anaesthesia. This avoids the problems associated with general anaesthesia in the seriously ill patient. They are inserted by the renal physician who is subsequently responsible for shunt care.

A wrist shunt inserted into the radial artery and the cephalic vein is the preferred site. This can be completed in less than half an hour with a minimum of surgical skill and a straight Silastic–Teflon shunt devised by C. T. Flynn[48] is used at our centre (see Figure 6). However, if there is a possibility of acute on chronic renal failure, it may be preferable to insert an ankle shunt to keep the wrist vessels for the formation of an arteriovenous fistula, and if, as is often the case, forearm vessels have been used for other ward or intensive care procedures, then a standard Ramirez[49] shunt may be placed at the ankle in the posterior tibial artery and long saphenous vein. Occasionally, neither upper nor lower limbs are suitable. Under these circumstances access can be obtained by inserting catheters into the inferior vena cava via the femoral vein[50, 51] or into the superior vena cava via the subclavian vein. More recently, we have used a single catheter inserted into a great vein and effected dialysis using a unipuncture control apparatus[52].

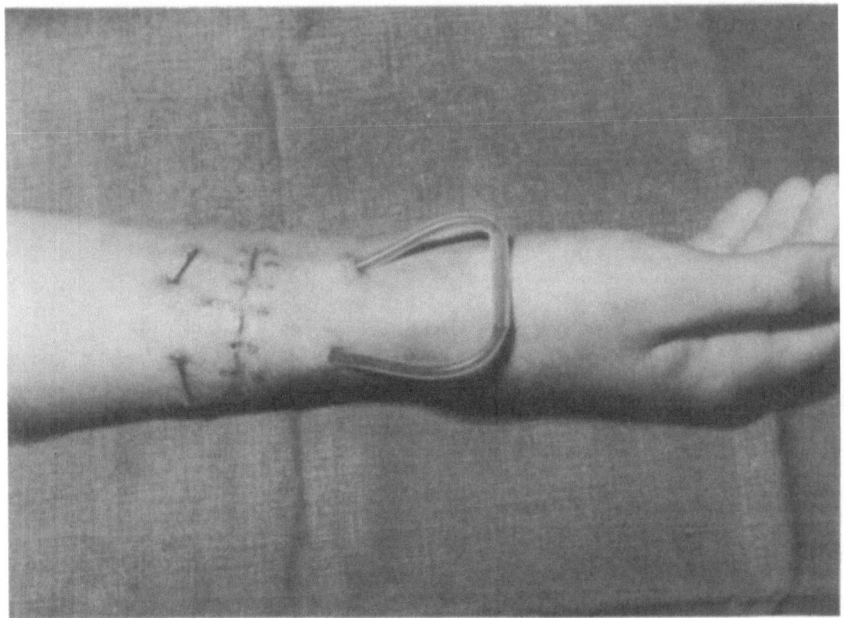

Figure 6   A straight Silastic wrist shunt

Frequency of dialysis

The frequency of dialysis will be governed by the rate of catabolism and the requirement to remove fluid.

It has been shown that maintenance of the blood urea below 200 mg/100 ml (approximately 33 mmol/l) reduces dramatically the incidence of 'uraemic' complications[53, 54]. Particularly in the hypercatabolic patient, dialysis should be scheduled to allow sufficient nutritional intake[55]. This almost invariably means daily dialysis.

Nutrition in acute renal failure

The importance of nutrition in the management of the patient with acute renal failure cannot be overemphasized (Figure 7). Failure to remember this

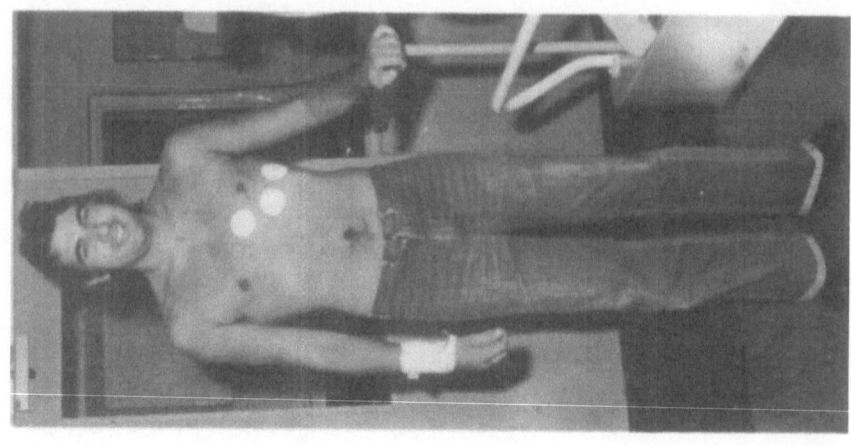

(b)

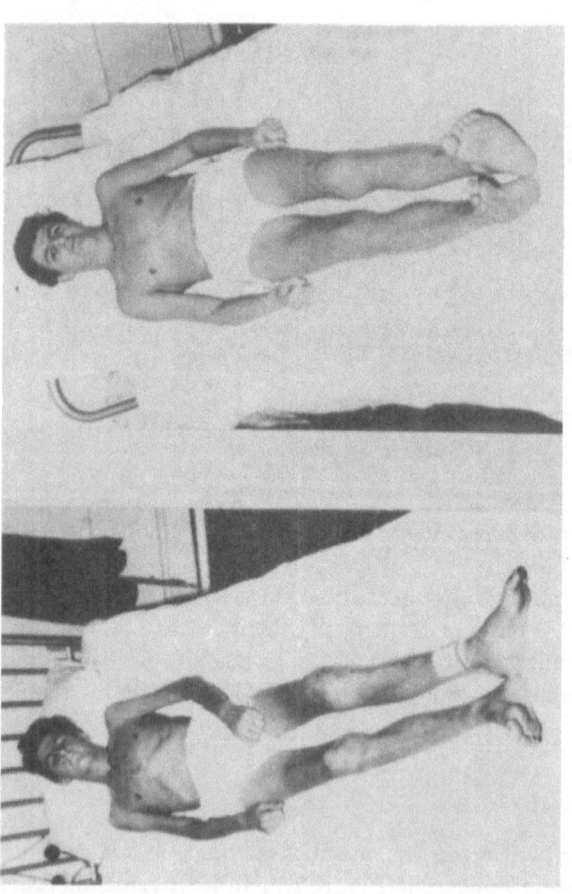

(a)

Figure 7 (a) These pictures were taken before the use of total parenteral nutrition in the management of acute renal failure. The picture on the left shows a young man after 6 weeks oliguria at the onset of diuresis. The right-hand picture shows him 6 weeks later and demonstrates how much muscle mass he lost during his acute illness. (b) This picture shows a young man on the day after removal of his central feeding line. He had just completed 6 weeks haemodialysis for acute renal failure and was parenterally fed

will lead to increasing endogenous protein breakdown, a rapidly rising blood urea, and a severe negative nitrogen balance. The consequences of a severe negative nitrogen balance are well known. Of particular importance to the patient are diminished wound healing[56,57] and a decreased resistance to infection[58]. Cellular and humoral immunity are depressed both by the negative nitrogen balance and the uraemic state.

Infection is the major cause of death in acute renal failure[59-61]. In Lordon's series[61], it accounted for 72% of deaths. It thus behoves us to attempt to improve the patients' resistance to infection, in an effort to improve their prognosis.

The attention to adequate nutrition, supplemented by frequent dialysis, has reduced the mortality of post-traumatic acute renal failure patients in our own series from 66% to 36%. This dramatic improvement in survival has also been seen by Abel and his associates[62].

If patients can be fed orally, then this avoids the use of central lines and is clearly the method of choice. Patients should be allowed a free diet and a fluid intake of up to 1.5 l/day. Dialysis should be tailored to cope with this regime, rather than reducing nutrition to suit the dialysis schedule.

Most patients who suffer acute renal failure, however, are unable to tolerate oral feeding, either because of intestinal ileus, anorexia, nausea and vomiting, or poor gastrointestinal absorption. Under these circumstances, the use of total parenteral nutrition is vital.

A detailed account of intravenous nutritional management is excellently described by Lee[63]. This section will therefore be confined to some of the more salient and important features.

Energy is provided using dextrose and Intralipid as the substrates. Nitrogen is provided as a synthetic crystalline amino acid solution. Insulin is given, both to control the blood sugar level and also for its anabolic effects. Hinton[64] demonstrated in patients with severe burns that, during glucose and insulin infusion, there was a fall in the catabolic rate of protein from approximately 300 g to 130 g daily. To provide 300 g of protein daily is difficult, but to provide 130 g is quite possible.

We have found that the administration of insulin by continuous infusion, using a pump, allows smoother and safer control than adding a bolus to the dextrose solution. The correct dose is estimated by frequent blood glucose estimations, but, as a guide, this usually lies between one and five units per hour.

Triglyceride metabolism is deranged in acute renal failure, and, until the uraemia is well controlled by dialysis, fat solutions may accumulate in the blood. A simple way of estimating whether or not fats are being efficiently metabolized is to examine a sample of plasma prior to dialysis (at least 4 hours postinfusion). If the plasma is clear, then utilization is satisfactory.

There are many amino acid solutions available and it is a matter of personal preference which one is used. Vamin (Kabi-Vitrum) provides a good balanced amino acid profile. Synthamin-17 (Baxter-Travenol) allows the administration of 17 g of nitrogen for only 1 litre of fluid, thus reducing the amount of 'space' that has to be made by ultrafiltration on dialysis. This preparation has been criticized because of the glycine content, but we have demonstrated that the glycine is easily metabolized and that a good plasma amino acid profile is produced after infusion[65].

The nutritional requirements of each patient will require individual assessment, but, except in the most catabolic of situations when vast amounts of nitrogen may be needed, the following balanced regime is usually satisfactory and is presented as a guideline:

> 50 ml of 50% dextrose hourly (+ soluble insulin 1–5 units/h)
> 1 l Synthamin-17 over 12 h, and
> 500 ml Intralipid 20% over 12 h.

This will provide about 12.5 MJ (3000 kcal) and 17 g of nitrogen between dialyses. Insulin should be given as described above.

The combination of dialysis and total parenteral nutrition will rapidly lead to severe folate deficiency and so folate supplements must be given from the start. This is best given as calcium leucovorin 3–6 mg intravenously daily.

Water-soluble vitamins are also lost on dialysis and require replacement. Alternate day Parenterovite is usually sufficient.

Phosphate deficiency may occur and the deficit should be calculated and replaced with Neutral Phosphate solution (Boots).

Deficiency of trace metals rarely provides a serious clinical problem in these patients, but if deficiencies should occur, they can be replaced using readily available commercial preparations such as Addamel (Kabi-Vitrum).

Appropriate electrolyte solutions will need to be given to replace gastro-intestinal or fistula losses.

Albumin and blood are best given over dialysis when the appropriate intravascular volume can be provided by ultrafiltration to prevent fluid overload.

Having established efficient dialysis and paid due attention to the nutritional requirements of the patient, if he remains hypercatabolic, what other features should be explored to determine the cause?

The causes of hypercatabolism in acute renal failure

The principal causes of hypercatabolism are:

(1) Gastrointestinal bleeding
(2) Infection
(3) Drugs
(4) Injured tissue

(5) Metabolic response to injury

(6) Inadequate feeding.

Their diagnosis and management will be considered in turn.

(1) *Gastrointestinal bleeding.* The mechanism whereby gastrointestinal haemorrhage increases the catabolic rate, as measured by a rapid rise in the blood urea, is by delivering a massive protein meal to the gut for digestion. It is a common problem in patients with acute renal failure. Kennedy et al.[66] described haemorrhage severe enough to be a problem in management in 12% of their series. In over 50% of these it was responsible for death.

In our own experience, it occurs most frequently in the septic hypercatabolic patient. Like Jungers[67] and Kerr[68], we have found, by using upper gastrointestinal endoscopy, that the commonest causes are either duodenal ulcer or multiple gastric erosions. In 1976, we were privileged to use intravenous cimetidine in a patient with hypercatabolic acute renal failure and serious gastrointestinal haemorrhage due to multiple gastric erosions. There was a dramatic response; the patient ceased bleeding and recovered from his acute renal failure. Since then, all hypercatabolic patients have been treated prophylactically with cimetidine and gastrointestinal bleeding on our unit has become a rarity. The recommended dose is 100 mg intravenously every 8 hours.

There is another more serious form of gastrointestinal bleeding seen in acute renal failure. The patients are invariably septicaemic and have usually suffered disseminated intravascular coagulation. The lining of the gastrointestinal tract is velvety in appearance with multiple small bleeding sites. There is a continuous sanguineous ooze and the condition is usually fatal, though the occasional patient will respond to ethamsylate.

(2) *Infection.* Despite the advent of new antibiotics, infection remains, not only a major problem as a complication of acute renal failure, but also the prime cause of death[59,61,66]. All patients should be considered to be infected until proved otherwise. Blood cultures should be taken as soon as the patient is seen and at regular intervals thereafter. Catheters left in the bladder 'just to see how the patient is doing' are to be condemned. When diuresis commences, this is more than obvious (to the nurses who deal with the bed linen even if not to the doctor!). Catheters left in a dry bladder invite infection, and, all too often in the past, the onset of diuresis has been accompanied by a Gram-negative septicaemia from a urinary infection.

The increased susceptibility to infection in acute renal failure[69] requires that strict sterile procedures must be adhered to at all times when handling shunts or intravenous lines. If an unexplained fever occurs, for which no other cause can be found, then the central feeding line should be removed, cultured, and a new one inserted at another site, as this may often be the source of infection.

Candida infection is extremely common and is the cause of the 'uraemic' mouth. Regular oral toilet with nystatin is an important part of management in eliminating yet another source of infection.

Patients with peritonitis, seen mainly in surgical and post-traumatic cases, have fared extremely badly in the past[61,66,70]. This is still true, but it has been our experience, and that of others[71], that the recent widespread use of metronidazole, both prophylactically and therapeutically, against the *Bacteroides* species is helping to reverse this trend.

Pulmonary infection was the most important cause of death in Allwall's early series[59]. With good physiotherapy and antibiotic treatment, we seem to have overcome this problem in many cases and we now find the major pulmonary cause of death to be 'shock lung'. The combination of acute renal failure and 'shock lung' appears to be particularly lethal and we have only treated four survivors out of 20 cases.

The use of antibiotics will be discussed in a separate section.

(3) *Drugs.* The catabolic effects of tetracycline have been known for some time[72]. Despite the warnings given by Philips and his colleagues[73] of its danger in renal failure, patients with acute renal failure continue to be transferred to renal units under treatment with this drug. If a situation exists where a drug of the tetracycline group is mandatory, then doxycycline should be prescribed as this has been shown to not cause a rise in the blood urea[74].

The other group of drugs which require special mention in this section are the steroids. Obviously there are situations where their use is lifesaving, but their metabolic effects and consequences should be borne in mind when they are prescribed.

(4) *Injured tissue.* The continued presence of injured tissue is commonly a cause of a high catabolic rate. There is no substitute for early and complete debridement in post-traumatic cases. There is, however, a natural reluctance on the part of many surgeons to remove limbs, especially in the young, if there is any question of viability. Ischaemic, damaged tissue must be removed early if these patients are to survive. In patients who are severely burned, with acute renal failure, survival is poor[75]. We could only find 11 reported survivors in the world literature and described a further four[76]. Seven of these 15 patients survived following limb amputations. One case complicated by gas gangrene and toxic myocarditis is described in detail[77]. The author is convinced that several more post-traumatic and burned patients could have survived with a more aggressive approach to removal of large areas of non-viable tissue.

(5) *Metabolic response to injury*. The metabolic responses to injury in terms of negative nitrogen balance and its effects have already been discussed. Allison[78] points out that the approximate daily calorie and protein losses of patients with no food intake are extremely high. He quotes 2–4000 kcals (8.4–16.7 MJ) and 75–150 g protein for a post-operative patient, and 4–6000 kcals (16.7–25.1 MJ) and 100–400 g protein for a patient with major burns. This is mediated by secretion of large amounts of catabolic hormones, in particular cortisol[79], adrenaline[80], growth hormone[81] and glucagon[82]. The anabolic hormone, insulin, is initially suppressed[83], but, after a few days, levels may become supranormal with end organ resistance[83].

In the patient with normal renal function, this response is relatively short lived, possibly because these hormones are degraded and excreted by the kidney. In acute renal failure this response tends to continue. There is little one can do at present to counteract the metabolic responses apart from providing adequate nutrition, although the use of insulin and glucose in these patients will reduce protein catabolism and make feeding much more effective[63].

Before leaving this section, it should be remembered that if all the remediable causes of increased catabolic rate listed above have been excluded but the patient remains catabolic, then the feeding regime should be reassessed and adjusted as necessary.

Antibiotics in acute renal failure

Most antibiotics can be used with safety in patients with acute renal failure, provided the prescriber has a full knowledge of the mode of excretion and their potential hazards. Tetracycline has already been discussed. Drugs such as colistin and amphotericin B are well known nephrotoxic agents and should be avoided.

The toxic effects of the aminoglycosides on the eighth cranial nerve are much more likely to occur in the renal failure situation as the elimination of this group of antibiotics is almost entirely through the kidneys. Particular attention must be paid to dosage and monitoring of blood levels. Charts relating dose and frequency of administration to renal function are available from the manufacturers, but this does not obviate the requirement for measurement of plasma levels. They should merely be used as a guide. Blood should be taken for both peak and trough levels. The trough level is taken just prior to the administration of the next dose and peak levels at 15 min after the dose if given intravenously and at 1 h if given intramuscularly. Peak levels should not exceed 10 µg/ml for gentamycin and trough levels should be maintained below 2 µg/ml. The rate of clearance of gentamycin by haemodialysis is in the order of 24 ml/min. Our own practice is to give a dose of gentamycin post-haemodialysis and then to adjust this on a daily basis according to plasma levels. If peak levels are satisfactory but trough levels high, adjustment of the dose interval is necessary. Amikacin peak levels should be maintained below 20 µg/ml.

The cephalosporins, apart from cephaloridine, have not been shown to be nephrotoxic[84]. However, their combination with gentamycin may be nephro-toxic[85]. The combination of the cephalosporin group with diuretics also enhances nephrotoxicity.

The penicillins are safe, though it is wise to reduce the dosage as accumulation may cause an encephalopathy. The high sodium content of some of the injectable penicillins must also be borne in mind.

Our antibiotic policy at present for most patients whilst awaiting culture results is to give a combination of amikacin and metronidazole. Amikacin is chosen because of its much wider safety margin between therapeutic and toxic levels. If the infection is clearly staphylococcal from a wound or shunt site, then flucloxacillin or fucidic acid are the drugs of choice.

Treatment of underlying condition

The absence of urine should never allow one to lose sight of the underlying condition which was responsible for causing the acute renal failure. The renal function will not improve until this is corrected. The natural reluctance to undertake further surgical procedures must be overcome. With modern dialysis techniques and regional heparinization, surgery can be planned within a few hours of dialysis, and dialysis can be repeated following the operation, without fear of bleeding, if necessary.

Modern anaesthesia is extremely safe and can be performed with a minimum of drugs. Particular care should be taken to prevent hypoxia, and drugs known to cause hypotension should be avoided.

The management of acute renal failure is a team effort with full recovery of the patient as the central goal. Good co-operation between the specialities gives the best chance of attaining this aim.

Management of the diuretic phase

The onset of the diuretic phase is heralded by an increase in urine output. Although this is a time of great excitement, it is no time for complacency. The kidney is unable to conserve water, sodium and potassium, and the patient may rapidly become fluid- and electrolyte-depleted. Strict attention to fluid and electrolyte balance is therefore vital. A fall in postural blood pressure is, in our experience, the best sign that sodium supplements are required. These can either be given as intravenous saline if the patient is unable to take oral fluids or as Slow-Sodium tablets (10 mmol/tab) if this is practical. A falling serum potassium is a satisfactory marker of impending depletion and indicates that replacement is required (Table 1).

Table 1 Management of the diuretic phase

Fluid balance
Maintain urine output at 3–4 l/day
Do not give 500 ml plus the previous day's output, as this will lead to excessive urine volumes
    and electrolyte losses

Salt balance
Record lying and standing blood pressures. If postural falls in blood pressure occur, give salt
    supplements. In those patients who cannot stand or sit up, balance sodium intake/output

Potassium
Measure serum potassium daily and give supplements as required

Urinary infection
Culture the urine daily and treat infection early

Nutrition
Ensure continuing attention to nutrition. If normal feeding is difficult, maintain parenteral
    feeding

The urinary concentrating mechanism is the last of the kidney's functions to recover and may take several months before it is efficient enough to prevent nocturia. The patient should be warned of this as it can cause great anxiety. He must also be told to maintain a fluid intake not less than 3 l/day to prevent dehydration and its compromising effects on renal function.

When to stop dialysis therapy

Despite a rising urinary output in the early diuretic phase, until this reaches about 2.5 l/day, the blood urea will continue to rise. Intermittent dialysis will continue to be necessary to prevent the blood urea from rising above 33 mmol/l. The serum creatinine always falls before the blood urea and is a useful sign that dialysis will soon no longer be necessary.

Recovery of renal function

In patients who have suffered acute tubular necrosis, the blood urea and serum creatinine levels will gradually return to normal. However, a slight reduction in glomerular filtration rate or concentrating ability is to be expected in the majority[86]. This is unimportant in terms of patient health and managemen Failure to achieve normal blood urea and serum creatinine levels suggests that either there was pre-existing renal disease or partial cortical necrosis has occurred. This is an uncommon occurrence, but we have seen it occur in patients who have suffered obstetric accidents, acute pancreatitis and severe disseminated intravascular coagulation. A renal biopsy will confirm the diagnosis.

Prognosis of acute renal failure

The prognosis of acute renal failure is very much dependent on the precipi-tating cause. Obstetric cases show the best figures[87], with an overall survival of 90%, whereas burns cases[75] carry a mortality of 90%. In 1972, Dr C. T. Flynn sent a questionnaire to all renal units in the United Kingdom. The figures that he obtained for mortality remain the most up to date overall picture that is available[87]. The overall mortality in this series was 43%. The breakdown was as follows: medical, 36%; surgical, 53%; trauma, 50%; obstetric, 10%; others, 46%.

Overall mortality must be judged in perspective. With better antenatal care there has been such a decline in obstetric cases of acute renal failure that this good prognostic group no longer weights the statistics. The increasing awareness of the possibility of renal failure, better attention to resuscitation and the advent of intensive care units has avoided renal failure in many patients who would have been sent to us even 5 years ago. Renal failure is now being seen as a late complication in the seriously ill patient due to sepsis or nephrotoxic drugs. This is in contrast to the cases seen due to poor resuscitation of primary shock, and the prognosis is necessarily much worse because of the underlying condition.

It has been stated before that more attention should be paid to adequate nutrition to help reduce the mortality rate of acute renal failure[88]. The improvement in our own figures for post-traumatic renal failure from 66% to 36% are a testament to this.

Table 2 shows the changing mortality at our own centre for cases admitted over the two periods 1958–1967 and 1968–1977. The major difference in management between these two periods was the use of more intensive dialysis and a stricter control of nutrition in the latter group.

Table 2   Mortality—admitted cases

	1958–1967	1968–1977
Medical	35.5%	20.2%
Surgical	55.5%	40.4%
Obstetric	18.8%	20.0%
Overall	44.0%	32.3%

The failure to show an improvement in the battle casualties of Vietnam[61], compared with those of Korea, was amost certainly related to insufficient administration of nutrition.

I am sure that the only way in which mortality can be improved is by better understanding of the metabolic problems of acute renal failure, daily dialysis, strict attention to nutritional requirements and fully co-ordinated team work within the intensive care unit.

PLASMA EXCHANGE IN ACUTE RENAL FAILURE

Plasma exchange is a therapeutic measure whereby the patient's plasma is exchanged for either whole or fractionated plasma[89].

The application of this technique is relatively new in the management of acute renal failure and this section will review the current 'state of the art' and give an account of some of the recently published results.

Much of the pioneering work in this field has been performed at the Hammersmith Hospital, London. It is the author's belief that, until more data are available, patients requiring this form of therapy should be treated in centres fully conversant with this technique so that the results can be fully evaluated.

The principle behind plasma exchange is to remove auto-antibodies and immune complexes and so reduce the inflammatory response. The concomitant depletion of complement components may improve the clearance of immune complexes by the reticulo-endothelial system[90]. Furthermore, replacement of the patient's plasma with PPF will lead to defibrination[91]. As fibrin is probably important in crescent formation[92], then defibrination may also help to ameliorate the tissue injury response.

The technique may be carried out either by hand or automatically using a cell separator. For a description of methods employed to effect plasma exchange, the reader is referred to the review by Pinching[89].

It follows from what has been written about the principles of plasma exchange that theoretically diseases caused by circulating antibodies or immune complexes might be expected to respond to this therapy.

The two disease groups that have been well studied and where results seem particularly promising are Goodpasture's syndrome and rapidly progressive glomerular nephritis. This latter group includes cases of Wegener's granulomatosis and polyarteritis nodosa.

Goodpasture's syndrome

Goodpasture's syndrome is usually caused by an antibody to the glomerular basement membrane, which is also directed against the alveolar basement membrane in the lung. The disease is characterized by glomerular nephritis and pulmonary haemorrhage. Progression to renal failure may be rapid and Wilson and Dixon's series[93] in 1973 showed that, out of 32 patients, only four escaped death or long-term renal substitution therapy.

Lockwood and his colleagues[91] reported seven cases treated by a combination of cytotoxic drugs, steroids and intensive plasma exchange. There was an improvement in renal function in three cases who had still retained some function at the start of treatment. The four cases who were anuric at the start of treatment showed no improvement in renal function.

A recent review of the treatment of Goodpasture's syndrome[94] shows that there are now 17 patients recorded who have been treated by plasma exchange. One case has no follow-up details[95], but, of the remaining, eight have survived without recourse to long-term substitution therapy. They all showed improvement in renal function, and their latest reported serum creatinine levels range from 1.0 to 2.6 mg/dl.

The use of steroids and immunosuppression in these cases appears to be important in causing a secondary reduction in antibody levels by decreasing the lymphocyte pool[94]. It does, however, make evaluation of pure plasma exchange difficult in this disease. Nonetheless, if we compare the latest results[94] with those of Wilson and Dixon's original series[93], there is little doubt of the tremendous benefit to these patients of the use of plasma exchange.

In the context of acute renal failure, there is now a clear role for plasma exchange in those patients in the early stages who are not yet anuric. They should be transferred rapidly to centres where plasma exchange therapy is available. Even in those patients who are anuric, there appears to be a secondary benefit in terms of survival even if there is no improvement in renal function. Lockwood[91] showed that the use of plasma exchange rapidly controlled severe pulmonary haemorrhage. It seems difficult, therefore, in the light of the promising results to date, to deny any patient with Goodpasture's syndrome the benefit of plasma exchange in experienced hands.

Rapidly progressive glomerular nephritis

Lockwood and his colleagues[96] followed up their studies on Goodpasture's syndrome[91] with a paper describing the results of plasma exchange and immunosuppression in the treatment of fulminating immune-complex crescentic nephritis. Nine patients were treated and only one, who was anuric at presentation, did not show any improvement in renal function. Perhaps the best evidence for the efficacy of plasma exchange comes from this paper. Using the C1q binding assay for the detection of circulating immune complexes, they showed a fall in C1q binding after plasma exchange in five out of eight patients. In three patients, this rose again after stopping plasma exchange and was accompanied by a decline in renal function in two of these. Circulating immune complexes fell after restarting plasma exchange and this was associated with an improvement again of renal function.

It appears, therefore, on the observations to date that there is clearly a role for plasma exchange in those patients with immune-complex-mediated rapidly progressive glomerular nephritis. Again, however, total anuria bodes ill for recovery of renal function.

For the future we look forward to more publications on the use of plasma exchange in patients with rapidly declining renal function. In particular, its use in acute renal failure due to multiple myeloma looks promising in the three patients reported recently[97], and complements the previous work of

Feest and his colleagues[98]. Whether plasma exchange will solve some of our problems with acute lupus nephritis and transplant rejection remains to be seen in the light of controlled trials.

References

1 Whelton, A. and Donadio, J. V. (1969). Post-traumatic acute renal failure in Vietnam. *Johns Hopkins Med. J.*, **124**, 95

2 Robson, J. S. (1977). Pathogenesis of acute renal failure. In *Recent Advances in Intensive Care*.

3 Kerr, D. N. S. and Elliot, R. W. (1974). The pathogenesis of acute renal failure. In Flynn, C. T. (ed.) *Acute Renal Failure*. (Lancaster: MTP)

4 Andreucci, V. E. (1977). Pathophysiology of acute renal failure. In Robinson, Hawkins and Vereerstraeten (eds.) *Proceedings of the European Dialysis and Transplant Association*. Vol. 14. (Pitman Medical)

5 Yorke, W. and Nauss, R. W. (1911). The mechanism of the production of suppression of urine in Blackwater fever. *Ann. Trop. Med. Parasitol.*, **5**, 287

6 Bywaters, E. G. L. and Dible, J. H. (1942). The renal lesion in traumatic anuria. *J. Pathol. Bacteriol.*, **54**, 111

7 Pusey, C. D., Flynn, C. T. and Winfield, C. R. (1977). Acute renal failure in heat exhaustion. *J. R. Army Med. Cps.*, **123**, 88

8 Jaenike, J. R. (1969). Micropuncture study of methaemoglobin-induced acute renal failure in the rat. *J. Lab. Clin. Med.*, **73**, 459

9 Cirksena, W. J. (1971). In Gessler, M., Schroder, K. and Weidinger, H. (eds.) *Pathogenesis and Clinical Findings with Renal Failure*, p. 105. (Stuttgart: Georg Thieme)

10 Oken, D. E., Arce, M. L. and Wilson, D. R. (1966). Glycerol induced haemoglobinuric acute renal failure in the rat. 1. Micropuncture study in the development of oliguria. *J. Clin. Invest.*, **45**, 724

11 Flanigan, W. J. and Oken, D. E. (1965). Renal micropuncture study of the development of anuria in the rat with mercury-induced acute renal failure. *J. Clin. Invest.*, **44**, 449

12 Munck, O. (1958). *Renal Circulation in Acute Renal Failure*. (Oxford: Blackwell Scientific Publications)

13 Oliver, J., MacDowell, M. and Tracy, A. (1951). The pathogenesis of acute renal failure associated with traumatic and toxic injury. Renal ischaemia nephrotoxic damage and the ischemuric episode. *J. Clin. Invest.*, **30**, 1305

14 Bank, N., Mutz, B. F. and Aynedjian, H. S. (1967). The role of leakage of tubular fluid in anuria due to mercury poisoning. *J. Clin. Invest.*, **46**, 695

15 Flamembaum, W., McDonald, F. D., Di Bona, G. F. and Oken, D. E. (1971). Micropuncture study of renal tubule factors in low dose mercury poisoning. *Nephron*, **8**, 221

16 Mason, J. and Thurau, K. (1975). *Proc. Int. Congr. Nephrol. (Florence)*, p. 592. (Basel: Karger)

17 Trueta, J., Barclay, A. E., Daniel, P. M., Franklin, K. J. and Pritchard, M. M. L. (1947). *Studies of the Renal Circulation*. (Oxford: Blackwell Scientific Publications)

18 Goormaghtigh, N. (1945). Vascular and circulatory changes in renal cortex in the anuric crush syndrome. *Proc. Soc. Exp. Biol. Med.*, **59**, 303

19 Brown, J. J., Gleadle, R. I., Lawson, D. H., Lever, A. F., Linton, R. L., MacAdam, R. F., Prentice, E., Robertson, J. I. S. and Tree, M. (1970). Renin and acute renal failure: studies in man. *Br. Med. J.*, **1**, 253

20 Henry, L. N., Lane, C. E. and Kashgarian, M. (1968). Micropuncture studies of the pathophysiology of acute renal failure in the rat. *Lab. Invest.*, **19**, 309

21 Flamembaum, W., McNeil, J. S., Kotchen, T. A., Lowenthal, D. and Nagle, R. B. (1973). Glycerol induced acute renal failure after acute plasma renin activity suppression. *J. Lab. Clin. Med.*, **82**, 587

22 Schnermann, J., Wright, F. S., Davis, J. M., von Stackelberg, W. and Grill, G, (1970). Regulation of superficial nephron filtration rate by tubulo-glomerular feedback. *Pflugers Arch.*, **318**, 147

23 Cortney, M. A., Nagel, W. and Thurau, K. (1966). Micropuncture study of the relationship between flow rate through the loop of Henle and sodium concentration in the distal tubule. *Pflugers Arch.*, **287**, 286

24 Mason, J. (1976). Tubulo-glomerular feedback in the early stages of experimental acute renal failure. *Kidney Int.*, **10**, S106

25 Torres, V. E., Romero, J. C., Strong, C. G., Wilson, D. M. and Walker, V. R. (1974). Renal prostaglandin E during acute renal failure. *Prostaglandins*, **8**, 353

26 Oken, D. E. (1976). Local mechanisms in the pathogenesis of acute renal failure. *Kidney Int.*, **10**, S94

27 Vitsky, B. H., Suzuki, Y., Strauss, L. and Churg, J. (1969). The haemolytic–uraemic syndrome. A study of renal pathologic alterations. *Am. J. Pathol.*, **57**, 627

28 Robson, J. S., Martin, A. M., Ruckley, V. A. and MacDonald, M. K. (1968). Irreversible post-partum renal failure. A new syndrome. *Q. J. Med.*, **37**, 423

29 Linton, A. L., Gavras, H., Gleadle, R. I., Hutchinson, H. E., Lawson, D. H., Lever, A. F., MacAdam, R. F., McNicol, G. P. and Robertson, J. I. S. (1969). Microangiopathic haemolytic anaemia and the pathogenesis of malignant hypertension. *Lancet*, **1**, 1277

30 Menon, I. S., Dewar, H. A. and Newell, D. J. (1968). Role of the kidney in fibrinolytic activity of blood. *Lancet*, **1**, 785

31 Wardle, E. N. (1975). Endotoxinaemia and the pathogenesis of acute renal failure. *Q. J. Med.*, **44**, 389

32 Spink, W. W., Raddin, J., Zak, S. J., Peterson, M., Starzecki, B. and Seljeskog, E. (1966). Correlation of plasma catecholamine levels with haemodynamic changes in canine endotoxin shock. *J. Clin. Invest.*, **45**, 78

33 Flynn, C. T. (1974). Treatment of acute renal failure. In Flynn, C. T. (ed.) *Acute Renal Failure*. (Lancaster: MTP)

34 Cantarovitch, F., Locatelli, A., Fernandez, J. C., Perez Loredo, J. and Cristhof, J. (1971). Frusemide in high doses in the treatment of acute renal failure. *Postgrad. Med. J.*, **47** (Suppl.), 13

35 Dawson, J. L. (1968). Acute post operative renal failure in obstructive jaundice. *Ann. R. Coll. Surg.*, **42**, 163

36 Barry, K. G. and Malloy, J. P. (1962). Oliguric renal failure: evaluation and therapy by the intravenous infusion of mannitol. *J. Am. Med. Assoc.*, **179**, 510

37 Thurau, K. (1964). Renal haemodynamics. *Am. J. Med.*, **36**, 698

38 Graber, I. G. and Sevitt, S. (1959). Renal function in burned patients and its relationship to morphological changes. *J. Clin. Pathol.*, **12**, 25

39 Saltissi, D., Pusey, C. D. and Rainford, D. J. (1981). Acute interstitial nephritis. (In preparation)

40 Eliahou, H. E. and Bata, A. (1965). The diagnosis of acute renal failure. *Nephron*, **2**, 287

41 Cattell, W. R., McIntosh, C. S., Moseley, I. F. and Kelsey, F. (1973). Excretion urography in acute renal failure. *Br. Med. J.*, **2**, 575

42 Mahaffy, R. G., Matheson, N. A. and Caridis, D. T. (1969). Infusion pyelography in acute renal failure. *Clin. Radiol.*, **20**, 320

43 Cattell, W. R. (1975). Acute renal failure. In Jones, N. F. (ed.) *Recent Advances in Renal Disease*. (London: Churchill Livingstone)

44 Britton, K. E. and Brown, N. J. G. (1971). In *Clinical Renography* (London: Lloyd Luke)

45 Joffre, F., Sablayrolles, J. L., Ecoiffier, J., Suc, J. M. and Putois, J. (1975). Etude systematique des temps nephrographiques au cours de l'urographie intraveineuse 2e partie: Aspects pathologique. *Ann. Radiol.*, **18**, 623

46 Rainford, D. J. (1977). The immediate care of acute renal failure. *Anaesthesia*, **32**, 277

47 Flynn, C. T. (1967). Peritoneal dialysis in hypercatabolic acute renal failure. *Lancet*, **1**, 129

48 Flynn, C. T. (1970). Some aspects of renal damage following trauma. *Proc. R. Soc. Med.*, **63**, 563

49 Ramirez, O., Swartz, C., Onesti, G., Mailloux, L. and Brest, A. N. (1966). The winged in line shunt. *Trans. Am. Soc. Artif. Intern. Organs*, **12**, 220

50 Shaldon, S., Chiandussi, L. and Higgs, B. (1961). Haemodialysis by percutaneous catheterisation on the femoral artery and vein with regional heparinisation. *Lancet*, **2**, 857

51 Shaldon, S., Silva, H., Pomeroy, J., Rae, A. I. and Rosen, S. M. (1964). Percutaneous venous catheterisation and reusable dialysers in the treatment of acute renal failure. *Trans. Am. Soc. Artif. Intern. Organs*, **10**, 133

52 Kopp, K. F., Gutch, C. F. and Kolff, W. J. (1972). Single needle dialysis. *Trans. Am. Soc. Artif. Intern. Organs*

53 Teschan, P. E., Baxter, C. R., O'Brien, T. F., Freyhof, J. N. and Hall, W. H. (1960). Prophylactic haemodialysis in the treatment of acute renal failure. *Ann. Intern. Med.*, **53**, 5

54 Parsons, F. M., Hobson, S. M., Blagg, C. R. and McCracken, B. H. (1961). Optimum time for dialysis in acute renal failure—Description and value of an improved dialyser with large surface area. *Lancet*, **1**, 129

55 Silva, H., Pomeroy, J., Rae, A. I., Rosen, S. M. and Shaldon, S. (1964). Daily haemodialysis in hypercatabolic acute renal failure. *Br. Med. J.*, **2**, 407

56 Hartzell, J. B., Winfield, J. M. and Irvin, I. L. (1941). Plasma vitamin C and serum protein levels in wound disruption. *J. Am. Med. Assoc.*, **116**, 669

57 McDermott, F. T., Nayman, J. and DeBoer, W. R. G. M. (1968). The effect of acute renal failure upon wound healing: histological and autoradiographic studies in the mouse. *Ann. Surg.*, **168**, 142

58 Sako, W. S. (1942). Resistance to infection as effected by variations in the proportions of protein, fat, and carbohydrate in the diet. *J. Paediatr.*, **20**, 475

59 Allwall, N. (1963). *Therapeutic and Diagnostic Problems in Acute Renal Failure.* (Stockholm: Scandinavian University Books)

60 Smith, L. H. Jr, Post, S., Teschan, P. E., Abernathy, R. S., Davis, J. H., Gray, D. M., Howard, J. M., Johnson, K. E., Klopp, E., Munday, R. L., O'Meara, M. P. and Rush, B. F. (1955). Post-traumatic renal insufficiency in military casualties. II. Management, use of an artificial kidney, prognosis. *Am. J. Med.*, **18**, 187

61 Lordon, R. E. and Burton, J. R. (1972). Post-traumatic renal failure in military personnel in South East Asia. *Am. J. Med.*, **53**, 137

62 Abel, R. M., Beck, C. H., Abbott, W. M., Ryan, J. A., Barbett, J. O. and Fischer, J. E. (1973). Improved survival from acute renal failure after treatment with intravenous essential L-amino acids and glucose: results of a prospective, double-blind study. *N. Engl. J. Med.*, **288**, 695

63 Lee, H. A. (1978). The nutritional management of renal disease. In Dickerson, J. W. T. and Lee, H. A. (eds.) *Nutrition in the Clinical Management of Disease.* (London: Edward Arnold)

64 Hinton, P., Allison, S. P., Littlejohn, S. and Lloyd, J. (1971). Insulin and glucose to reduce catabolic response to injury in burned patients. *Lancet*, **1**, 767

65 Rainford, D. J. and Philips, M. (1979). Unpublished data

66 Kennedy, A. C., Burton, J. A., Luke, R. G., Briggs, J. D., Lindsay, R. M., Allison, M. E. M., Edward, N. and Dargie, H. J. (1973). Factors affecting the prognosis in acute renal failure. *Q. J. Med.*, **165**, 73

67 Jungers, P., Maillard, J. N., Bienayme, J., Glaser, P. and Mery, J. Ph. (1967). Haemor-rhagies digestives par ulcerations gastro-duodenales au course de l'insufficance renale aigue. A propos de cinq cas operes et gueris. *Proc. Eur. Dialysis Transplant Assoc.*, 4, 301

68 Kerr, D. N. S. (1972). Acute renal failure. In Black, D. (ed.) *Renal Disease.* (Oxford: Blackwell Scientific Publications)

69 Montgomerie, J. Z., Kalmanson, G. M. and Guze, L. B. (1968). Renal failure and infection. *Medicine (Baltimore)*, 47, 1

70 McGeown, M. (1974). In Flynn, C. T. (ed.) *Acute Renal Failure*, p. 130. (Lancaster: MTP)

71 Price, D. (1979). Personal communication

72 Shils, M. E. (1963). Renal disease and the metabolic effects of tetracycline. *Ann. Intern. Med.*, 58, 389

73 Philips, M. E., Eastwood, J. B., Curtis, J. R., Gower, P. E. and de Wardener, H. E. (1974). Tetracycline poisoning in renal failure. *Br. Med. J.*, 2, 149

74 Little, P. J. and Bailey, R. R. (1970). *NZ Med. J.*, 72, 183

75 Cameron, J. S. and Miller-Jones, C. M. H. (1967). Renal function and renal failure in badly burned children. *Br. J. Surg.*, 54, 132

76 Davies, D. M., Brown, J. M., Bennett, J. P., Pusey, C. D. and Rainford, D. J. (1979). Acute renal failure in burns. *Scand. J. Plast. Reconstr. Surg.*, 13, 189

77 Davies, D. M., Brown, J. M., Bennett, J. P., Rainford, D. J., Pusey, C. D., Chesshire, A. and Maw, D. S. J. (1979). Survival after major burn complicated by gas gangrene, acute renal failure and toxic myocarditis. *Br. Med. J.*, 1, 718

78 Allison, S. P. (1972). The metabolic response to injury. *Medicine*, 11, 730

79 Cope, O., Nathanson, I. T., Rourke, G. M. and Wilson, H. (1943). Metabolic observations on shock. *Ann. Surg.*, 117, 937

80 Halme, A., Pekkarinen, A. and Turonen, M. (1957). On the excretion of noradrenaline, adrenaline, 17-hydroxy-corticosteroids and 17-keto-steroids. *Acta Endocrinol.*, 24 (Suppl.), 32

81 Ross, H., Johnson, I. D. A., Welborn, T. A. and Wright, A. D. (1966). Effect of abdominal operation on glucose tolerance and serum levels of insulin, growth hormone and hydro-cortisone. *Lancet*, 2, 563

82 Aguilar-Parada, E., Eisentraut, A. M. and Unger, R. H. (1969). Effects of starvation on plasma pancreatic glucagon in normal man. *Diabetes*, 18, 717

83 Allison, S. P., Hinton, P. and Chamberlain, M. J. (1968). Intravenous glucose tolerance, insulin and free fatty acid levels in burned patients. *Lancet*, 2, 113

84 Perkins, R. L., Apicella, M. A., Lee In-Sung, Cuppage, F. E. and Saslaw, S. (1968). Cephaloridine and cephalothin: comparative studies of potential nephrotoxocity. *J. Lab. Clin. Med.*, 71, 75

85 Fillastre, J. P., Laumonier, R., Humbert, G., Dubois, D., Metayer, J., Delpech, A., Leroy, J. and Robert, M. (1973). Acute renal failure associated with combined gentamycin and cephalothin therapy. *Br. Med. J.*, 2, 396

86 Briggs, J. D. B., Kennedy, A. C., Young, L. N., Luke, R. G. and Gray, M. J. B. (1967). *Br. Med. J.*, 3, 513

87 Flynn, C. T. (1974). Treatment of acute renal failure. In Flynn, C. T. (ed.) *Acute Renal Failure.* (Lancaster: MTP)

88 Editorial (1973). Prognosis of acute renal failure. *Br. Med. J.*, 1, 435

89 Pinching, A. J. (1978). Plasma exchange. *Br. J. Hosp. Med.*, 20, 552

90 Czop, J. and Nussenzweig, V. (1976). *J. Exp. Med.*, 143, 615

91 Lockwood, C. M., Rees, A. J., Pearson, T. A., Evans, D. J., Peters, D. K. and Wilson, C. B. (1976). Immunosuppression and plasma-exchange in the treatment of Goodpasture's syndrome. *Lancet*, 1, 711

92 Churg, J., Morita, T. and Suzuki, Y. (1973). In Kincaid-Smith, P., Mathew, T. H. and Becker, E. L. (eds.) *Glomerular Nephritis, Morphology, Natural History and Treatment*, p. 677. (New York: Wiley)

93 Wilson, C. B. and Dixon, F. G. (1973). Anti-glomerular basement membrane antibody-induced glomerulonephritis. *Kidney Int.*, 3, 74

94 Rosenblatt, S. G., Knight, W., Bannayan, G. A., Wilson, C. B. and Stein, J. H. (1979). Treatment of Goodpasture's syndrome with plasmapheresis. *Am. J. Med.*, 66, 689

95 Depner, T. A., Chaffin, M. E., Wilson, C. B. and Gulyassy, P. F. (1975). Plasmapheresis for severe Goodpasture's syndrome (abstract). *Kidney Int.*, 8, 409

96 Lockwood, C. M., Rees, A. J., Pinching, A. J., Pussell, B., Sweny, P., Uff, J. and Peters, D. K. (1977). Plasma exchange and immunosuppression in the treatment of fulminating immune-complex crescentic nephritis. *Lancet*, 1, 63

97 Misiani, R., Remuzzi, G., Bertani, T., Licini, R., Levoni, P., Crippa, A. and Mecca, G. (1979). Plasmapheresis in the treatment of acute renal failure in multiple myeloma. *Am. J. Med.*, 66, 684

98 Feest, T. G., Burge, P. S. and Cohen, S. L. (1976). Successful treatment of myeloma kidney by diuresis and plasmapheresis. *Br. Med. J.*, 1, 503

2

Chronic renal failure

V. E. Andreucci

Nephrologists may be very proud to have developed excellent techniques for replacing renal function and to have improved renal graft survival to such an extent that the kidney is the only organ for which transplantation is now a routine. Unfortunately, the same cannot be said concerning the conservative management of chronic renal failure (CRF), defined as the use of therapeutic measures other than dialysis or transplantation. When renal function is impaired because of chronic renal disease, GFR slowly and progressively declines, leading inexorably to dialysis or death. Undoubtedly chronic uraemia *per se* contributes to this progression through such factors as the intrarenal deposition of either uric acid, secondary to hyperuricaemia, or calcium salts, secondary to high plasma calcium × phosphorus product, and the renal damage induced by urinary tract infections which are so frequently asymptomatic, or by hypertension, which may itself be caused by CRF. Even though the correction of hypertension, the adequate treatment of urinary infections and well-balanced dietary measures cannot avoid the evolution of chronic uraemia, they may slow its progression[1-3].

Whilst awaiting methods to treat the underlying pathological causes of CRF, the aim of the conservative management must be to delay this progression, to correct the metabolic disorders and to blunt the extrarenal injuries that result from the deterioration of renal function.

CAUSES OF CHRONIC RENAL FAILURE

Chronic renal failure is the end result of damage to both kidneys arising from a multiplicity of causes. Whatever the original cause is, either glomerular or tubulo-interstitial, either congenital or acquired, all may lead to a progressive loss of functioning nephrons until the development of the clinical state 'uraemia'.

The major causes of CRF are listed in Table 1. According to the Registry of the European Dialysis and Transplant Association (EDTA)[4], of 10233 patients coming to either renal dialysis treatment (RDT) or renal transplantation in the year 1978, chronic glomerulonephritis was responsible for the renal failure in 32.7%, interstitial nephritis in 20.9%, cystic kidney disease in 9.2%, multi-system disease in 8.5%, renal vascular disease in 8.3%, drug nephropathy in 3.0% and heredo-familial renal disease in 2.8%. Although as many as 10.5% of all cases of CRF were classified as of uncertain aetiology, the incidence of chronic glomerulonephritis is still overestimated[5], since glomerulonephritis is usually diagnosed as the primary renal disease when a progressive deterioration of renal function cannot be attributed to other known causes of CRF.

Table 1 Causes of chronic renal failure

Primarily glomerular disease	Glomerulonephritis
	Collagen disease: disseminated lupus erythematosus; polyarteritis (periarteritis nodosa) glomerulonephritis*; Wegener's granulomatosis; primary systemic sclerosis (scleroderma); thrombotic thrombocytopenic purpura; anaphylactoid purpura (Schönlein–Henoch syndrome)
	Subacute bacterial endocarditis
	Diabetic glomerulosclerosis
	Amyloidosis
Primarily tubulo-interstitial disease	Pyelonephritis
	Tuberculosis
	Obstruction of the urinary tract: prostatic obstruction, urolithiasis (bilateral renal stones); congenital urogenital pathology (urethral valves; vesicoureteral reflux; neurogenic bladder)
	Analgesic (phenacetin) nephropathy
	Gouty nephropathy
	Nephrocalcinosis
	Myeloma kidney
	Radiation nephropathy
Primarily vascular disease	Malignant hypertension
	Non-malignant hypertension
	Caval and/or bilateral renal vein thrombosis
	Renal polyarteritis (periarteritis nodosa)*
	Bilateral cortical necrosis
Heredo-familial renal disease	Alport's syndrome
	Fabry's disease
	Polycystic kidney disease
	Nephronophthisis
	Oxalosis

This list is not exhaustive
*Two renal lesions may occur (separately or together) in polyarteritis nodosa: (a) a form of glomerulonephritis and (b) an arteritic lesion involving the arcuate and interlobular arteries[6]

PATHOPHYSIOLOGY AND CLINICAL MANIFESTATIONS OF CHRONIC RENAL FAILURE

Water metabolism

Nocturia is one of the earliest symptoms in CRF. The normal diurnal rhythm of urine output (the mechanism of which is not known but may be related to a greater ADH secretion at night) is lost; thus the volume passed during the night exceeds the daytime total. Presumably this is because the reduced blood perfusion of the diseased kidneys is improved at rest in bed, while the concentrating effect of the presumably greater ADH secretion at night is offset by the impaired responsiveness of the uraemic cortical collecting tubules to vasopressin (recently demonstrated in uraemic rabbits by Fine et al.[7]).

Daily urine volume is not reduced until the end stage; it is frequently more than 2000 ml/day (with a pale urine due to a diminished excretion of urochromogen), despite the significant reduction in functioning nephrons. In the uraemic environment, this is due to:

(a) The increased plasma concentration of filtrable but poorly reabsorbable solutes, such as urea, sulphate, phosphate, etc., which will result in an osmotic diuresis in the residual nephrons, accounting for the greater urine excretion per nephron with a concentration fixed at the same osmolality as plasma (the so-called isosthenuria).

(b) The increased filtration rate per single surviving nephron, due to compensatory hypertrophy, which will further contribute to the osmotic diuresis.

(c) The expansion of extracellular volume which is a peculiarity of CRF and will suppress the fractional tubular reabsorption of filtrate.

(d) The increased secretion of parathyroid hormone (PTH), due to secondary hyperparathyroidism, which will suppress the tubular reabsorption of phosphate and presumably of sodium.

Because of these mechanisms, water and solute output in renal failure is maintained unchanged despite the progressive reduction of functioning nephrons.

The ability to concentrate urine is lost mainly because of the osmotic diuresis due to the increased solute excretion of each nephron[8-10] and because of the hyporesponsiveness of the uraemic kidneys to vasopressin. Recent in vitro studies by Fine et al.[7] have demonstrated a vasopressin unresponsiveness of isolated cortical collecting tubules of uraemic rabbits. This tubular defect may limit the ability of the kidneys to concentrate the urine both directly by impairing the diffusion of water out of the collecting tubules and indirectly by reducing the recycling of urea[7,11]. If urea is not concentrated in the cortical collecting tubules by water abstraction, it cannot diffuse from the lumen of the papillary collecting ducts into the papillary interstitium down its concentration gradient, and thus it cannot create a hypertonic medullary interstitium, according to Kokko and Rector's theory of countercurrent multiplication system for urine concentration[12]. Intrarenal disturbances, such as presence of exudate and scarring, disturbances of renal blood flow and, mainly, destruction of juxtamedullary nephrons, may all contribute to the defect in producing the hypertonic urine. A thirsty normal subject may excrete urine with an osmolality approximately four times greater than that of plasma (i.e. up to 1200 mmol/kg water); with the fall in GFR, maximum urine osmolality soon approaches that of plasma. Thus, in the uraemic patient with solute excretion of 600 mmol/day, 1 l of water must be excreted with every 400 mmol of solutes, leading to an obligatory diuresis of approximately 1.5 l despite water deprivation[13,14].

The intrarenal lesions may be greater at medullary level in those cases of CRF secondary to chronic pyelonephritis or to special conditions, such as medullary cystic disease, amyloid disease of the renal medulla and urinary tract obstruction[15]. Indeed, these conditions may account for the occurrence of polyuria sometimes observed in CRF.

In CRF, the ability to dilute the urine is maintained long after impairment of the concentrating ability, and it is frequently normal until very low degrees of renal function. The diluting ability of the surviving nephrons of uraemic patients (a fairly good estimate of which is given by the millilitres of solute-free water excreted per 100 ml glomerular filtrate) is expected to be greater than normal because of the functional adaptation of residual nephrons to the uraemic environment. The expansion of extracellular volume will significantly increase salt delivery to Henle's loop (the site where solute-free water is generated because of solute reabsorption without water), creating an increase in free water generation. The latter, however, does not increase because the same ECV expansion that is the main factor for increasing distal delivery (through a suppression in proximal tubular reabsorption) will suppress, at approximately the same extent, salt reabsorption at the ascending limb of Henle's loop (Figure 1).

The ability to excrete a water load, however, is impaired much earlier, even when the urine may still become hypotonic. This is due to the very low number of functioning nephrons, as shown by the following example.

P.S., a 40-year-old male patient, had stable CRF secondary to glomerulonephritis. Creatinine clearance was 10.9 ml/min and blood urea 161 mg/100 ml while on a protein intake of 40 g/day with 5 g/day of salt in the diet. His diluting capacity was studied under the influence of a maximal sustained water diuresis by measuring the minimal urinary molarity (U_{mol}), maximal urinary flow (V) and free water clearance (C_{H_2O}). The values obtained by our study were referred to 24 h and C_{H_2O} was corrected to normal renal mass by assuming that creatinine clearance was a reasonable estimate of residual functioning nephrons (Table 2). Thus, while maximal urinary flow was 3.73 ml/min with a U_{mol} of 193 mmol/l (P_{mol} of 295 mmol/l), C_{H_2O} was

1.289 ml/min. When C_{H_2O} was expressed per 100 ml of glomerular filtrate, a value of 11.83 ml/min was obtained, comparable to C_{H_2O} of normal subjects at equivalent rates of solute excretion[16]. If we assume now that a normal subject, with a GFR of 120 ml/min, has the same solute excretion (1037 mmol/24 h), P_{mol} (295 mmol/l) and C_{H_2O} per 100 ml of GFR (11.83 ml/min), the solute-free water excreted in 24 h will be 20442 ml (rather than

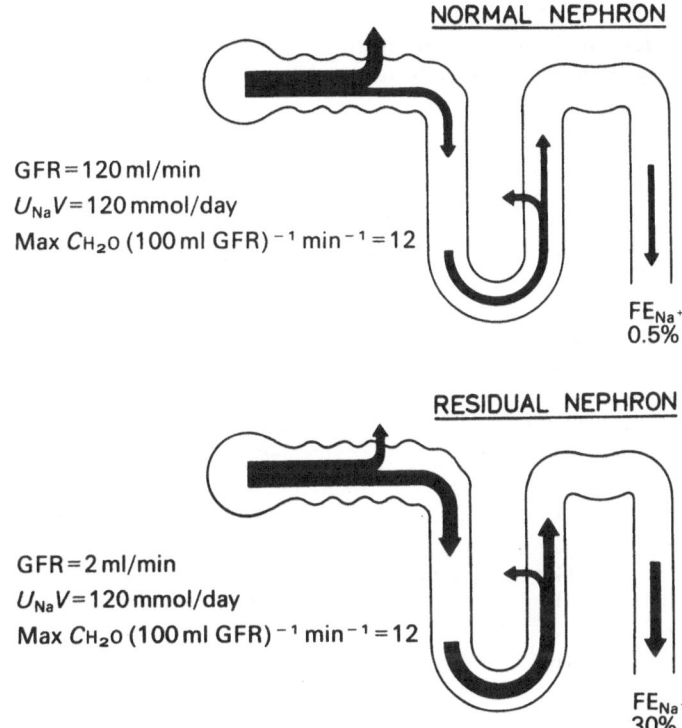

Figure 1 Residual nephrons in a uraemic patient with a GFR of 2 ml/min may excrete up to 30% of filtered sodium (FE_{Na^+}) (compared with 0.5% in normal nephrons), so that overall sodium excretion can be maintained despite a significant reduction in the nephron population. An extracellular volume (ECV) expansion, due to the uraemic condition, may account for this adaptation of surviving nephrons by suppressing proximal tubular reabsorption. The increased salt delivery to the distal nephron, however, does not increase free water formation because ECV expansion will also suppress sodium reabsorption at approximately the same extent in the ascending limb of Henle's loop

1857 ml of the uraemic patient, P.S.). If we add this solute-free water to the isotonic fraction of urine volume (3515 ml/day) necessary to excrete the 1037 mmol (obligatory water excretion should be 1 l every 295 mmol solute), the final urine volume will be 23957 ml/day which will dilute the 1037 mmol solute to 43 mmol/l. This minimal urinary molarity is what we expect from a normal subject during maximal water diuresis. The greater value of the minimal urinary molarity during maximal water diuresis in the uraemic patient by comparison with normal subjects (193 against 43 mmol/l), despite comparable $C_{H_2O}/100$ ml GFR, is due to the reduction in the nephron population so that the solute-free water excreted in 24 h that should dilute the isotonic obligatory urine is much less than in normal subjects. The danger of i.v. infusion of large amounts of water, in the form of 5% or 10% glucose, is therefore obvious. The inability of surviving nephrons to excrete the water load will cause overhydration. Similarly, physicians should invite uraemic patients to drink only when thirsty rather than forcing them to drink as much as possible.

Table 2 Diluting capacity of a uraemic patient during maximal sustained water diuresis compared with theoretical values of a normal subject with identical solute excretion, plasma concentration and free-water clearance per 100 ml glomerular filtrate

		Patient P.S.	*Normal subject*
GFR	ml/min	10.9	120
	ml/24 h	15696	172800
$U_{mol}V$	mmol/min	0.72	—
	mmol/24 h	1037	1037
P_{mol}	mmol/l	295	295
C_{mol}	ml/min	2.441	—
	ml/24 h	3515	3515
C_{H_2O}	ml/min	1.289	—
	ml min^{-1} (100 ml GFR)$^{-1}$	11.83	11.83
	ml/24 h	1857	20442
V	ml/min	3.73	—
	ml/24 h	5372	25957
U_{mol}	mmol/l	193	43

Sodium metabolism

In each nephron of normal mammals, tubular reabsorption of sodium is linked to GFR so that a relatively constant proportion of filtered sodium is reabsorbed. This phenomenon, well investigated by micropuncture techniques[17], is termed glomerulotubular balance and is biologically very important to prevent large changes in sodium excretion with slight changes in GFR. In CRF, glomerulotubular balance is reset at a very different level, thus allowing for the maintenance of external sodium balance despite significant reduction in nephron population. In other words, even in CRF, the general rule that what goes in must come out otherwise it is retained in the body is not changed. Hence, if sodium intake is maintained but nephron population is reduced, the fraction of filtered sodium reabsorbed by each residual nephron must be reduced (despite a normal or even greater filtration rate in that nephron) in proportion to the reduction in functioning nephrons.

In a subject with normal renal function, 0.5–1.0% of the filtered sodium is excreted in the urine. If sodium intake is maintained constant, the reduction in nephrons with an associated fall in overall sodium excretion will result in expansion of extracellular fluid volume, since sodium retention will lead to water retention to keep the concentration of body fluids constant. This imbalance between sodium intake and excretion is, however, transitory since ECV expansion will decrease sodium reabsorption in the remaining functioning nephrons to an extent sufficient to compensate for the decrease in the number of nephrons. The increase in overall sodium excretion will again balance sodium intake; however, the price paid for this is a permanent expansion of ECV, necessary to maintain a permanent increase in the

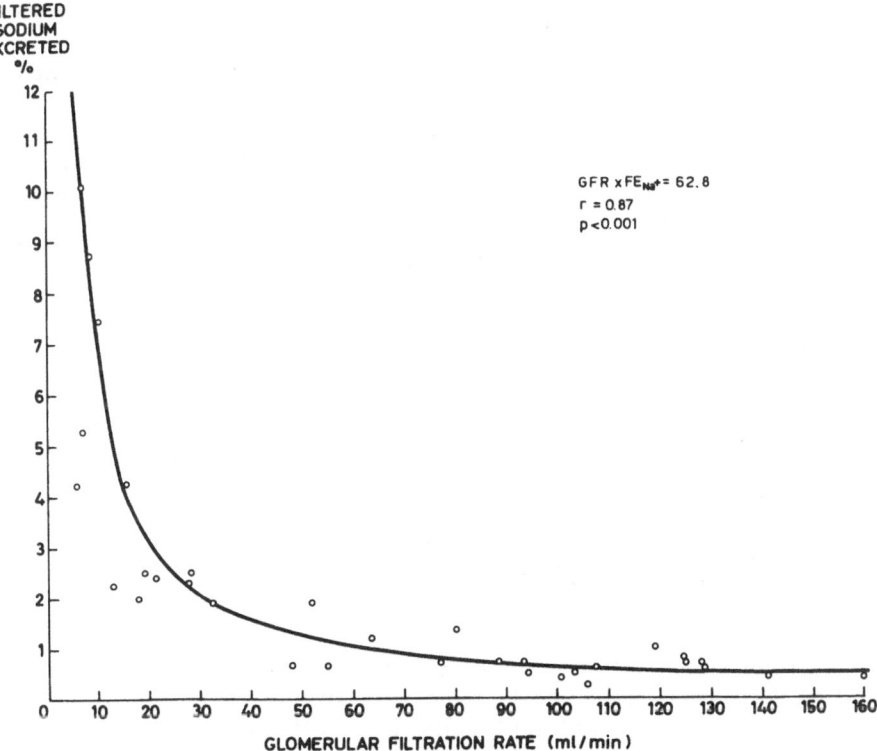

Figure 2 Fractional excretion of filtered sodium (FE_{Na^+}) in 33 patients with normal renal function or various degrees of chronic renal failure. FE_{Na^+} appears to increase exponentially with the fall in creatinine clearance so that the creatinine clearance × FE_{Na^+} product remains constantly equal to 62.8. The variation observed when creatinine clearance is less than 80 ml/min is due to a variation in salt intake between 3 and 5 g/day in different patients

sodium excretion per nephron. As further nephron destruction occurs, transient sodium retention will again take place, further expanding the ECV, and, in this way, increasing sodium excretion in the surviving nephrons so that an external balance is again achieved. It is therefore evident that, with a progressive fall in GFR, it is not necessary to reduce sodium intake, since the external balance will be maintained by a progressive decrease in fractional sodium reabsorption in the surviving nephrons through a progressive expansion of ECV. The fractional excretion of filtered sodium will, in fact, increase exponentially with the fall in GFR, as shown in Figure 2. The magnitude of this ECV expansion is evident when patients with advanced CRF begin regular dialysis treatment; their weight will decrease after a few dialyses because of the loss of water and salt, and urine output will simultaneously fall, clearly showing that a considerable amount of their body mass was due to excess salt and water.

The extent of the adaptation of the residual nephron population to the uraemic environment is shown by the following representative example (Table 3). In the patient P.S. with a GFR of 10.9 ml/min and serum sodium concentration of 135 mmol/l the external sodium balance was maintained,

Table 3 Fractional excretion of Na^+ in a uraemic patient (P.S., a 40-year-old male patient, 57 kg body weight) at different Na^+ intakes compared with theoretical values of a normal subject with the same Na^+ intakes

Subject	GFR (ml/min)	Serum Na^+ (mmol/l)	Filtered load of Na^+ (mmol/day)	Excretion rate of Na^+ (mmol/day)	FE_{Na^+} (%)
NaCl intake of approximately 5 g/day					
Patient P.S.	10.9	135	2118.96	85	4.01
Normal subject	120	135	23 328.00	85	0.37
NaCl intake of approximately 12 g/day					
Patient P.S.	10.9	135	2118.96	210.24	9.92
Normal subject	120	135	23 328.00	210.24	0.90

both while on 5 g salt intake (85 mmol Na^+) per day and while on 12 g salt intake (204 mmol Na^+) per day; the fractional excretion of filtered Na^+ (FE_{Na^+}) was 4.01% and 9.92% respectively. If we assume that a normal subject, on the same salt intake, has a GFR of 120 ml/min and the same serum concentration of sodium, the external sodium balance is maintained by a FE_{Na^+} of 0.37% and 0.90% respectively. In other words, in response to an identical 13% increase* in ECV, the fraction of filtered sodium excreted by a surviving nephron of the uraemic patient P.S. (residual nephron

---

*At a salt intake of 12 g, if sodium is absorbed iso-osmotically as sodium chloride, 204 mmol of Na^+ will enter ECV, expanding the latter by approximately 1.5 l; since the body weight of patient P.S. was 57 kg, his ECV was approximately 11.4 l. Hence, the addition of 1.5 l would represent 13% ECV expansion.

population one-eleventh of normal) is 11 times greater than that by a nephron of a normal subject (100% functioning nephrons). Hence the renal response to a given ECV expansion is 'magnified' in the uraemic condition[18].

The mechanism by which ECV expansion is responsible for the decrease in tubular reabsorption of sodium by surviving nephrons in a stepwise fashion is not clear. Physical factors as well as a still unidentified natriuretic hormone have been suggested by different investigators. Intrarenal redistribution of blood flow in a situation where many nephrons are no longer perfused despite a relatively maintained overall renal perfusion may account for this different ('magnified') behaviour of the surviving nephrons in uraemic patients in comparison with the nephrons of normal subjects. It is also possible that the effect of ECV expansion on tubular reabsorption is greater in subjects already expanded (i.e. uraemic patients) than in non-expanded normal subjects.

Should the adaptation of residual nephrons to the uraemic environment not exist, a uraemic patient with a GFR of 10.9 ml/min and sodium intake of 12 g/day would retain as much as 185 mmol/day (being 0.90% excretion of a filtered load of only 19 mmol), and that would correspond to the retention of more than 1.25 l of isotonic saline solution each day.

Despite this ability of the surviving nephrons to maintain external sodium balance while on normal salt intake, there is an upper limit (the 'ceiling') as well as a lower limit (the 'floor') of the amount of sodium that may be excreted in the urine in CRF[14]. A normal subject may increase salt excretion to even more than 20 g/day. The maximal rate of salt excretion is reduced in CRF, but does not represent a problem (i.e. it does not require salt restriction in the diet) until a GFR as low as 2 ml/min. At this level of renal function, salt retention will take place if the salt intake exceeds 7–8 g/day[13]; in other words, despite the still quite large tubular Na^+ reabsorption, the latter may not be depressed to less than 60% of the filtered load[19]. Obviously, unnecessary i.v. saline infusions in uraemic patients may easily induce salt retention and oedema formation because of this ceiling for sodium excretion. Similarly, oedema may occur in uraemic patients, even though on restricted salt intake, when either nephrotic syndrome or congestive heart failure co-exist.

It is well known that a normal subject on a salt-free diet may reduce sodium excretion, within 4 to 5 days, to 1–2 mmol/day. This capability is lost in CRF. For unexplained reasons, uraemic patients have an obligatory sodium excretion that has been shown[20] to range between 15 and 30 mmol/day when GFR is lower than 10 ml/min. This means that salt depletion will occur if sodium intake is maintained lower than 1–2 g/day in advanced renal failure. The osmotic diuresis typical of CRF and the excretion of poorly reabsorbable anions, such as sulphate and phosphate, which requires the excretion of an accompanying cation, may partially account for this obligatory sodium loss. This mechanism, however, does not explain why patients with nephrotic syndrome or congestive heart failure may excrete urine virtually free of sodium despite advanced renal failure.

In summary, uraemic patients with a GFR less than 10 ml/min may modulate their sodium excretion, in accordance with sodium intake, in the range between 20–30 mmol/day and 120–170 mmol/day. If this is the rule, however, it is not uncommon to see patients in CRF with a tendency to either retain or lose sodium. Indeed, gradual retention of sodium, without oedema, is the main factor responsible for the hypertension so frequently present in uraemic patients. The salt-dependent nature of this hypertension is shown by its correction after dialysis (Figure 3). The condition should be treated by high-ceiling diuretics such as furosemide, bumetanide or, better, muzolimine[21] (Figure 4).

Other uraemic patients have a tendency to lose sodium with the consequent fall in blood pressure, contraction in ECV and worsening of renal function. A mild negative sodium balance may be asymptomatic and may be accompanied by increase in aldosterone secretion (thus causing a tendency to hypokalaemia) and normal blood pressure. It has been even suggested that a urinary leak of sodium should always be suspected when blood pressure is normal in uraemic patients[22]. Severe sodium loss in the urine may rapidly worsen renal failure, with severe hypotension, thirst and anorexia. This represents the so-called 'salt-losing nephritis', usually secondary to chronic urinary obstruction, polycystic kidney disease, phenacetin nephropathy and chronic pyelonephritis with urinary infection[22]. This condition of urinary salt leaks requires sodium supplements.

It must be stressed that a deficit of sodium is frequently accompanied by an equivalent loss of water, so that salt depletion is not reflected by changes in serum sodium concentration, whilst hyponatraemia usually reflects changes in hydration (i.e. retention of water in excess of salt). However, when salt depletion is particularly severe and ECV contraction assumes more significant proportions, the initial priority of maintaining a normal osmolality is sacrificed in order to minimize the further fall in extracellular fluid volume; thus, water is retained through an increased secretion of ADH[23]. In the latter condition, hyponatraemia occurs, reflecting a severe volume deficit.

Phosphate metabolism

Serum concentration of phosphate is maintained within the normal range in CRF until glomerular filtration rate has fallen to approximately 25–30 ml/min ('regulation with limitation'[14]). This is possible, without modification of phosphate intake with the diet, because of the progressive reduction in tubular reabsorption of phosphate in a stepwise fashion, similar to that which occurs in sodium metabolism. The mechanism of this adaptation of phosphate excretion to reduced nephron population is quite peculiar; there

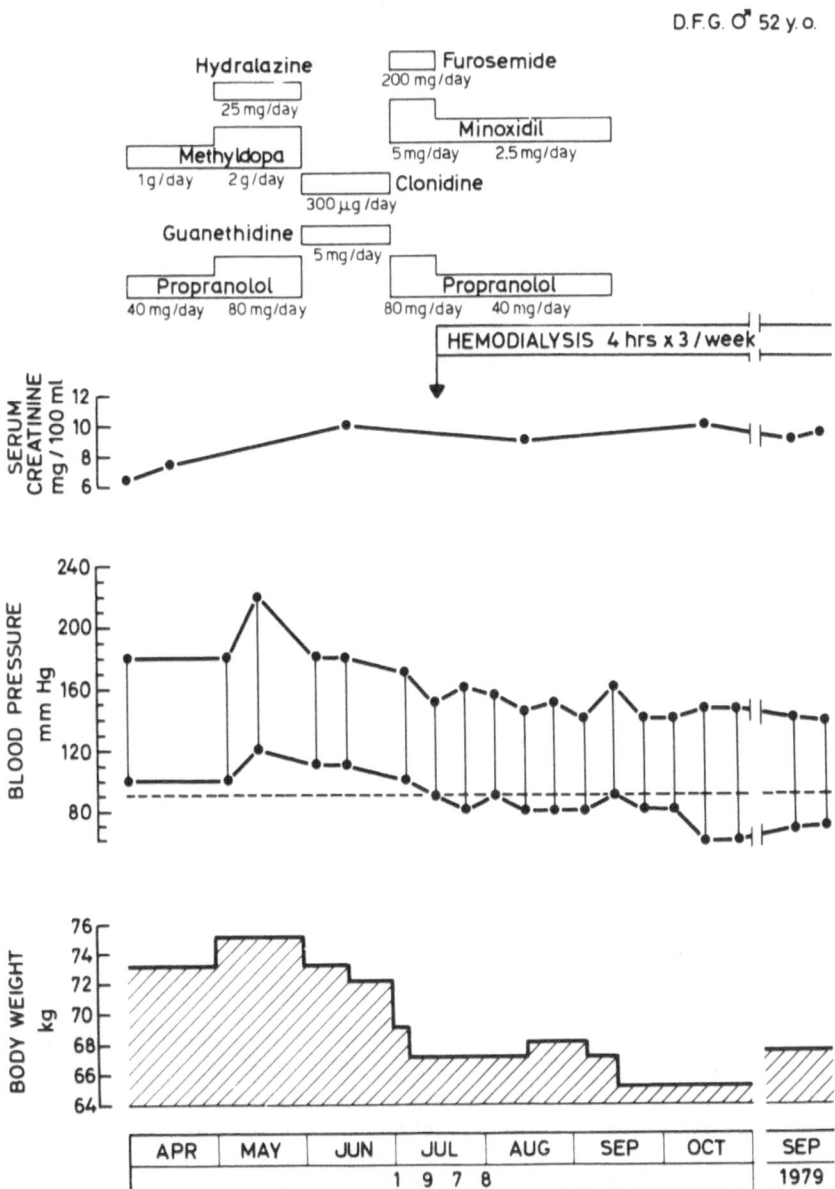

Figure 3 D.F.G., a 52-year-old male patient, was admitted because of far-advanced CRF, low urine output, oedema and hypertension unresponsive to treatment with conventional anti-hypertensive drugs. Only when regular haemodialysis treatment was started did blood pressure fall significantly (without further need for antihypertensive drugs), with a simultaneous fall in body weight due to correction of salt retention by dialysis ultrafiltration. The rise in body weight observed recently is due to the improved nutritional status (i.e. increase in 'dry weight') of the patient

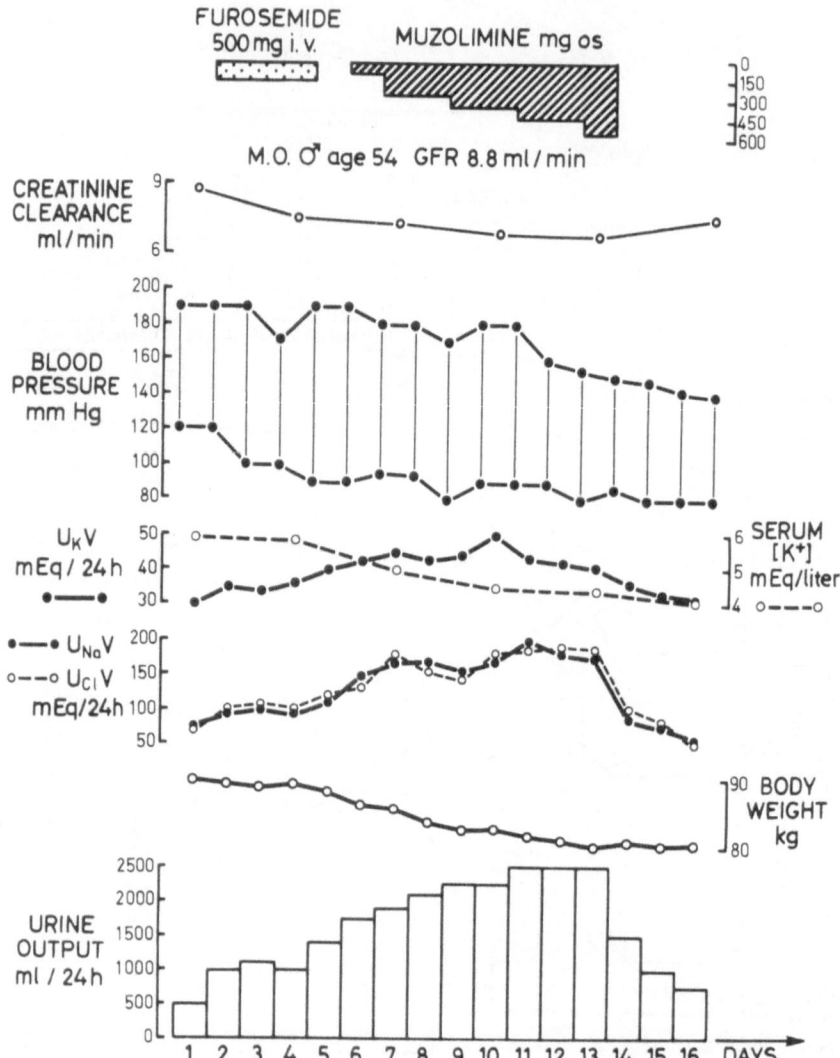

Figure 4 M.O., a 54-year-old male patient with a creatinine clearance of 8.8 ml/min, low urine output, oedema and hypertension (190/120 mmHg), was treated with high-ceiling diuretics, furosemide 500 mg i.v. daily and then muzolimine at increasing oral doses up to 580 mg/day. The increase in sodium excretion (up to 200 mmol/24 h) and in urine output (up to 2500 ml/24 h) and the fall in body weight were associated with a normalization in blood pressure

is evidence to support the view that it involves the activity of parathyroid glands.

Even in normal subjects it has been demonstrated that phosphate absorbed in the gut increases serum phosphate concentration, and even this slight hyperphosphataemia results in (a) an increase in filtered load of phosphate, and (b) a reciprocal fall in serum ionized calcium*. The fall in serum ionized calcium represents a stimulus for parathyroid glands to release parathyroid hormone (PTH)[24]. PTH reduces reabsorption of phosphate (in a condition of increased filtered load), and the resulting increase in phosphate excretion normalizes (i.e. reduces to fasting levels) both serum phosphate and ionized calcium concentration, and finally parathyroid gland activity[25].

This system appears to operate in a similar manner after a reduction in nephron population[26–29]. If phosphate intake is maintained at a constant level, as the number of functioning nephrons is reduced, some phosphate is retained and serum phosphate concentration rises, thereby increasing the filtered load of phosphate in residual nephrons. The reciprocal fall in serum ionized calcium results in PTH secretion[24], which in turn reduces tubular reabsorption of phosphate in the still functioning nephrons (in which the filtered load is increased); thus, the phosphate retained because of the reduction in nephron population will be excreted by surviving nephrons, normalizing serum phosphate concentration. The normalization of serum ionized calcium concentration abolishes the stimulus for hypersecretion of PTH. But the drop in PTH level again results in a fall in phosphate excretion, with the resulting tendency to phosphate retention and hypocalcaemia. The result of this condition is a permanent increase in the level of PTH activity which maintains an increased fractional excretion of filtered phosphate in surviving nephrons in order to prevent a recurrence of the hyperphosphataemia and hypocalcaemia. Serum phosphate concentration and serum ionized calcium concentration remain normal despite the drop in nephron population. Hence, PTH levels remain permanently elevated. Further reduction in the nephron population will initiate the same sequence resulting in a further increase in PTH level. Thus, as renal function decreases, phosphate excretion per residual nephron increases, so that external balance is maintained. The consequence ('trade-off') of this increase, however, is hyperparathyroidism (secondary hyperparathyroidism). This mechanism will maintain[14] the serum concentration of phosphate within normal range until GFR values of about 25–30 ml/min; with a further reduction in overall GFR, the mechanism will keep working, but, if phosphate intake is not reduced, hyperphosphataemia will necessarily result[18]. Thus, our patient P.S., for example, had a GFR of 10.9 ml/min: with a phosphate intake of about 700 mg/day and a serum concentration of phosphate of 4.9 mg/100 ml, the filtered load of phosphate was 769 mg/day (Table 4). To maintain the external balance, phosphate excretion had to be 700 mg/day, which represents 91.03% of the filtered load. Should the GFR of this patient fall to 5 ml/min, with a phosphate serum concentration of 4.9 mg/100 ml, the filtered load would be 353 mg/day (condition *a* in Table 4). Hence, even with

---

*Extracellular fluid is supersaturated with respect to bone mineral; hence any increase of serum phosphate will result in increased deposition of phosphate and calcium in bones.

a fractional excretion of phosphate of 100%, if phosphate intake is maintained at about 700 mg/day, as much as 347 mg/day will be retained. Phosphate retention will cause an increase in serum concentration of phosphate to a value (at least 9.73 mg/100 ml) that allows the maintenance of the external balance (with 100% fractional excretion of phosphate in condition b of Table 4). The logical consequence of what we have said is the need for a lower phosphate intake[14].

Table 4 Fractional excretion of phosphate in a uraemic patient with maintained external balance and theoretical values of phosphate excretion if GFR falls to 5 ml/min to demonstrate that hyperphosphataemia (condition b) is necessary for maintaining external balance

Patient or condition	Phosphate intake (mg/day)	GFR (ml/min)	Serum phosphate (mg/100 ml)	Filtered load of phosphate (mg/day)	Excretion rate of phosphate (mg/day)	Fractional excretion of phosphate (%)	Phosphate retention (mg/day)
P.S.	700	10.9	4.90	769	700	91.03	0
a	700	5.0	4.90	353	353	100.00	347
b	700	5.0	9.73	700	700	100.00	0

Undoubtedly secondary hyperparathyroidism in CRF is partly due to acquired resistance to the normal action of vitamin D which results in malabsorption of calcium from the intestine[30,31]. However, this is only a secondary factor which appears in advanced CRF[32,33]. The primary factor which increases the activity of parathyroid glands is the tendency to retain phosphate, which appears even when GFR is reduced to only 60 ml/min.

In favour of this 'trade-off hypothesis', suggested by Bricker and his group, are:

(a) The demonstration of a marked increase in serum PTH levels in CRF, with values 10–20 times normal, and far exceeding the levels observed in primary hyperparathyroidism[34-37].

(b) The progressive increase in PTH levels, with the fall in GFR, in dogs maintained on a diet containing 1200 mg of phosphorus per day but not in dogs on a diet with less than 100 mg of phosphorus per day[27].

(c) The demonstration of an inverse linear relationship between serum phosphate and ionized calcium in uraemic dogs on high phosphate intake with a simultaneous positive correlation between the fall in ionized calcium concentration and the rise in immunoreactive PTH (iPTH)[38].

(d) The prevention of the rise in iPTH in uraemic animals with the reduction of phosphate intake in direct proportion to the fall in GFR[28,38], especially when the contribution of vitamin D 'resistance' in the induction of secondary hyperparathyroidism was abolished by 25-OHD$_3$ supplements[39].

(e) The observation that, while a normal subject may usually maintain the external balance of phosphate by excreting about 15% of the filtered load, in advanced CRF, with the same phosphate intake, fractional excretion of phosphate may exceed 90% of the filtered load in order to maintain the external balance[40-42].

If phosphate reabsorption is inhibited in fasting uraemic patients due to chronic hyperparathyroidism, after ingestion and absorption of phosphate, further stimulation of parathyroid glands will occur with a consequent further increase in phosphaturia. The hyperphosphaturic effect in response to phosphate intake is, however, greater in the uraemic patients than in normal subjects receiving the same phosphate intake. This 'magnification phenomenon' seems to be accounted for by a greater increase in serum phosphate levels, and consequently a greater reciprocal fall in serum ionized calcium, as well as by a greater sensitivity of the residual nephrons of uraemic patients to the phosphaturic effect of parathyroid hormone[18].

Calcium metabolism

Chronic renal failure is characterized by multiple disturbances in calcium metabolism, despite the almost normal external calcium balance. This relatively normal calcium balance is accounted for by a very low urinary calcium excretion (less than 60 mg/day and sometimes even less than 10 mg/day)[22,43,44] in a condition of severe malabsorption of calcium from the intestine. Plasma calcium concentration may therefore be normal or, more frequently, low.

Multiple mechanisms may account for the alteration in calcium homeostasis in CRF: (a) malabsorption of calcium, (b) alteration in vitamin D metabolism, (c) relative deficiency of calcitonin, and (d) secondary hyperparathyroidism.

Malabsorption of calcium

A marked impairment of the intestinal absorption of calcium in chronic renal failure is well established. The intestinal defect in calcium absorption, usually detectable when creatinine clearance is lower than 40 ml/min (serum creatinine greater than 2.5 mg/100 ml in the adult man), is restricted to the proximal small intestine, i.e. duodenum and upper jejunum[45,46] which represent the vitamin D-dependent transport sites. Calcium absorption is apparently normal in more distal sites[45], where the process is passive and not dependent on vitamin D. Indeed, calcium absorption becomes normal[47] when calcium intake is augmented to 4–10 g/day. Uraemic patients are instead unable to adapt to the low dietary calcium intake that usually occurs[48] with low-protein diets, since intestinal adaptation to diets deficient in calcium should occur in the duodenum and upper jejunum[46]. The pathogenesis of calcium malabsorption in CRF is still uncertain. The major factor is the alteration in vitamin D metabolism. The increase in potassium concentration in intestinal juice, demonstrated in uraemic patients with secondary hyperaldosteronism, further compromises enteric absorption of calcium because of the interference of potassium with calcium transport[49].

Alteration in vitamin D metabolism

In man vitamin D has two sources:

(1) Endogenous production in the epidermal layer of skin where the provitamin 7-dehydrocholesterol is converted to vitamin D_3 by ultraviolet irradiation.

(2) The diet, both vitamin D_3 (cholecalciferol) and vitamin D_2 (ergocalciferol) being absorbed primarily from the duodenum and jejunum.

Both endogenous and dietary vitamin D are metabolized in the liver to 25-hydroxylated derivatives, i.e. 25-hydroxycholecalciferol (25-OHD_3) and 25-hydroxyergocalciferol (25-OHD_2).

25-OHD_3 represents the major circulating form of vitamin D and has been shown to stimulate enteric absorption of calcium, increase bone reabsorption, and enhance the proximal renal tubular reabsorption of sodium, calcium and phosphate (the effect on phosphate excretion being antagonistic to the phosphaturic effect of PTH). 25-OHD_3 is hydroxylated by the kidney to either 1,25-dihydroxycholecalciferol (1,25-$(OH)_2D_3$), under the influence of PTH, or 24,25-dihydroxycholecalciferol (24,25-$(OH)_2D_3$). The latter is further hydroxylated to 1,24,25-$(OH)_3D_3$, which exerts its biological activity by promoting the intestinal absorption of calcium. The chief vitamin D metabolite, with maximal biological activity, is 1,25-$(OH)_2D_3$, which controls the intestinal transport of calcium (it is more than twice as effective as 25-OHD_3) and the reabsorption of bone (it is some 100 times as effective as 25-OHD_3)[50].

The well-recognized vitamin D resistance in CRF, although not yet completely clarified, has been attributed mainly to interference in the normal production of the biologically active vitamin D metabolite. The demonstration that even small doses of 1,25-$(OH)_2D_3$ enhance intestinal calcium absorption and raise the serum calcium concentration in uraemic patients, while intermittent haemodialysis is unable to reverse calcium malabsorption and intestinal resistance to vitamin D, is consistent with the assumption that the reduction in functional renal mass (and consequently of the 1-hydroxylase activity) in the uraemic state results in decreased synthesis of 1,25-$(OH)_2D_3$. On the basis of the demonstrated stimulating effect of parathyroid hormone on the hydroxylation of 25-OHD_3 to 1,25-$(OH)_2D_3$, secondary hyperparathyroidism observed early in CRF is, in theory, expected to compensate for the decreased $1,25$-$(OH)_2D_3$ synthesis anticipated by the loss of renal mass. This is not the case, since serum levels of $1,25(OH)_2D_3$ are very low or even undetectable in uraemic patients[50]. It should be stressed, however, that although $1,25$-$(OH)_2D_3$ is the vitamin D_3 metabolite with maximal biological activity in regulating intestinal absorption of calcium and in remodelling bones, the renal conversion of 25-OHD_3 to $1,25$-$(OH)_2D_3$ does not appear to be an obligatory condition for the vitamin D effect at the intestinal and bone levels[51]. Indeed, vitamin D_3 is effective in raising serum calcium in anephric patients[52]. On the other hand, another dihydroxy-vitamin D metabolite, $24,25$-$(OH)_2D_3$, increases bone reabsorption and enhances the effect of $1,25$-$(OH)_2D_3$ on bone[53,54]. We may therefore conclude that the progressive osteomalacia (rickets in children) observed in untreated uraemic patients is accounted for by:

(1) Decreased $1,25$-$(OH)_2D_3$ synthesis due to reduction in renal mass, or to persistent metabolic acidosis and/or hyperphosphataemia (which are known to interfere with 1-hydroxylase activity)[55,56].
(2) The decreased biological availability of 25-OHD_3 because of poor nutrition, inadequate sunlight exposure and/or impaired hepatic hydroxylation of vitamin D_3 in the uraemic condition[50,57,58].
(3) Probably the retention of some unidentified substance which prevents the action of vitamin D metabolites on the bone[22].

Relative deficiency of calcitonin

It has been recently suggested that a relative deficiency of calcitonin, in conditions of increased PTH activity, may have a possible role in the pathogenesis of renal bone disease. Thus, Kanis et al.[59] have shown that uraemic patients with normal serum concentrations of alkaline phosphatase* exhibit a positive correlation between serum immunoreactive PTH (iPTH) and serum immunoreactive calcitonin, whereas uraemic patients with increased serum alkaline phosphatase and increased serum iPTH show a negative relation between the two hormones. Since calcitonin has been shown to inhibit intestinal absorption of phosphate[61], its deficiency may favour phosphate absorption and contribute to hyperphosphataemia and associated hypocalcaemia[62].

---

*The plasma concentration of alkaline phosphatase is generally used as a marker of bone turnover. Alkaline phosphatase is elaborated by osteoblasts[60] and from the latter it enters the peripheral circulation. In skeletal disorders in which osteoblastic activity increases, plasma alkaline phosphatase rises in proportion to the rise of the osteoblast number in bone biopsies; hence the measurement of plasma concentration of alkaline phosphatase may also represent a marker of bone reabsorption.

Secondary hyperparathyroidism

As nephrons are lost, the fall in overall GFR will result in a rise in plasma inorganic phosphate, but this is blunted by the secondary hyperparathyroidism which follows the reciprocal fall in ionized calcium concentration of extracellular fluid. When GFR is reduced to 20% of normal values, hyperphosphataemia and hypocalcaemia will occur, further stimulating parathyroid activity. Calcium malabsorption will provide an additional stimulus to parathyroid glands as well as the decreased response to calcitonin.

The biological effects of parathyroid hormone are not limited, however, to the inhibition of phosphate reabsorption in the renal tubule. It also maintains the concentration of soluble calcium in the extracellular fluid within the normal range. This is primarily due to its direct action on bone mineral by mobilization of calcium from the skeleton, and secondarily by increasing the conversion of $25\text{-}OHD_3$ to $1,25\text{-}(OH)_2D_3$ which stimulates intestinal calcium absorption[63]. Extracellular-fluid calcium, in turn, regulates the secretion of PTH and eventually its biosynthesis, for increased concentrations of extracellular calcium suppress, and decreased concentrations stimulate, hormone release. The responses of parathyroid glands to extracellular-fluid calcium levels are relatively fast. A modulation of an intracellular degradative pathway in the parathyroid glands may account for the rapid regulation of the amounts of parathyroid hormone available for secretion before the biosynthesis rate is changed to the extent required to meet secretory demands[64].

Thus, summarizing, PTH has the following effects:

(a) Mobilization of calcium and phosphate from bones;
(b) Stimulation of $25\text{-}OHD_3$ to $1,25\text{-}(OH)_2D_3$ conversion which will result in a rise of intestinal calcium absorption;
(c) Inhibition of phosphate reabsorption by renal tubules.

These effects lead to increased calcium in extracellular fluid without simultaneous increase in phosphate concentration, since the renal tubular effect of PTH (effect (c)) will offset the phosphate mobilization from bones (effect (a)). In advanced renal failure, however, the filtered load of phosphate is so reduced that even with a massive inhibition of tubular reabsorption of phosphate by PTH (effect (c)), the resulting phosphaturic effect will not be sufficient to match the effect of PTH in mobilizing phosphate from the bones (effect (a)) into the extracellular fluid[22]. Thus, in advanced renal failure, secondary hyperparathyroidism will contribute to an increase plasma phosphate. It is interesting that in advanced renal failure, plasma calcium concentration is low despite secondary hyperparathyroidism. This may be explained if the stimulation of the $25\text{-}(OH)D_3$ to $1,25\text{-}(OH)_2D_3$ conversion is ineffective in compensating for the decreased synthesis of $1,25\text{-}(OH)_2D_3$ due to loss in renal mass. Alternatively, the relatively constant hypocalcaemia of uraemic patients, despite the sometimes astronomical levels of PTH, may result from a kind of parathyroid hormone resistance[22]. It should be stressed, however, that the low serum concentration of calcium is an indispensable condition for the high levels of PTH. Should hypercalcaemia occur, parathyroid glands would be suppressed and PTH levels would fall, except for the existence of primary and 'tertiary' hyperparathyroidism.

In the average uraemic patient with secondary hyperparathyroidism, PTH secretion can be suppressed when the serum calcium is acutely increased[53]. In some patients, however, calcium infusion cannot suppress PTH secretion because of hyperplasia of parathyroid tissue[65]. These patients have hypercalcaemia and serum iPTH levels five to ten times higher than those high levels observed in most uraemic patients with normal or low serum calcium concentrations[35]. Only long-term (several months) regimens with low phosphate and high calcium can reverse this syndrome[66]. This functional relative autonomy of the hyperplastic parathyroid glands in chronic renal failure has been termed 'tertiary' hyperparathyroidism[35,67,68].

Renal osteodystrophy

Osteomalacia, osteitis fibrosa, osteosclerosis and (more rarely) osteoporosis, i.e. the skeletal abnormalities that occur in CRF, have been included in the general term 'renal osteodystrophy'. The prominence of one or other of these different bone lesions in uraemic patients is extremely variable, depending on factors such as geography, original kidney disease, duration of renal failure, diet and type of therapy. It has been stated that only chronic long-standing renal failure with urinary sodium leak (and therefore without hypertension), such as chronic pyelonephritis with recurrent infections, polycystic kidney disease, medullary cystic disease and chronic obstructive uropathy, is commonly associated with symptomatic bone disease[69].

Secondary hyperparathyroidism, abnormal metabolism or action of vitamin D and perhaps metabolic acidosis, with consequent buffering activity of bones, appear to be the main factors involved in the aetiology of renal osteodystrophy. However, the final effect is to cause decalcification of bones. Whether this decalcification is due only to negative calcium balance or, more probably, to redistribution of calcium within the bone, is still a matter of discussion[22].

Osteomalacia

Osteomalacia (rickets in children) is defined as a delay in the rate of skeletal mineralization which will result in an excess of unmineralized bone collagen[62]. In certain parts of the world, such as Europe and Asia, osteomalacia represents the main abnormality of renal osteodystrophy, while in North

America and Australia it is less common. The difference is probably related to the variation in dietary habits, exposure to sunshine and vitamin D supplements.

A low plasma calcium × plasma phosphorus product may result in osteomalacia by preventing calcium phosphate deposition into osteoid. This must be borne in mind when treating hyperphosphataemia with phosphate-binding gels, because they may cause an excessive fall in plasma phosphate with a consequent fall in the plasma calcium × plasma phosphorus product. The occurrence of defective skeletal mineralization in uraemic patients with a high calcium × phosphorus product in the plasma, and the improvement which may occur with large doses of vitamin D without changes in the calcium × phosphorus product[70,71], clearly show that uraemic osteomalacia is primarily related to vitamin D deficiency or resistance[72].

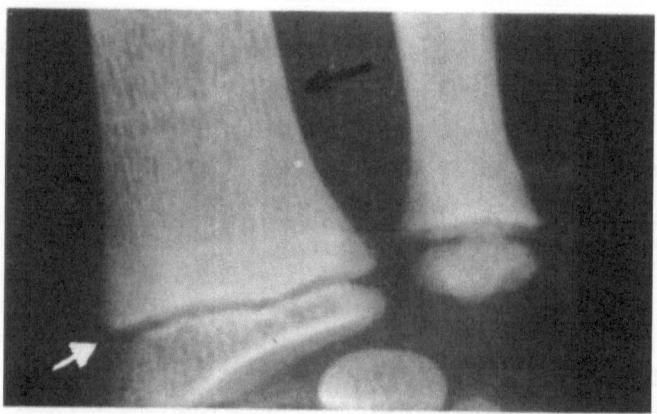

Figure 5   Pseudo-fracture (Looser's zone; upper arrow) in a patient with renal failure

Only 10% of patients with terminal renal failure have symptomatic osteodystrophy[73]. The symptoms are mainly referable to osteomalacia and are characterized by generalized aching (especially in the pelvis when the patient walks), proximal myopathy, severe weakness and, in children, bone deformities, such as genu valgum, and retardation of growth[69]. Only a small percentage of uraemic patients with histological changes of osteomalacia also have radiographic evidence of it[65] in the form of decreased bone density. The radiological finding is non-specific, since it also occurs in secondary hyperparathyroidism and osteoporosis[74]. The only radiological sign that is pathognomonic of osteomalacia is the 'pseudo-fracture' or 'Looser's Zone' (Figure 5). This is a linear band of lower density, perpendicular to the bone surface, usually seen in the pubic rami, the lower ribs, the inferior angle of the scapula and the metatarsal shafts[74]. In children, the defective mineralization of bones due to chronic uraemia may result in the radiographic features of rickets.

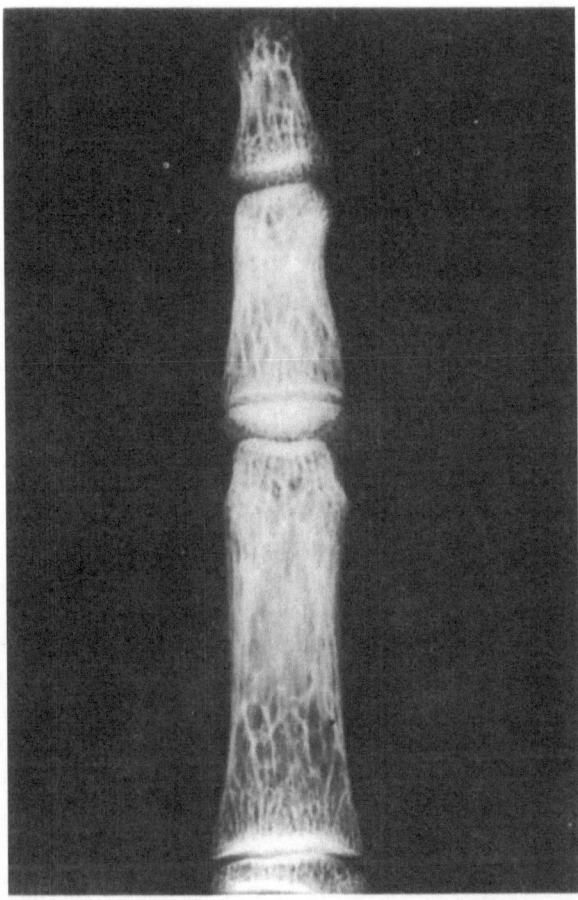

Figure 6 Exaggerated cortical striations due to enhanced bone resorption in the phalanges of the hand of a uraemic patient with secondary hyperparathyroidism

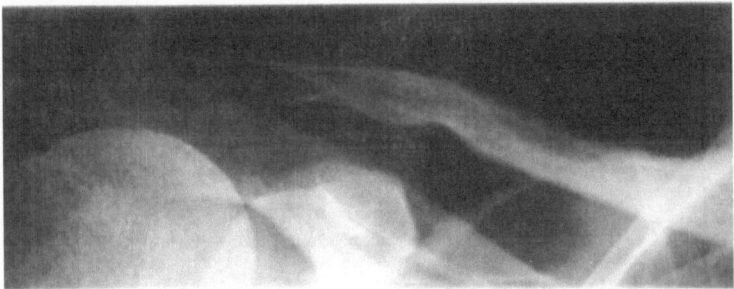

Figure 7 Erosion of the right clavicle in a uraemic patient with secondary hyperparathyroidism

Osteitis fibrosa

Since untreated chronic uraemia is invariably characterized by secondary hyperparathyroidism, osteitis fibrosa is a common feature of renal osteodystrophy, being the expression of increased osteoclastic activity (induced by PTH) that results in erosive lesions of the skeleton. The histological features of osteitis fibrosa include: woven bone collagen (the immature form of skeletal collagen), a great number of osteoclasts and osteoblasts, peritrabecular marrow fibrosis and an excess of osteoid[62]. Although most uraemic patients have histological evidence of secondary hyperparathyroidism in bone biopsies, only 50% of them also have radiological evidence of it[75]. The latter includes:

(1) Bone resorption (Figure 6) and, in particular, subperiosteal resorption quite common in the phalanges of hands and feet, but also in the medial margin of the tibia;

(2) The erosion of the distal ends of the clavicles (Figure 7), the inferior surface of the ribs, femur, tibia, ulna and mandible, and the sites of muscle insertions (e.g. ischial tuberosities);

(3) A mottled 'ground-glass' or 'salt and pepper' appearance of the skull (Figure 8);

(4) The large but rare cystic-like lesions, due to the so-called 'brown tumours' (because of haemosiderin deposition), usually localized in long bones (Figure 9), ribs, metacarpals, phalanges and skull[62,74]. The cystic-like lesions due to secondary hyperparathyroidism appear quite different from those observed in patients with oxalosis (Figure 10).

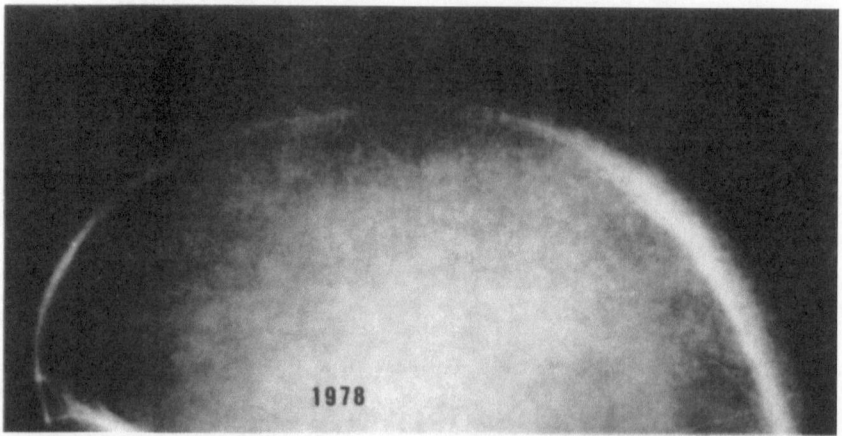

Figure 8 'Ground-glass' or 'salt and pepper' appearance of the skull in a uraemic patient with secondary hyperparathyroidism. The enhanced cortical resorption and the areas of increased trabecular density give rise to the typical granularity on X-ray

The action of PTH on bones releases calcium and phosphorus from the skeleton with a consequent rise in their plasma concentrations and secondary deposition in osteomalacic areas[72]. However, despite calcium release from bones, the plasma calcium concentration remains normal or, more frequently, below normal. Hypercalcaemia greater than 12 mg/100 ml in uraemic patients should suggest the possibility that (primary) hyperparathyroidism has caused renal failure rather than the reverse[22].

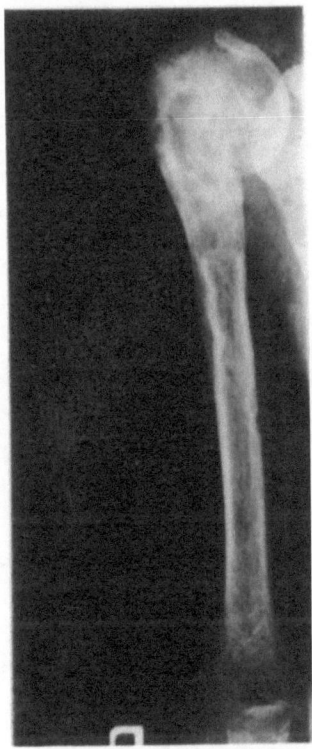

Figure 9   Severe cortical and medullary cystic-like lesions with pathological bone fracture in an adult with uraemia

Osteosclerosis

Osteosclerosis, which is characterized radiologically by an increase in bone density, may be the most frequent bone lesion in advanced chronic uraemia, especially in children[76-78]. It is usually overlooked because it does not cause symptoms, fractures or bone deformities[62]. Its usual location is in the axial skeleton, and on X-ray there is a characteristic 'rugger jersey sign' of horizontal bands of increased bone density at the upper and lower borders of the vertebral bodies alternating with horizontal bands of lower density[62,69,74].

Although osteosclerosis seems to be due to a relative decrease in osteoclastic activity, it has been attributed to a raised concentration of circulating parathormone[22,62,79,80].

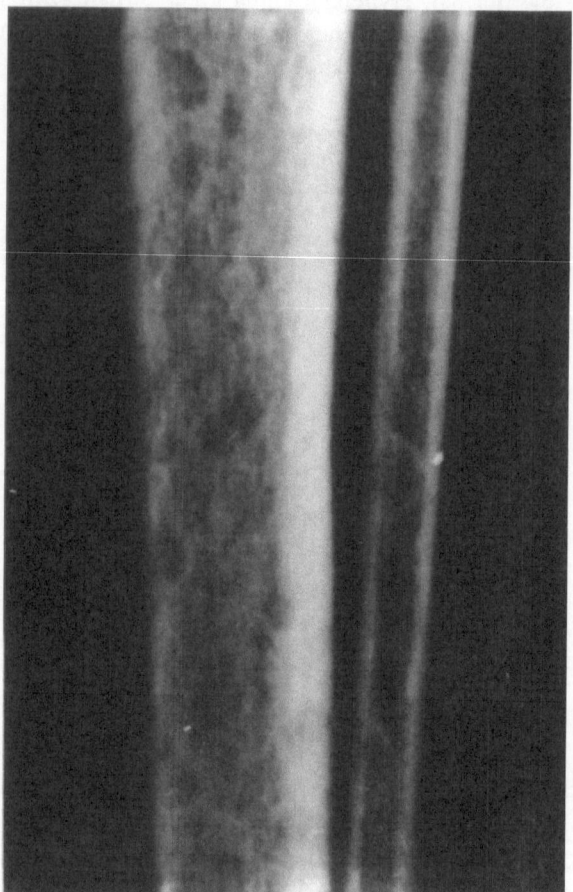

Figure 10 Cystic-like lesions due to oxalate deposits (observed in bone biopsy preparations) in a young patient with chronic uraemia secondary to hereditary oxalosis

Osteoporosis

Osteoporosis is a decreased mass of normally mineralized bone which shows radiologically as decreased skeletal density. It is quite a rare component of renal osteodystrophy, and is undoubtedly facilitated by immobilization, calcium deficiency and chronic protein depletion, in addition to those factors which in normal patients over 50 years old cause senile osteoporosis[72,74].

Undoubtedly the increased use of bone biopsies for diagnostic purposes has made possible the identification of different components of renal osteodystrophy and the prominence of some of them in individual cases.

Bone biopsies in uraemic patients will be of great help in the future for better understanding of the extent of deleterious effects on bones of factors such as metabolic acidosis or the demonstrated aluminium deposition in uraemic bones[81] secondary to the extensive use of aluminium-containing phosphate binders.

Metastatic calcification in extraosseous tissues

When serum concentration of total calcium and phosphorus is such that the Ca (mg/100 ml) × P (mg/100 ml) product exceeds 65–70, metastatic calcification in soft tissues may occur[44]. Conger et al.[82], however, have not observed any difference between Ca × P product in uraemic patients with and without metastatic calcifications. Hence, other factors, such as pH and circulating inhibitors of calcification, which may be removed by peritoneal dialysis but not by haemodialysis, may play an important role in the genesis of metastatic calcifications in chronic uraemia[83, 84].

Calcium phosphate deposition may take place in many extraosseous tissues and organs, causing more or less important symptoms:

(1) The epithelial layer of the sclera[84–87];
(2) The sclerocorneal border (band keratopathy)[84–87];
(3) The cornea and superficial layers of the interpalpebral bulbar conjunctiva, frequently causing hyperaemia (the 'red eyes' picture) and occasionally the sensation of 'foreign body'[84–87];
(4) The synovial fluid and periarticular tissues, with the appearance of an acute arthritis quite similar to hyperuricaemic gout (known as 'pseudo gout')[22, 88], usually involving interphalangeal joints of the hands, knees, ankles, elbows and shoulders[84];
(5) Muscles near the joints causing pain[84, 89];
(6) The stomach[84, 89];
(7) The kidneys[84, 89];
(8) The lungs and heart, causing breathlessness, atrio-ventricular conduction abnormalities, fibrillation and possibly sudden death[69, 84, 89–91];
(9) The blood vessels[89, 92, 93] (Figure 11);
(10) The brain[94];
(11) The skin, with calcium deposits in the dermis, in the hair follicles and in sebaceous glands, but never in sweat glands. When surrounded by a reactive fibrosis in the skin, it may cause pruritus[84, 95, 96].

Itching is, indeed, a frequent complaint of patients with advanced CRF and becomes even more frequent when RDT is started. It may be generalized, but it is usually more severe in certain areas, such as the back or extensor extremities, being exacerbated at night or during dialysis[97]. Proposed mediators of this cutaneous sensation are histamine, endopeptidases, kinins and prostaglandins[97]. The specific aetiology is not known. It was initially attributed to toxic effects of uraemia on small cutaneous nerve endings, then to increased number of mast cells in the skin, to abnormal function of sweat glands due to fibrosis, and finally to secondary hyperparathyroidism, since it may disappear after parathyroidectomy[73,95,97-99]. It is more likely to be due to high plasma calcium × phosphorus product which results in calcium phosphate deposition in the skin[22].

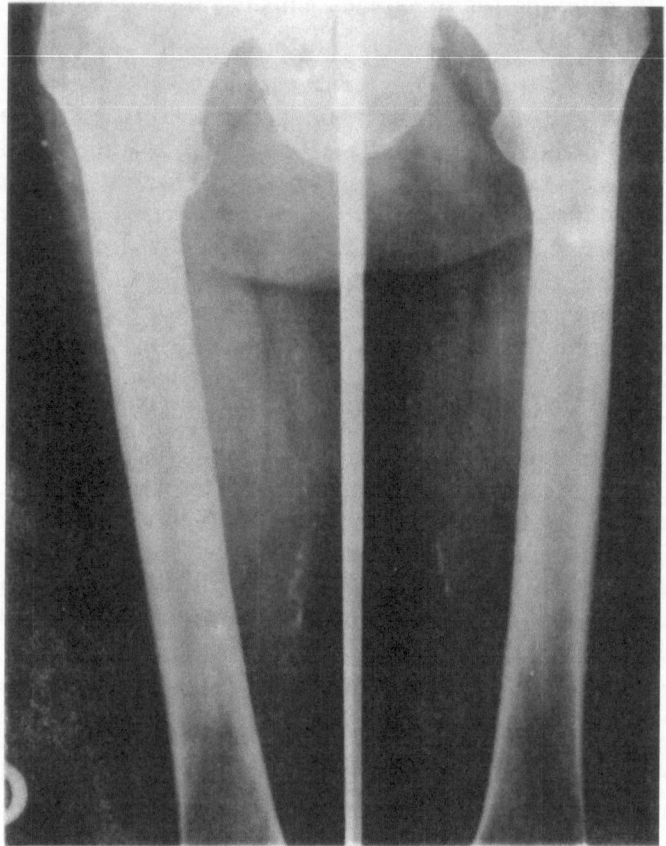

Figure 11   Vascular calcification in a patient with chronic uraemia

Indeed, calcium salt deposition in renal tissue requires further discussion. While it is reasonable that the underlying renal disease may continue to destroy renal tissue in some cases of CRF, the inexorable downhill course of all cases of CRF is still unexplained. In a retrospective study, Walser and his co-workers[100] have recently shown that the progression of CRF was slowed when the Ca × P product was maintained at subnormal values. Similar preliminary results have been obtained by the same authors in a prospective study in which the progression of CRF was slowed by dietary phosphate restriction and/or treatment with phosphate binders. It has therefore been postulated that the increase in plasma phosphorus that follows the fall in GFR causes secondary hyperparathyroidism and an increase in Ca × P product, and that both may lead to deposition of amorphous calcium phosphate in the mitochondria, causing death of renal cells. The further fall in GFR will further initiate the cycle, which may be interrupted by lowering plasma phosphorus[100].

It has been demonstrated that there are two different kinds of metastatic calcifications:

(1) Visceral (heart, lung, muscle) calcifications are amorphous or micro-crystalline compounds of magnesium witlockite[89,101] and calcium pyrophosphate[102];

(2) Non-visceral (periarticular and subcutaneous) and arterial calcifications are hydroxyapatite.

Since Mg is an integral part of visceral calcification, it may play an important role in its formation[89,103]. Since non-visceral calcification is prevented by lowering serum P concentration[88], visceral calcification may be prevented by lowering serum Mg concentration[89].

Various investigators have demonstrated that excess PTH enhances calcium deposition in soft tissues and that parathyroidectomy is quite efficient in preventing soft tissue calcification in experimental uraemic animals[93,94] and in decreasing soft tissue content of calcium in uraemic patients[96].

Potassium metabolism

More than 80% of the ingested potassium (normal daily potassium intake ranges between 50 and 90 mmol) is normally excreted by the kidneys. In CRF, however, despite a loss of up to 90% of the renal mass and maintenance of a normal potassium intake, serum potassium concentration is stabilized within or slightly above the upper limit of normal range (5–5.5 mmol/l). This implies a progressive adaptation of those mechanisms which are involved in the regulation of potassium homoeostasis. Undoubtedly, the kidneys play a key role in this adaptation phenomenon since potassium excretion with the urine is maintained at a normal level despite a progressive fall in GFR[104]. Since most of the urinary potassium in normal subjects derives from tubular secretion, renal adaptation in CRF is based more on increased tubular secretion than on decreased tubular reabsorption of filtered potassium[105]. This adaptive increase in potassium secretion in CRF has been located in the most distal part of the nephron (mainly collecting ducts) and is based on increased activity of Na–K-ATPase* in the medulla[105–107]. Normal levels of aldosterone are necessary, however, since long-term treatment with spironolactone in CRF may induce decreased potassium secretion and hyperkalaemia[108], and persistent hyperkalaemia may occur when hypoaldosteronism complicates CRF[109]. It should be stressed that the increased delivery of filtrate to the distal nephron is characteristic of surviving nephrons in CRF and represents another factor that favours potassium secretion by making more sodium available for cation exchange. Thus excessive restriction of salt intake may lead to hyperkalaemia[110].

When GFR falls below 5 ml/min, faecal excretion of potassium (normally 20% of the ingested potassium) is significantly increased, making an important contribution to potassium homoeostasis[108,111,112]. Whether this enhanced faecal potassium output is due to reduced intestinal water reabsorption, to hyperaldosteronism or to an augmented level of Na–K-ATPase in the colonic mucosa has not yet been elucidated[105]. It must be stressed, however, that this enteric adaptation occurs at an advanced stage of CRF when serum potassium rises above normal limits. The intestinal tract is a potential source of considerable potassium loss during the whole of the progressive course of CRF, as shown by the serious potassium deficits produced by protracted diarrhoea[105].

Serum potassium, however, is not an adequate index of body potassium stores. The latter may be reduced in uraemic patients in three conditions recently termed[105] as:

(a) 'Potassium deficiency', which is cellular loss of potassium in the face of a normal 'potassium capacity' (as defined by Scribner and Burnell[113]). It may be corrected by potassium supplements and is due to potassium loss, for example by vomiting.

(b) 'Potassium depletion', which is an expression of cellular loss of potassium that cannot be corrected by potassium supplements. This loss is due to an impaired ability of the cells to maintain normal potassium content. It has been attributed to reduced membrane Na–K-ATPase activity because of uraemic toxins and is corrected by chronic haemodialysis[114].

(c) 'Pseudodepletion', which is diminished 'potassium capacity'[113] due to a reduction in total muscle mass, while the cellular concentration of potassium is normal and potassium supplements are useless[105,115]. Pseudodepletion is usually observed in malnourished uraemic patients on inadequate protein diets and/or insufficient calorie intake.

---

*Sodium–potassium activated adenosine triphosphatase (Na–K-ATPase) is an essential enzyme for the active transport of sodium out of and potassium into the cells. At the renal level, peritubular uptake of potassium is mediated by the membrane Na–K-ATPase[105].

Despite the adaptive ability of uraemic patients, hyperkalaemia may occur during the whole of the progressive course of CRF because of several events that are summarized below[105].

1. Alteration in intra–extracellular distribution of potassium

It has been demonstrated that changes in acid–base balance may modify serum concentration of potassium independently of total body potassium through a redistribution of potassium ions across the cellular membrane. Metabolic acidosis, so frequently observed in CRF, causes a shift of K^+ into the extracellular fluid and increases serum potassium concentration by 0.6 mmol/l every 0.1 units change in extracellular pH (the opposite phenomenon occurs in alkalosis[113,116]). Similar effects have been described following the infusion of arginine hydrochloride in CRF, since arginine (like other cationic amino acids) enters the cells and displaces potassium[117,118]. It is therefore evident that intravenous infusions of arginine may be very dangerous in advanced CRF. Finally, acute increases in blood glucose may cause efflux of cellular potassium, leading to severe hyperkalaemia, presumably secondary to the sudden increase in serum osmolality[105] observed in uraemic diabetics with acute hyperglycaemia[119].

2. Alteration in renal adaptation

As previously mentioned, normal levels of aldosterone are necessary for renal adaptation. Hence, hyperkalaemia may occur in hypoaldosteronism, which is sometimes observed in CRF, particularly in diabetic patients when it is usually secondary to hyporeninaemia[120–124]. Similarly, hyperkalaemia may occur following long-term treatment with spironolactone. Finally, tubular unresponsiveness to mineralocorticoids has been suggested as a cause of hyperkalaemia in some cases of CRF[125,126].

3. Potassium loads

Exogenous potassium comes from food (meat, fruits, fruit juices, green vegetables, etc.), some antibiotics (such as potassium salt of penicillin) and intravenous infusion of solutions containing potassium salts. Banked blood transfusions may contain excessive potassium and it has been reported that a potassium concentration of over 30 mmol/l occurs in banked blood over 10 days old. This is due to potassium migration from red blood cells into plasma[127].

Similarly, excessive catabolism, secondary to infections, trauma or high fever, may cause massive release of endogenous cellular potassium. It has been calculated that 2.7 mmol of potassium per gram of nitrogen is liberated from tissue breakdown[128].

Both exogenous and endogenous potassium loads may cause severe hyperkalaemia by overwhelming the renal adaptive capacity of uraemic patients whose residual functioning nephrons are constantly working close to their maximum ability for potassium secretion[105]. In advanced renal failure, when the urine volume falls below 500 ml/day, serious hyperkalaemia (i.e. serum potassium concentration greater than 7.0 mmol/l) may occur and dialysis becomes necessary. Severe hyperkalaemia must be treated immediately because severe cardiac arrhythmia and arrest may occur when the serum concentration of potassium exceeds 7.5–8.0 mmol/l.

Acid–base balance

Acid–base balance in healthy subjects

Most of the carbohydrate and fat metabolized in the human body is completely burned to carbon dioxide (CO_2) and water. Since CO_2 is excreted by the lungs (approximately 20 000 mmol/day in normal adults), this metabolic pathway does not result in H^+ accumulation in body fluids. Only a small fraction of carbohydrate and fat is incompletely oxidized to organic acids, thus contributing to the generation of fixed (i.e. non-volatile) acid end products of metabolism. The main source of fixed acid end products of metabolism is protein, through the oxidation of the sulphur-containing amino acids to sulphuric acid and the oxidation and hydrolysis of phosphoproteins to phosphoric acid[129].

It has been calculated that fixed acid generation is approximately 1 mmol/kg body weight in normal adults[130]. In children and infants it is much greater, reaching 2 and even 3 mmol/kg body weight because of hydrogen ion release following calcium deposition in new bone formation[131–133]. All of these fixed acids are normally excreted by the kidneys.

The generation of fixed acids would readily decrease the pH of body fluids were it not for very sophisticated buffering mechanisms. The first of these mechanisms occurs practically instantaneously and is a true chemical buffering. Body fluids contain several buffer systems that minimize the deviation of pH resulting from addition of strong acids (or bases). These include bicarbonate, phosphate and proteins of plasma, and intracellular fluids, and haemoglobin of the red blood cells. The buffer activity of body fluids is demonstrated in the bicarbonate–carbonic acid system of plasma, which is the body fluid most accessible for analysis. Thus the pH of plasma (that in healthy subjects is maintained close to 7.4) is defined by the Henderson–Hasselbalch equation:

$$pH = 6.1 + \log \frac{[NaHCO_3]}{\text{dissolved } CO_2 + [H_2CO_3]} \tag{1}$$

$$\nwarrow \quad \downarrow \quad \uparrow$$
$$CO_2 + H_2O$$

This is a very peculiar buffer system, since its acid component (the denominator of equation (1)) is a gas that is constantly formed in the body as a metabolic end product and whose excretion is readily modulated by respiratory exchange[134]. Thus the addition of strong acid (e.g. H_2SO_4 or NaH_2PO_4) to body fluids will induce a bicarbonate consumption as a consequence of the following reactions:

$$H_2SO_4 + 2NaHCO_3 \rightarrow Na_2SO_4 + 2H_2CO_3 \qquad (2)$$
$$\downarrow$$
$$2H_2O + 2CO_2$$

$$NaH_2PO_4 + NaHCO_3 \rightarrow Na_2HPO_4 + H_2CO_3 \qquad (3)$$
$$\downarrow$$
$$H_2O + CO_2$$

There will be, therefore, a fall in plasma bicarbonate concentration (the numerator of equation (1)). Any change in blood pH will be minimized by the CO_2 excretion of the lungs, i.e. the accelerated respiratory exchange (due to the rise in P_{CO_2} and the fall in blood pH) will readily reduce the tension of CO_2 (the denominator of equation (1)) so that the $[NaHCO_3]/[H_2CO_3]$ ratio will be normalized and, consequently, the pH will return to the initial normal value.

The second buffering mechanism may be called 'biological buffering' and consists of ionic (anionic and cationic) shifts across cell membranes in order to protect extracellular pH[129]. Exchange of anions (HCO_3^- and Cl^-) seems to be restricted to red blood cells and renal tubular cells, while the exchange of cations (Na^+, K^+ and perhaps Ca^{2+}) involves muscle cells and bone[134]. If acids are added to the extracellular fluid, some (almost half) of the H^+ will be buffered in the extracellular compartment (chemical buffering). More H^+ (almost half) will diffuse across cell membranes into the cells, either with an accompanying anion (e.g. Cl^-) or, more commonly, in exchange for intracellular Na^+ or K^+[135]. The net result will be the removal of some acid from the extracellular compartment in order to minimize any deviation of extracellular pH from normal. Similarly, i.v. infusion of bicarbonate solution will be followed by diffusion of part (half) of HCO_3^- into the cells[136]. This biological buffering mechanism is very important indeed and takes 2 to 4 hours to be accomplished[129].

The third buffering mechanism is a physiological buffering by respiratory adaptation[129]. As mentioned previously, the chemical buffering of strong acids by the bicarbonate–carbonic acid system, while consuming plasma bicarbonate, will generate excess carbon dioxide. This process will therefore cause a rise in CO_2 tension (P_{CO_2}) and a fall in blood pH (because of the fall in the $[HCO_3^-]/[H_2CO_3]$ ratio). The central chemoreceptors located in the medullary respiratory centres are particularly sensitive to changes both in P_{CO_2} and in pH so that both the increase in P_{CO_2} and the fall in pH will promote pulmonary ventilation. Respiratory buffering is a fast mechanism occurring within a few minutes.

The fourth buffering mechanism is a physiological buffering by renal adaptation[129]. It is a rather slow mechanism and may take hours or days to be accomplished. The kidneys combat acidosis by two tubular processes, bicarbonate reclamation and bicarbonate regeneration. Bicarbonate reclamation is the complete tubular reabsorption of all filtered bicarbonate, a condition necessary for maintaining the plasma bicarbonate concentration. It takes place mainly (85–90%) in the proximal tubule but also in the distal tubule. It is a somewhat 'indirect' reabsorption (see Figure 12), since Na^+ of the filtered $NaHCO_3$ is exchanged with secreted H^+ derived, within the tubular cells, from the following reaction (accelerated by the enzyme carbonic anhydrase, CA)

$$\overset{CA}{CO_2 + H_2O \rightleftharpoons H_2CO_3 \rightleftharpoons H^+ + HCO_3^-} \tag{4}$$

Thus the process of bicarbonate reclamation may be summarized in the following reaction:

$$\underset{\substack{\text{(tubular} \\ \text{lumen)}}}{NaHCO_3} + \underset{\substack{\text{(tubular} \\ \text{cell)}}}{H_2CO_3} \rightarrow \underset{\substack{\text{(tubular} \\ \text{lumen)}}}{H_2CO_3} + \underset{\substack{\text{(peritubular} \\ \text{fluid)}}}{NaHCO_3} \tag{5}$$

The aim of this reaction is to move $NaHCO_3$ from the tubular lumen to the peritubular fluid; the H_2CO_3 formed in the tubular lumen readily dissociates to $CO_2 + H_2O$ (reaction (4)) under the influence of luminal carbonic anhydrase[137]. Bicarbonate reclamation alone is not sufficient to prevent bicarbonate depletion since, as mentioned earlier, bicarbonate in body fluids is continuously dissipated by the buffering action of strong acids with the bicarbonate–carbonic acid system; thus, one molecule of H_2SO_4 will dissipate two molecules of $NaHCO_3$ (see reaction (2)) and one molecule of NaH_2PO_4 will dissipate one molecule of $NaHCO_3$ (see reaction 3)). Hence the need for a bicarbonate regeneration that implies acidification of the urine (Figure 12); i.e. the $NaHCO_3$ dissipated for buffering purpose is regenerated by the distal tubules of the kidneys according to the following reactions:

$$\underset{\substack{\text{(tubular} \\ \text{lumen)}}}{Na_2HPO_4} + \underset{\substack{\text{(tubular} \\ \text{cell)}}}{H_2CO_3} \rightarrow \underset{\substack{\text{(tubular} \\ \text{lumen)}}}{NaH_2PO_4} + \underset{\substack{\text{(peritubular} \\ \text{fluid)}}}{NaHCO_3} \tag{6}$$

The filtered Na_2HPO_4 within the tubular lumen is transformed into NaH_2PO_4 by exchanging one of its sodium ions for one secreted hydrogen ion (this is derived from reaction (4)). Hence, one molecule of $NaHCO_3$ is regenerated for each molecule of Na_2HPO_4 that has been filtered (i.e. reaction (6) will reverse reaction (3)).

$$\underset{\substack{\text{(tubular} \\ \text{lumen)}}}{Na_2SO_4} + \underset{\substack{\text{(tubular} \\ \text{cell)}}}{2H_2CO_3} + \underset{\substack{\text{(tubular} \\ \text{lumen)}}}{2NH_3} \rightarrow \underset{\substack{\text{(tubular} \\ \text{lumen)}}}{(NH_4)_2SO_4} + \underset{\substack{\text{(peritubular} \\ \text{fluid)}}}{2NaHCO_3} \tag{7}$$

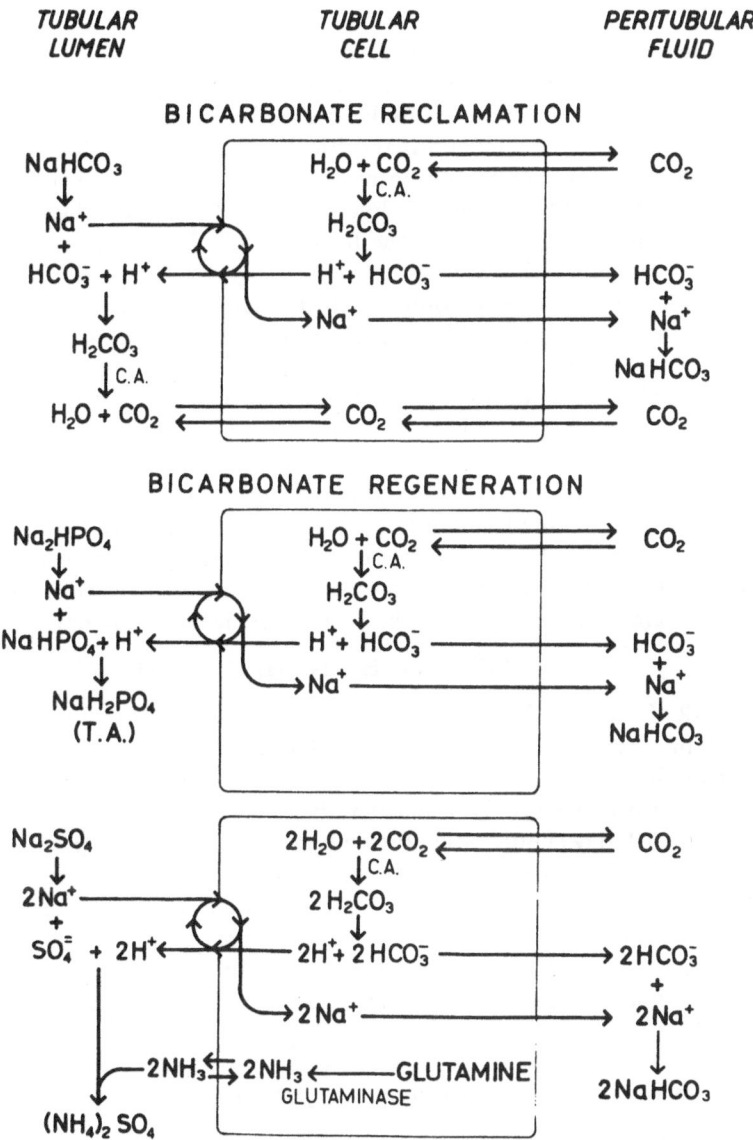

Figure 12 Bicarbonate reclamation and regeneration along the nephron

The filtered Na_2SO_4 within the tubular lumen is transformed into $(NH_4)_2SO_4$ by exchanging both of its sodium ions ($2Na^+$) for two secreted hydrogen ions ($2H^+$) (that are derived from reaction (4)), the latter being buffered by ammonia ($2NH_3$) formed in the tubular cells (mainly from deamination of glutamine) and then diffused to the tubular lumen. Two molecules of

$NaHCO_3$ are therefore regenerated for each molecule of Na_2SO_4 that has been filtered (i.e. reaction (7) will reverse reaction (2)).

Both processes (bicarbonate reclamation and bicarbonate regeneration) are based on H^+ secretion by tubular cells. Most of this H^+ (i.e. approximately 4500 mmol/24 h in a normal subject with a GFR of 120 ml/min and plasma bicarbonate concentration of 26 mmol/l) is secreted solely for reclaiming all filtered bicarbonate, while as little as 1.5–2% of all secreted H^+ will reach the urine, mainly in the form of buffered phosphate and ammonium ions (NH_4^+).

The net urinary acid excretion (i.e. the kidney's total excretion of H^+) is given by the titratable acid (TA) plus ammonium (NH_4^+) minus bicarbonate (whose excretion in healthy subjects is negligible). Titratable acid is represented by the hydrogen ions present in the urine both as free acid compounds and incorporated in the buffers of the urine. It is equivalent to the amount of NaOH necessary to bring the urine pH to that of blood. Obviously a low urinary pH does not necessarily mean a high rate of acid excretion, since a small amount of a strong acid will lower the pH very slightly in a well-buffered urine but quite considerably in a poorly buffered urine[134]. Titratable acidity is almost completely due to phosphate, the titration being accomplished on the basis of the following reaction:

$$NaH_2PO_4 + NaOH \rightarrow Na_2HPO_4 + H_2O \qquad (8)$$

When all of the NaH_2PO_4 has reacted, addition of NaOH will raise the pH (ammonia is so alkaline[129] that titration to blood pH does not free hydrogen ions from NH_4^+).

In a healthy subject on a normal diet, the total quantity of acid excreted in the urine each day should equal the daily generation of fixed (non-volatile) acid. Thus, it approximates to 1 mmol/kg body weight in normal adults[130] (i.e. about 40–70 mmol/day) and 2–3 mmol/kg body weight in children and infants[131]. In normal adults, half or somewhat more than half of the urinary H^+ is excreted as NH_4^+, the remainder as TA. In infants[138,139], who have a low excretion rate of phosphate buffer, almost all H^+ is excreted as NH_4^+.

Alteration in acid–base balance in uraemic patients

When GFR falls to 20 ml/min or less, a mild metabolic acidosis occurs with a slight fall in plasma bicarbonate concentration. This is due to reduced efficiency of the renal buffering mechanism, in particular to an impaired ability to excrete hydrogen ions, and, therefore, to regenerate bicarbonate.

Ammonium excretion. The most striking and frequent abnormality in uraemic patients is the impaired urinary excretion of ammonium ions. Ammonia (NH_3) is formed within the tubular cells by deamination of glutamine (and other amino acids). It is a base, soluble in lipids and readily diffusible across cell membranes down a concentration gradient. Hence, it may easily diffuse from the tubular cells, where it is formed, into both the tubular lumen and the peritubular capillaries. The amount diffusing into the peritubular blood is inversely proportional to that diffusing into urine[22]. Once in the tubular lumen, ammonia (NH_3) combines with hydrogen ions (H^+), becoming ammonium ions (NH_4^+) whose diffusibility is low; hence NH_4^+ cannot diffuse back across the renal tubular cell membrane and is excreted in the urine with an accompanying anion. This process maintains a low concentration of ammonia within the tubular lumen and favours further passive ammonia diffusion from the tubular cells. The consequent fall in intracellular concentration represents an important stimulus for further ammonia generation from glutamine[22].

It is therefore evident that many factors may influence urinary ammonium output:

(1) Tubular secretory rate of H^+: reduced secretion will reduce NH_4^+ formation within the tubular lumen. This, in turn, will decrease NH_3 diffusion into the lumen and consequently its intracellular generation.

(2) Urine pH: it has been demonstrated that urinary ammonium output is inversely related to urine pH[140].

(3) Blood pH: metabolic acidosis, induced in healthy subjects (with normal GFR) by ammonium chloride administration (NH_4Cl is metabolized to urea and HCl, making the extracellular fluid acidic), will increase NH_4^+ excretion without corresponding changes in urine pH[129].

(4) Quantity of glutamine (and other amino acids) available for ammonia generation: the administration of supplementary amino acid substrates during chronic acidosis will significantly raise the excretion rate of ammonium ions[141].

(5) Renal tubular cell mass generating ammonia: a reduction in this cell mass will limit the amount of ammonia that can be generated[140].

The most simple explanation for the reduced excretion of NH_4^+ in CRF is that the damaged renal tubular cells have lost their ability to generate NH_3 at a normal rate. Experimental studies in dogs by Bricker and his co-workers[142,143] argue against such an explanation, since the excretion of ammonium ions per unit of glomerular filtrate ($U_{NH_4^+} \cdot V/GFR$) by a diseased (pyelonephritic) kidney was much greater after the removal of the contralateral healthy kidney (i.e. in uraemic condition) than before (i.e. in non-uraemic condition) because the fall in GFR by the experimental kidney is compensated by the normal or even greater GFR of the contralateral healthy kidney. Similar supernormal ammonium output per millilitre of GFR has been observed in humans with CRF[144]. The uraemic environment therefore raises the ability of the diseased kidney to generate NH_3 (presumably because metabolic acidosis induces an adaptation of the ammonia synthetic system) and in turn to excrete NH_4^+. This renal adaptation, however, is not sufficient to compensate for the reduction in functioning renal tissue. Even though NH_3 generation by renal tubular cells of surviving nephrons is greatly increased, the surviving nephrons are so few in number that overall ammonia generation may be inadequate for H^+ buffering and consequently absolute ammonium output will be quite low. For example, assuming that a normal subject of 70 kg body weight, with a GFR of 120 ml/min, is excreting 1 mmol/kg body weight of H^+, half of which (i.e. 35 mmol/day) is as NH_4^+, the excretion rate of NH_4^+ will be 0.29 mmol/ml of glomerular filtrate per day. In a uraemic patient with a GFR of 4 ml/min, NH_4^+ excretion may increase up to 4 mmol (ml of GFR)$^{-1}$ day^{-1}, but this large amount of NH_4^+ excretion per unit of glomerular filtrate will result in an overall NH_4^+ excretion of only 16 mmol/day, a quantity obviously insufficient to contribute significantly to H^+ excretion.

Titratable acid (TA) excretion. The titratable acid excretion (i.e. the excretion of phosphate-buffered hydrogen ions) is usually well preserved in CRF as long as total phosphate excretion is maintained. The reduction in the number of functioning nephrons is compensated by a greater titratable acid excretion per unit of glomerular filtrate ($U_{TA} . V$/GFR), since phosphate excretion per nephron is also increased because of greater PTH activity (see 'Phosphate metabolism', p. 42). Only qhen a uraemic patient is fed with low-protein diet is the availability of phosphate buffer in the tubular fluid reduced. The addition of phosphate binder medications to a low-protein diet will further reduce intestinal absorption of phosphate and consequently phosphate excretion. In this condition, overall titratable acid excretion decreases to the extent that phosphate excretion is reduced.

Bicarbonate reclamation. In uraemic patients, plasma bicarbonate concentration is reduced when GFR is lower than 20 ml/min. Urine pH in this situation is normally acid (usually less than 5.0)[145,146], clearly showing that bicarbonate reclamation is complete and that urinary bicarbonate loss is not contributing to the maintenance of uraemic metabolic acidosis. Nevertheless, in some cases, an increase in plasma bicarbonate concentration to within the normal range may cause the fractional excretion of plasma bicarbonate to rise from a normal value of less than 1% to as much as 20%. This bicarbonate leak will impair the acidification of urine[147], whose pH will fall below 5.5 only when plasma bicarbonate concentration is lower than 20 mmol/l. Hence, bicarbonate reclamation may also be impaired in CRF. This defect (a Type II or proximal renal tubular acidosis) is usually not detectable at low plasma bicarbonate levels but becomes evident when bicarbonate concentration is normalized. In such cases it appears to be difficult to normalize blood bicarbonate by exogenous administration of base.

In chronic uraemia, the ability of diseased kidneys to secrete H^+ (a process necessary for bicarbonate reclamation) is obviously reduced because of the severely reduced number of surviving nephrons. Whether this reduction in functioning nephrons is directly responsible for the overall reduction in H^+ secretion, or only indirectly through the increased fractional excretion of Na^+ (due either to ECV expansion or to a natriuretic hormone)[148,149] or through secondary hyperparathyroidism[22,129,150-153] has not yet been settled.

Metabolic acidosis. In uraemic patients, hydrogen ion generation from metabolism is comparable to that of normal subjects as long as protein intake is not restricted. Phosphate intake is usually normal, thereby allowing the maintenance of a normal titratable acid excretion despite the reduction in nephron population. The excretion of ammonium ions by each nephron is greatly increased, but the severe reduction in functioning nephrons will make such renal adaptation inadequate. The overall urinary ammonium output will be lower than normal and insufficient to contribute significantly to the maintenance of the H^+ external balance. Consequently, the rate of H^+ excretion and bicarbonate regeneration is much lower than the rates of H^+ generation and bicarbonate utilization for buffering[154]. A mild metabolic acidosis will result with a slight fall in plasma bicarbonate concentration. When uraemic patients are fed with low-protein diets, the generation of fixed (non-volatile) acid is reduced (every 10 g of protein provides 7 mmol of H^+[110]), but the simultaneous fall in urinary phosphate excretion (due to lower phosphate intake) will reduce the rate of titratable acid excretion so that the external positive H^+ balance and metabolic acidosis will be maintained.

Uraemic metabolic acidosis is usually stable (unless a further deterioration of renal function occurs) despite a positive external balance for H^+ which would be expected to lead to progressive falls in pH and plasma bicarbonate concentration[147,154]. Hence, an extra buffering system must operate in chronic uraemia and it is a common opinion that this is apatite in bones[154-156]. The price paid for using this compensatory mechanism is decalcification of bones. As hydrogen ions enter bones and are buffered by carbonate and other calcium buffers in bone, calcium ions leave the bones and are excreted in the urine. It has been calculated that buffering 15 mmol of H^+ daily by bones results in nearly 50% bone calcium being lost in 3 years[157]. Uraemic acidosis may therefore significantly contribute to uraemic osteodystrophy by 'dissolving' bones.

Evaluation of metabolic acidosis

Standard bicarbonate and base excess. Acid–base disturbances may occur as the consequence of alterations in either respiratory or metabolic activity. Hyperventilation, by lowering P_{CO_2}, leads to respiratory alkalosis, while, conversely, hypoventilation results in respiratory acidosis through an increase in Pco_2. Alterations in the metabolic status of the patient will result in metabolic acidosis or alkalosis. Astrup and his co-workers[158] have suggested the measurement of 'standard bicarbonate' as a method for eliminating the respiratory component in the acid–base imbalance. The standard bicarbonate is the concentration of bicarbonate in an oxygenated blood sample once it has been equilibrated with CO_2 at a Pco_2 of 40 mmHg at 38 °C. Any deviation from the normal range of values (about 21–25 mmol/l) represents a metabolic change, 'base excess' and 'base deficit' being found in metabolic alkalosis and metabolic acidosis respectively. In the absence of both base excess and base deficit, the disturbance must be respiratory in origin.

Measurement of standard bicarbonate is now widely used for fast and simple evaluation of acid–base abnormalities. This method has, however, two very important disadvantages[129]. Firstly, carbon dioxide titration curves are different *in vitro* and *in vivo*, as clearly shown by Brackett *et al*.[159]. *In vivo*, the bicarbonate generated in the red blood cells at increasing Pco_2 distributes itself throughout the 'bicarbonate space' (which approximates to the total body water), whereas *in vitro* it is confined to the blood. Secondly, in long-standing acid–base imbalance, the renal buffering mechanism has already played an important role in adjusting the plasma bicarbonate concentration to the primary alteration of Pco_2: thus base excess and base deficit can be misleading terms, since they may not represent primary metabolic changes in acid–base balance, but just a normal physiological response to primary changes in Pco_2. For these reasons, we agree with Makoff[129] that standard bicarbonate measurement offers no advantages over analysis of acid–base balance by measurement of pH and Pco_2, and calculation of plasma bicarbonate concentration from the Henderson–Hasselbach equation.

Anion gap. The fall in bicarbonate concentration in the extracellular compartment, observed in metabolic acidosis, must be compensated by accumulation of other anions to satisfy the requirement for electroneutrality. The nature of this anion depends on GFR. When GFR is normal or only slightly reduced, the lower plasma bicarbonate is compensated by increased plasma chloride (hyperchloraemic metabolic acidosis), since more sodium is reabsorbed from the tubular fluid as sodium chloride. In uraemic metabolic acidosis, since GFR is low enough to induce retention of other anions, such as sulphate and phosphate, the drop in plasma bicarbonate concentration is compensated by these usually unmeasured anions that belong (together with proteins and organic acids) to the so-called 'anion gap'. The anion gap is calculated as:

$$([Na^+]_P + [K^+]_P) - ([Cl^-]_P + [HCO_3^-]_P) = \text{anion gap}$$

and, in healthy subjects, it is usually equal to 16 mmol/l (if $[Na^+]_P =$

140 mmol/l, $[K^+]_P = 4$ mmol/l, $[Cl^-]_P = 102$ mmol/l and $[HCO_3^-]_P = 26$ mmol/l).

In hyperchloraemic metabolic acidosis, the anion gap is normal (i.e. about 16 mmol/l), the lower plasma bicarbonate concentrations (e.g. 14 mmol/l rather than 26 mmol/l) being compensated for by a greater plasma chloride concentration (114 mmol/l rather than 102 mmol/l in the example if $[Na^+]_P = 140$ mmol/l and $[K^+]_P = 4$ mmol/l).

In the uraemic metabolic acidosis, the anion gap is increased (e.g. to 28 mmol/l when plasma bicarbonate is 14 mmol/l, if $[Na^+]_P = 140$ mmol/l, $[K^+]_P = 4$ mmol/l, while $[Cl^-]_P$ remains equal to 102 mmol/l); this wide gap is accounted for by an increased plasma concentration of phosphate and sulphate.

Calculation of the anion gap may help in identifying the possible causes of metabolic acidosis. Thus, a normal anion gap is observed in metabolic acidosis secondary to diarrhoea, draining fistulas, ammonium chloride administration, renal tubular acidosis and 'expansion' acidosis. A wide anion gap occurs in uraemic metabolic acidosis, diabetic ketoacidosis, lactic acidosis and following the ingestion of salicylate, methyl alcohol, paraldehyde and ethylene glycol[129].

Clinical manifestations of metabolic acidosis

The most evident clinical sign of metabolic acidosis is dyspnoea, characterized by an increase first in depth and then in frequency of respirations with the effort that is peculiar to the expiratory phase (Kussmaul breathing). This is the only symptom undoubtedly due to the acidosis[22]. In our experience, however, acidotic uraemic patients, suffering from nausea, retching and vomiting, may have these symptoms reversed by correction of metabolic acidosis with exogenous base administration in the form of intravenous $NaHCO_3$.

Uraemic acidosis inhibits growth in children, since mobilization of calcium salts from bone for buffering fixed acids leads to alteration in bone structure and interferes with growth[160–162].

The development of renal osteodystrophy may also be partly related to uraemic acidosis[156].

Uraemic toxicity

Uraemia is responsible for many abnormalities in the functional integrity of almost every organ. Most of these abnormalities have been attributed to unidentified 'uraemic toxins'. It has been clearly demonstrated that protein-poor diets decrease uraemic symptoms, especially in the gastrointestinal tract, suggesting that uraemic toxins derive mainly from protein catabolism. On the other hand, while carbohydrates and fats may be oxidized to carbon dioxide and water, which are excreted through the lungs and skin, many products of protein metabolism are not completely oxidized, and, being less volatile and diffusible, must be excreted by functioning kidneys[163]. Hence, when kidney function is lost, most organic compounds, mainly derived from protein metabolism, are retained.

The function of the kidneys is not limited to excretion of waste products and excess water and electrolytes, but is also involved in endocrine activities related to the regulation of blood pressure (e.g. renin), calcium homoeostasis (e.g. PTH) and erythropoiesis (e.g. erythropoietin). Therefore some uraemic symptoms may be secondary to endocrine disturbances, either directly related to the loss of functioning renal tissue or secondary to impaired homoeostasis[164].

Urea

Urea is the major nitrogenous end product of protein metabolism. After some initial observations in favour of a key role of urea in uraemic toxicity[8,165], there is much evidence that urea itself is not responsible for all the symptoms of uraemia. Oral or intravenous loads of urea (1 g/kg body weight) in hundreds of patients, with consequent increases in blood urea nitrogen (BUN) up to 140 mg/100 ml, did not lead to any toxic effects[166]. The addition of urea to dialysate to prevent changes in BUN in patients undergoing haemodialysis treatment could not offset the excellent clinical response to dialysis[167]. Finally, in our experience[168], a haemofiltration technique, used regularly substituted for RDT, did not allow the appearance of uraemic symptoms, but instead induced a better sense of well-being in uraemic patients, despite a blood concentration of urea as high as 359 mg/100 ml.

More recent clinical studies that tried to avoid the abrupt increase in blood urea concentration by addition of urea to the dialysate, gave different results from those reported earlier. Johnson et al.[169,170] have observed that long-standing high levels of BUN were accompanied by headache, nausea, vomiting, glucose intolerance and bleeding tendency. It should be stressed, however, that in these studies, neither cardiovascular nor neurological changes of uraemia were observed in relation to the increase in BUN[170].

We may therefore conclude that even if urea has some toxic effect, it may be considered as only a mild uraemic toxin[164], since it cannot explain all toxic manifestations in uraemic patients.

Guanidino compounds

The next major nitrogenous end products of protein metabolism are the guanidino compounds, which include guanidine, methylguanidine, dimethylguanidine, guanidinoacetic acid, guanidinosuccinic acid, 1,3-diphenylguanidine, creatine and creatinine. Some toxic effects have been attributed by many investigators to guanidino compounds which may account for uraemic toxicity, but many of these effects were obtained with concentrations much greater than those observed in sera of uraemic patients[163]. The rise in plasma creatinine is not considered to produce any symptoms but it is important as a guide to the level of renal function.

Ammonia

In uraemic patients, urea retention results in a large pool of circulating nitrogen. Part of retained urea (15–40% of the urea produced daily in normal subjects and possibly more in uraemic patients) is degraded to ammonia and carbon dioxide by intestinal bacteria[171]. Ammonia diffuses into portal blood from the intestinal tract and is transported to the liver, where it may be either resynthesized into urea or transaminated into amino acids and thus utilized for protein synthesis[172].

According to Walser[173], a small part of ammonia derived from urea is utilized for protein synthesis, the bulk of ammonia being resynthesized to urea. Only in the presence of congestive heart failure, and obviously in the condition of hepatic failure, may the livers of uraemic patients not metabolize ammonia normally, so that hyperammonaemia may occur[174].

In most uraemic patients, blood concentration of ammonia is either normal or often decreased[174]. This is because the ammonia excreted in the urine as well as blood ammonia is normally generated by the kidneys by deamination of glutamine and other amino acids; hence, as kidney function is lost, ammonia generation is reduced and blood ammonia is decreased.

Despite normal or decreased blood levels, elevated levels of ammonia in the gastrointestinal tract, as observed in severe uraemia, may cause stomatitis, gastritis, ulcerative enteritis and colitis[163].

Uric acid

Two-thirds of uric acid produced daily by a normal subject is usually excreted in the urine[175].

When renal function is impaired, the clearance of uric acid does not fall in proportion to the fall in GFR, so that, in patients with stable CRF, serum uric acid does not rise as early and to the same degree as blood urea does[176,177]. In non-gouty uraemic patients, serum uric acid is usually increased[22] when creatinine clearance is less than 20 ml/min. In advanced renal failure, however, hyperuricaemia may insidiously lead to a further fall in renal function, presumably through intrarenal urate deposition (Figure 13). Thus, it has been reported that kidneys from non-gouty uraemic patients contain tophaceous urate deposits[178]. In hyperuricaemia due to urate overproduction (as observed in patients with lymphoproliferative or myeloproliferative disorders, especially following radiation or chemo-therapy), there is rapid and progressive renal failure due to precipitation of uric acid crystals in the renal collecting system with consequent obstruc-tion[179].

It is therefore very important to treat hyperuricaemia of uraemic patients with allopurinol (e.g. 300 mg/day), possibly with associated alkali (Figure 13).

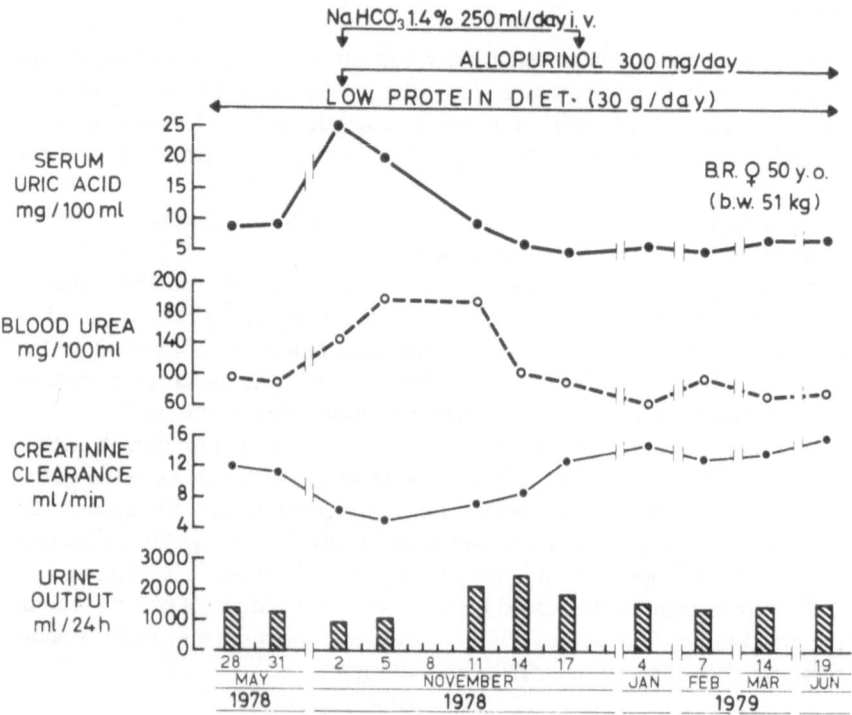

Figure 13 Effect of hyperuricaemia on renal function in a non-gouty normotensive uraemic patient. B.R., a 51-year-old female patient with CRF of unknown origin, was first observed in May 1978. At that time creatinine clearance was about 11–12 ml/min, urine output 1300–1500 ml/24 h and serum uric acid about 8 mg/100 ml. A high biological low-protein diet (0.6 g body weight^{-1} day^{-1}) without salt restriction was therefore started, with an intake of 0.15 MJ kg^{-1} day^{-1}. The patient was discharged when blood urea was approximately 90 mg/100 ml. She was lost to follow-up until November 1978, when anorexia and nausea were severe. Thus, severe hyperuricaemia was observed with a drop in both renal function and urine output and with an increase in blood urea (up to 198 mg/100 ml). The patient was not dehydrated and blood pressure was within the upper limits of normal range. Treatment with sodium bicarbonate infusion and allopurinol orally was started. Serum uric acid fell and then urine output increased significantly (up to 2.5 l) and creatinine clearance returned to the values of 6 months earlier. After a few days of high urine output, blood urea also returned to about 90 mg/100 ml. In June 1980, renal function, blood urea and urine output were still maintained at the values of May 1978, while serum uric acid was stabilized at about 7 mg/100 ml with a low protein diet and allopurinol

Parathyroid hormone (PTH)

According to Massry and his co-workers[180-182], PTH represents a major uraemic toxin, affecting the function of many organs through an increase in the cellular concentration of calcium, an alteration in the cellular membrane permeability, an exaggerated stimulation of cyclic AMP, an increase in protein catabolism and, therefore, an accumulation of nitrogenous compounds.

Undoubtedly, high blood levels of PTH play an important role in the pathophysiology of many disorders occurring in chronic renal failure.

It is well demonstrated that osteitis fibrosa due to hyperparathyroidism is an important component of renal osteodystrophy and that parathyroid-ectomy is usually associated with healing of it[74]. We have discussed the bone lesions of renal osteodystrophy in more detail in another section of this chapter. Another bone disorder which has been attributed to PTH is the aseptic necrosis of the femoral head. This severe complication has been observed particularly in patients with secondary hyperparathyroidism[183,184] independent of treatment with glucocorticoids[183]. Similarly, soft tissue necrosis has been attributed to calciphylaxis induced by secondary hyper-parathyroidism; healing follows parathyroidectomy[84,185,186].

Even metastatic calcification in extraosseous tissues may be due to secondary hyperparathyroidism, as mentioned in another section of this chapter. It has been suggested that by this mechanism (i.e. calcium depo-sition in the kidneys), PTH may contribute to the progression of renal damage[100].

Secondary hyperparathyroidism may play an important role in the genesis of anaemia in uraemic patients through the reduction in the amount of bone marrow which follows fibrosis of the bone marrow cavity induced by excess PTH[181] or through direct suppression of erythropoiesis by PTH[182]. PTH may therefore add to the main pathogenic factors of uraemic anae-mia[187]. In favour of this hypothesis is the observation that parathyroid-ectomy or suppression of the parathyroid glands with $1,25-(OH)_2D_3$ in uraemic patients is followed by reduction of fibrosis of the bone marrow cavity[188] and by improvement of anaemia[181,189].

It has been claimed that PTH plays an important role in the pathogenesis of uraemic hyperlipidaemia[190], itching[95,97-99] and even the sexual dysfunc-tion frequently observed in chronic uraemia[191,192]. Massry and his co-workers have, in fact, shown that impotence of uraemic patients may be reversed by parathyroidectomy or medical suppression of the activity of parathyroid glands[181,182].

EEG changes observed in chronic uraemia and neurobehavioural ab-normalities of uraemic patients, such as emotional lability, anxiety, sleep-lessness, physical restlessness and the inability to keep still, have been attributed to secondary hyperparathyroidism[69], presumably through an increase in calcium content of the brain[94,182,193–195]. Suppression of para-thyroid gland activity or parathyroidectomy were followed by normalization of EEG and remission of neurological symptoms[182]. More recently, even peripheral neuropathy has been shown to be related to an excess of PTH through the increase in calcium content of peripheral nerve. Thus, Goldstein et al.[196] have demonstrated that an increase in calcium content of the sciatic nerve occurred in dogs with experimental uraemia, but not in those previously thyro-parathyroidectomized, and that the administration of parathyroid extract to dogs with normal renal function increased nerve calcium. An inverse relationship was observed between the nerve calcium content and the motor nerve conduction velocity. More recently Avram et al.[197] have demonstrated that subtotal parathyroidectomy in chronic uraemic patients is followed by a clear improvement in motor nerve conduction velocity.

Urochromogens

Urochromogens are lipid-soluble pigments (lipochromes) that darken in the sunlight. In normal subjects they are excreted by the kidneys, accounting for the yellow colour of urine. In patients with CRF, urochromogens are retained and deposited in the subcutaneous fat. This accounts both for the pale aspects of their urine and for the characteristic dirty yellow pigmentation of their skin[22].

Other organic compounds: the 'middle molecules'

Other possible uraemic toxins include:

(a) Hormones (in addition to PTH), such as insulin, glucagon, growth hormone and gastrin, which accumulate in chronic uraemia. The exact role of these in uraemic toxicity is not well defined.

(b) Renin, which may be important in those seriously hypertensive patients whose kidneys produce an excess of this enzyme[164].

(c) Choline and other aliphatic amines (e.g. methylamine, dimethylamine, trimethylamine, ethanolamine), many of which are probably produced by bacterial action in the gut[198].

(d) Derivatives of the aromatic amino acids (phenylalanine, tyrosine and tryptophan), i.e. phenolic and hydroxyphenolic acids, aromatic amines and indolic compounds[163].

(e) Polyamines, and especially spermine (the plasma concentration of spermine is markedly increased in chronic uraemia[164]).

(f) Cyclic AMP, which may be involved in platelet defects of chronic uraemia[199].

(g) Myoinositol, which has been related to the uraemic peripheral neuropathy[164].

(h) The so-called 'middle molecules'.

According to the 'middle molecule' hypothesis (initially suggested on the basis of the clinical results of different dialysis strategies), patients with severe uraemia accumulate some as yet unidentified solutes of middle-sized molecular weight (300 to 5000). These are the 'middle molecules' which may exert toxic effects[200]. Bergstrom and his co-workers[201,202] have been able to demonstrate the existence of 'middle molecules' by gel chromatography and UV detection. We now know[203,204] that measurable plasma peaks (most often peak 7c) of 'middle molecules' are found in patients with CRF when their creatinine clearance falls below 15 ml/min.

The exact role of 'middle molecules' in uraemic toxicity has not yet been settled. It has been shown that patients with severe uraemic symptoms, such as malnutrition, fluid retention, peripheral neuropathy and pericarditis, have high plasma levels of 'middle molecules', whereas, in patients free of uraemic symptoms, plasma levels of these solutes are low[205]. More recent in vitro studies have given evidence that 'middle molecules' may significantly contribute to certain uraemic symptoms, such as anaemia, glucose intolerance, immunological deficiency, susceptibility to infections, bleeding tendency and peripheral neuropathy, but they cannot explain all of the clinical features of uraemia[164,206,207].

Middle molecules still need to be identified, but it should be stressed that many peptide hormones have a molecular weight within the middle molecule range or a little higher. These include insulin (mol. wt. 6000), glucagon (mol. wt. 3500), parathyroid hormone (mol. wt. 9500) and fragments of it, gastrin (mol. wt. 2000), calcitonin (mol. wt. 3400) and gastric inhibitory peptide (mol. wt. 5100). Even the so-called natriuretic factor which has been isolated by gel filtration from serum and urine of uraemic patients seems to be a peptide (mol. wt. < 1000)[207].

Further studies are undoubtedly necessary for better understanding of the nature of uraemic toxicity.

Carbohydrate metabolism

Patients with CRF show a moderate degree of carbohydrate intolerance: peripheral utilization of glucose is decreased primarily because of peripheral insulin resistance[208–210]. Furthermore, although basal insulin levels are normal or elevated[210], they do not increase normally in response to hyperglycaemia[211]. Since insulin is mainly metabolized by the kidney, the halflife of circulating insulin is prolonged in CRF[212]. This accounts for the decrease in requirements for insulin or oral hypoglycaemic agents in diabetic patients when renal failure develops[211]. The latter phenomenon, together with the disappearance of glycosuria with the fall in renal function (because of the higher threshold for glucose due to the fall in GFR), gives the patients the wrong impression of a complete recovery of their diabetes mellitus when they develop renal failure.

The impaired utilization of glucose in CRF leads to a decreased deposition of liver glycogen (due to decreased uptake of glucose by hepatic cells)[213]. Hence, the sensitivity to hypoglycaemic agents, including insulin, in uraemia is enhanced, not only because of decreased insulin metabolism, but also because less liver glycogen is available for utilization in response to hypoglycaemia[211]. For these reasons, it is very important to avoid (or limit) insulin when i.v. infusion of glucose solutions is needed in patients with CRF. Without this precaution, severe hypoglycaemia and even hypoglycaemic coma may occur, usually after the infusion.

Hypertriglyceridaemia

It has been observed that 40–60% of patients with moderate to severe CRF have hypertriglyceridaemia and increased pre-β-lipoprotein (VLDL)* concentration (type IV hyperlipoproteinaemia according to Fredrickson et al.[215]), which represents an important predisposing factor for the development of atherosclerosis and cardiovascular disease[214–222].

Uraemic hypertriglyceridaemia results both from increased production of triglyceride-rich VLDL by the liver and from decreased removal of triglycerides because of decreased lipoprotein lipase activity[214]. It is claimed that uraemic hypertriglyceridaemia is secondary to the alteration in carbohydrate metabolism in uraemia, since the high levels of triglycerides appear to be correlated with increased basal levels of insulin, secondary to the impaired glucose utilization. The liver may respond to the elevated basal insulin levels by increasing VLDL synthesis[211,214].

Post-heparin lipolytic activity is depressed in uraemia, suggesting reduced synthesis or release of lipoprotein lipase, and, consequently, reduced removal of triglycerides by peripheral tissues[211,214]. Since insulin is required for normal function of lipoprotein lipase, it has been claimed that the reduced lipoprotein lipase activity in uraemic patients results from the diminished insulin response characteristic of uraemia[211].

Anaemia in CRF

A moderate normochromic, normocytic anaemia is a constant feature of CRF. Its severity has been correlated with the level of BUN[223] and with the drop in creatinine clearance[224]. Figures 14 and 15 illustrate the fall in

---

*Triglyceride and cholesterol are lipids that circulate in plasma associated with phospholipids and proteins (apoproteins) in the so-called 'lipoproteins'. The proportion of protein and lipid (triglyceride, cholesterol and phospholipid) in each lipoprotein accounts for its size, density and electrophoretic migration. VLDL (or very low density lipoproteins) are lipoproteins of hepatic origin which migrate ahead of the β-globulins on paper electrophoresis: hence they are also called 'pre-β-lipoproteins'[214].

haemoglobin plotted against the rise in blood urea and against the fall in creatinine clearance in our patients with CRF. Several factors have been invoked in the pathogenesis of uraemic anaemia; they include haemolysis, decreased erythrocyte production and bleeding tendency.

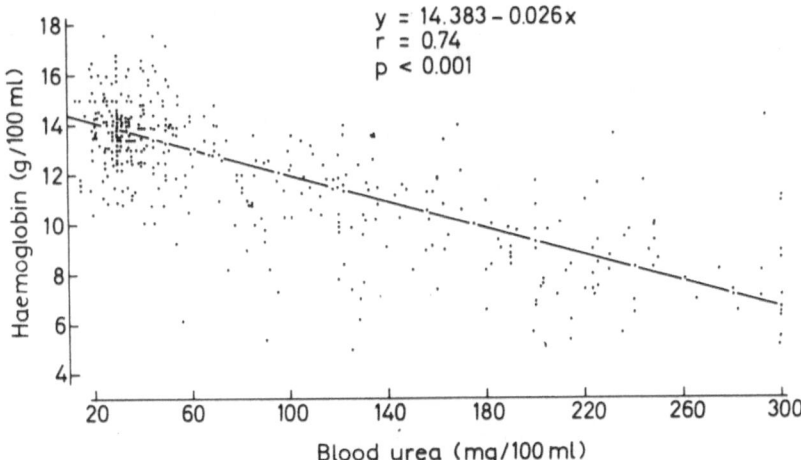

Figure 14 Relationship between blood urea and haemoglobin concentration in 400 non-dialysed patients with various degrees of chronic renal failure, hospitalized in the period 1977–1979

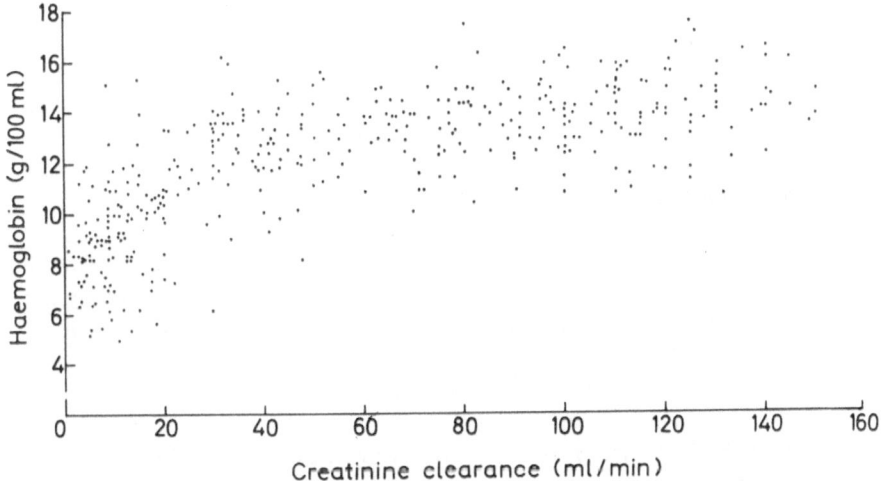

Figure 15 Relationship between creatinine clearance and haemoglobin concentration in 400 non-dialysed patients with various degrees of chronic renal failure, hospitalized in the period 1977–1979

Haemolysis

A shortening of the life span of red blood cells (RBC) has been demonstrated in about 70% of uraemic patients[225]. Cross-transfusion studies have shown that normal RBC have a shortened survival in uraemic recipients while the survival of uraemic RBC in healthy recipients is normal[225-227]. However, no specific 'toxin' that may be responsible for this reduced RBC life span has been detected in uraemic blood. According to Erslev and Shapiro[228], in addition to the uraemic environment, non-uraemic stress, such as hypertension or vascular lesions, may contribute to the increased haemolysis in uraemic patients.

Decreased erythrocyte production

The rate of haemolysis in uraemic patients is so mildly increased that it would easily be compensated for by normal bone marrow. Since a reduction in haematocrit occurs (with a proportional reduction in haemoglobin concentration and erythrocyte count), it is likely that decreased erythrocyte production is the major factor in uraemic anaemia[229]. This is demonstrated by:

(a) The normal (0.5–1.0%) or even subnormal reticulocyte count when correlated with the degree of anaemia.
(b) The inappropriately normal bone marrow smears (i.e. without compensatory increase in the number of erythroblasts despite the anaemia)[228,230].
(c) The ferrokinetic studies showing a reduction in plasma iron turnover and in the incorporation of iron into RBC[225,231].

This decreased erythrocyte production has been attributed both to an insufficient production of a specific hormone, the erythropoietin, by the uraemic kidneys and to a decreased responsiveness of uraemic bone marrow to erythropoietin.

RBC represent an organ whose main function is carrying oxygen from the lungs to the peripheral tissues and whose optimal size is maintained by the bone marrow in relation to the tissue's need for oxygen. It has been demonstrated that RBC production in response to low tissue oxygen tension is modulated by a humoral erythropoietic factor, erythropoietin[232,233]. Erythropoietin acts primarily on stem cells of bone marrow[234,235] and probably also on the earliest erythroblasts[236]. Its production has been located in the kidney; it seems that an oxygen sensor ('oxygenstat'), presumably located in the renal medulla, responds to oxygen deprivation by triggering erythropoietin production[237,238]. Since the erythropoietin-producing cells have been located in the juxtaglomerular apparatus[239-241] or in the glomeruli[242,243], a releasing substance, possibly a prostaglandin, has been suggested as an intermediary between the medullary oxygen sensor and the cortical erythropoietin production site[238]. However, the existence of such an intermediary has not been demonstrated. Neither has it been possible to extract erythropoietin from renal homogenate[237]. This has suggested two alternative hypotheses:

(a) The kidney releases an enzyme, the erythrogenin, that activates an erythropoietinogen produced by the liver[244].
(b) The kidney is producing an inactive form of the hormone that is activated by a plasma enzyme[245].

The demonstration by Erslev[246] of *in vitro* production of erythropoietin by kidneys from hypoxic animals perfused with a serum-free solution appears to contradict both hypotheses. It is possible that the kidneys usually release erythropoietin as it is being produced, without storing it. This may well explain why we are unable to extract it from renal tissue[228].

Subjects with normal renal function respond to any form of anaemia with increased production of erythropoietin and this is proportional to the fall in haematocrit. In contrast, the production of erythropoietin is not increased despite a significant drop in haematocrit[228] in almost all patients with CRF.

The inability of the failing kidney to respond to the increased demand for RBC by increasing erythropoietin production is probably associated with a decreased responsiveness of uraemic bone marrow to erythropoietin. The administration of erythropoietin to uraemic rats has been found to be less effective than when the hormone was given to normal rats[247], and similar results were observed in uraemic patients[248]. An important role of uraemic toxin(s) as erythropoietin inhibitor(s) has been postulated by some authors[249] but not confirmed by others[250,251]. On the other hand, this reduced responsiveness to erythropoietin may be simply accounted for by a reduction in red marrow availability due to fibrosis of the bone marrow cavity resulting from secondary hyperparathyroidism[182].

Undoubtedly there is also an extrarenal production of erythropoietin which has been located in the liver (hepatocytes or Kupffer cells)[252,253]. This production, however, is so limited (about 10% of the total) that anephric patients, despite adequate dialysis treatment, are always more anaemic than those patients with their own non-functioning kidneys in place. This is why bilateral nephrectomy, even in the absence of any urine output in dialysis patients, should be avoided whenever possible.

Bleeding tendency

The bleeding tendency is a frequent complication of advanced CRF. It has been attributed to abnormal platelet function, rather than to thrombocytopenia, since the latter is present in only 20% of uraemic patients and the platelet count is very rarely less than 50000 per cubic millimetre. This abnormality in platelet function is corrected by haemodialysis, peritoneal dialysis and renal transplantation.

The haemorrhagic tendency of uraemic patients may appear in the form of purpuric lesions, continuous slow blood loss from ulcers in the gastro-intestinal tract, frank melaena, haematemesis, gynaecological or nasal bleeding. Continuous blood leaks or severe blood losses may contribute to the uraemic anaemia. In these cases, oral or parenteral iron administration may be useful. After severe blood losses, transfusions of packed cells may become necessary.

Neurological disorders

Disorders of the central nervous system and peripheral nerve function frequently occur in the advanced stages of CRF.

Cerebral manifestations

Mental function may remain surprisingly good when the progression of CRF is slow. In contrast, rapid progression may cause severe mental disturbances[254–256].

Intellectual deterioration is the most frequent complication of chronic uraemia. Mental concentration and recent and remote memory are reduced, and the ability to focus or sustain attention is frequently impaired. Patients may have difficulty in expressing ideas in simple language and in making decisions. Euphoria, depression, apathy, anxiety, sleeplessness, emotional irritability, sluggishness, paranoid and compulsive personality changes may all occur in CRF. In the final stages, headaches, lassitude, muscular fatigue, weakness, daytime drowsiness and insomnia at night may be present. If dialysis treatment is not started, further deterioration of cerebral function will occur with disorientation, confusion, hallucinations, torpor, progressive lethargy and coma[22,255–257].

Epileptic convulsions may occur, either as an expression of hypertensive encephalopathy following a sudden increase in blood pressure in hypertensive patients, or, in non-hypertensive young patients, as a result of increasing blood urea concentrations[22].

Electroencephalographic changes usually occur with these clinical symptoms[194,254,258–260].

In addition to the behavioural disorders described, abnormal function of the nervous system may be manifest as neuromuscular and autonomic phenomena. The former may include slurred speech, fibrillary muscle twitching, muscle jerks and cramps, tics and hiccoughs. The latter include hypothermia, nausea, vomiting and sex organ dysfunction[256]. A high incidence of sexual impotence, as well as loss of libido, with reduced frequency of sexual intercourse in both men and women (in addition to disturbances in menstruation in women and spermatogenesis in men) have been reported in chronic uraemia. These are only partially corrected by dialysis. A multi-factorial origin of this dysfunction has been suggested, the factors involved including psychological depression, anaemia, hormonal imbalance, malnutrition, antihypertensive therapy and possibly the direct toxic effect of uraemia[261]. Promising results have been obtained[182] in impotence by suppressing parathyroid gland activity with $1,25-(OH)_2D_3$.

Finally, it should be stressed that some of these clinical disorders may be accounted for by endocrine disturbances. A functional state of hypothyroidism is almost constantly present in chronic uraemia (despite high blood levels of thyrotropin hormone[262]), and this may cause low body temperature, cold intolerance, dry skin, sallow complexion, muscular fatigue, anorexia, mental dullness, lethargy, hyporeflexia and pseudomyotonia[261]. In contrast, Massry suggests that secondary hyperparathyroidism, by raising brain calcium, is partly responsible for central nervous system aberrations in uraemia, with typical changes in the electroencephalogram that are reversed when the excess of PTH is abolished[94,194,195].

Peripheral neuropathy

Uraemic neuropathy was described more than a century ago, but its significance was largely unrecognized until the introduction of dialysis techniques, when RDT in chronic uraemia was often complicated by a severe progressive distal neuropathy[263,264]. The first substantial description referred to patients with severe CRF not treated by dialysis, so that the renal failure itself was considered responsible for the neuropathy[263,264].

Uraemic neuropathy is a symmetrical mixed motor and sensory polyneuropathy involving the distal portions of peripheral nerves. The first clinical manifestations appear at the lower extremities. Painful muscle cramps and peculiar creeping (deep in the muscles), crawling, pricking and itchy sensations, which are worse at rest and relieved by movement (the so-called 'restless legs syndrome')[265], have been considered early indications of uraemic neuropathy[254]. In 109 uraemic patients, however, Nielsen[266] found that cramps and/or restless legs were equally frequent in cases with and without evidence of neuropathy. Hence, these symptoms have been related to fluid and electrolyte disturbances[267]. Muscle cramps have been correlated with changes in potassium–calcium ratio[254], phosphate concentration in cerebrospinal fluid[268], with systemic hypomagnesaemia[269] and with removal of sodium chloride by haemodialysis[270] or diuretics. According to Teschan and Ginn[256], the clinical experience suggests that disturbances in the acid–base and electrolyte balance play an important role in the pathophysiology of muscle cramps and restless legs in many patients. In some patients, these symptoms are relieved by treatment of secondary hyperparathyroidism by administration of phosphate binding agents, calcium supplements or parathyroidectomy[256].

A relatively frequent sensory symptom related to peripheral neuropathy in advanced uraemia is paraesthesia in the form of a pricking, tingling, effervescent sensation which is sometimes painful, especially in the soles ('burning feet')[258,266,267].

All uraemic patients complain of more or less severe muscle weakness which may sometimes cause difficulty in walking and in negotiating stairs[256].

A number of uraemic patients have an asymptomatic neuropathy[267,271]. A common objective abnormality, and sometimes, in young patients, the only sign of neuropathy, is the depression or even loss of deep tendon reflexes, especially the Achilles reflex, but also patellar reflexes[256,266].

Nerve conduction velocity has been widely used in recent years as an index of peripheral nerve function. It is not, however, an adequate test for evaluating uraemic neuropathy.

Neuropathies may be subdivided into two types: the demyelinating neuropathies characterized by primary damage of the myelin sheath with relative preservation of the axons, and the neuropathies in which there is a progressive centripetal axonal degeneration of a 'dying back' type[272] with associated myelin breakdown. In the first type, nerve conduction velocity is relatively mildly affected, while, in demyelinating neuropathies, very low values are usually observed[267]. Although some authors have considered uraemic neuropathy as primarily demyelinative in type[273-275], most investigators agree today that in chronic uraemia the demyelination of peripheral nerve fibres is secondary to primary abnormalities of axons[267,276-280]. Histological studies in uraemic neuropathy have shown degeneration of nerve fibres in their distal portion and loss of large myelinated nerve fibres[263,264,277,280,281]. Electromyographic studies have clearly indicated signs of denervation and re-innervation in uraemic patients even when only slight clinical evidence of neuropathy was present[271,280]. In biopsies of the sural nerve of uraemic patients, not yet on RDT, observed in our unit, signs of demyelination (Figure 16) and remyelination were observed on teased single nerve fibre preparations[280]. The moderate degrees of reduction in both motor and orthodromic sensory nerve conduction velocity observed in uraemic patients is consistent with the expectation of neuropathy due to axonal degeneration[267,280]. It should be stressed, however, that nerve conduction velocity, being reduced in both demyelinated and immature regenerating fibres[281], cannot be used as an index of dialysis adequacy[280].

Another peripheral nerve abnormality in uraemic patients is a nerve conduction block (following an initial phase of hyperexcitability) during ischaemia with muscle paralysis and sensory loss[267].

The mechanisms responsible for uraemic neuropathy are not yet elucidated. After the initial suggestion of vitamin deficiency, many toxic factors, such as magnesium, guanidino compounds, myoinositol and middle molecules have been implicated. It has been recently shown that secondary hyperparathyroidism may play an important aetiological role through an increase in calcium content of the peripheral nerves[196].

At present, only successful renal transplantation is an effective treatment of uraemic neuropathy[266].

The appearance of uraemic neuropathy has also been suggested as one of the criteria for initiation of chronic maintenance haemodialysis. Preliminary results of a study on uraemic neuropathy carried out in our unit[280] have clearly shown that peripheral nerve damage takes place so early in the progression of CRF that it is quite impossible to suggest initiation of RDT on the basis of subclinical appearance of peripheral neuropathy[282].

Figure 16 Teased single fibre from the sural nerve of a patient with uraemic neuropathy showing segmental demyelination. (Courtesy of G. Caruso, Department of Clinical Neurophysiology, University of Naples)

Cardiovascular manifestations of chronic renal failure

Pathophysiology of uraemic hypertension

Hypertension is almost a constant feature of chronic renal failure, since it appears in as many as 80% of patients with advanced uraemia. The rise in systemic blood pressure may be either the cause (less frequently) or the consequence (very frequently) of renal disease, and, despite accurate clinical evaluation, the differentiation between primary renal disease with secondary hypertension and primary hypertension with consequent renal failure may be impossible because of considerable overlap between the two conditions.

Salt retention and extracellular volume expansion play a key role in the pathophysiology of hypertension secondary to chronic renal failure[283,284].

The proposed mechanism of this, which is today widely accepted, is shown in Figure 17. If functioning nephrons are lost and sodium intake maintained, the consequent retention of salt and water will cause expansion of the extracellular fluid volume (ECV) and increase in blood volume and venous return to the heart. An increase in cardiac output will result, which is *per se* responsible for a rise in blood pressure. As the autoregulation of peripheral blood flow becomes operative (because of the excessive blood flow to peripheral tissue that follows the increased cardiac output), vasoconstriction of peripheral arterioles takes place[285-287]; the resulting increase in total peripheral resistance will account for the persistent hypertension. In a steady state, the cardiac output returns to normal, since the autoregulatory peripheral vasoconstriction will normalize tissue blood flow and reduce the venous return to heart. The ECV expansion and increased renal perfusion[288-292] will

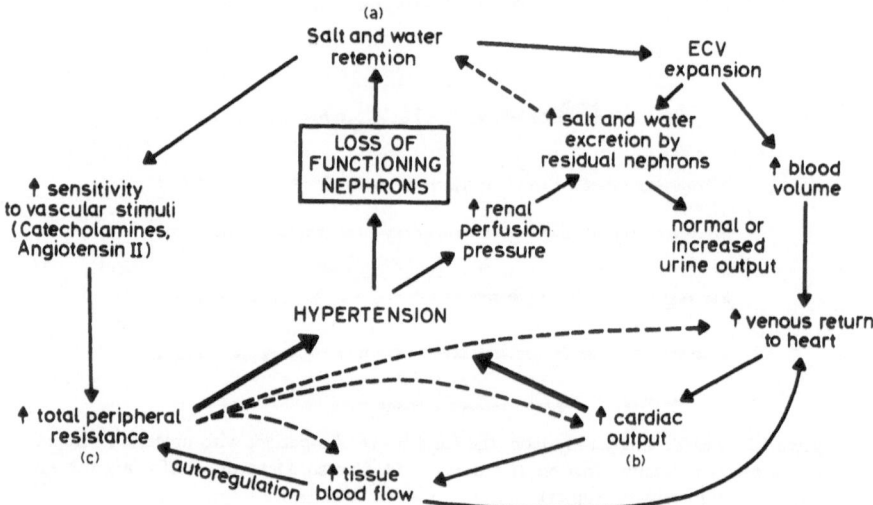

Figure 17 Proposed mechanism of uraemic hypertension and sites of action of dietary restriction of salt and diuretics (a), β-adrenergic blockers (b) and peripheral vasodilator drugs (c). (Dashed arrows indicate negative effects)

increase salt and water output of residual nephrons through a permanent reduction in tubular reabsorption of filtrate, so that the external sodium and water balance is restored to normal. The price paid for this is a persistent ECV expansion with hypertension[283,284,286,287,293,294]. Unfortunately, hypertension *per se* will damage the kidneys[294]. The further loss of functioning nephrons will expand further the extracellular fluid volume so that, in a stepwise fashion, untreated hypertension may become more and more severe as renal function deteriorates.

Although ECV expansion represents the main mechanism by which salt and water retention causes hypertension, a great deal of evidence has been produced on the effect of increased sodium and water in the arteriolar muscle cells[283]. Greater water content will thicken the wall of the vessel, reducing its elasticity and narrowing the lumen: the resulting effects will be greater vascular resistance and increased sensitivity to vascular stimuli, such as catecholamines[295-298]. On the other hand, excess sodium will increase vascular contractility and the sensitivity of the arteriolar wall to the normal blood levels of angiotensin II[299, 300] (Figure 17).

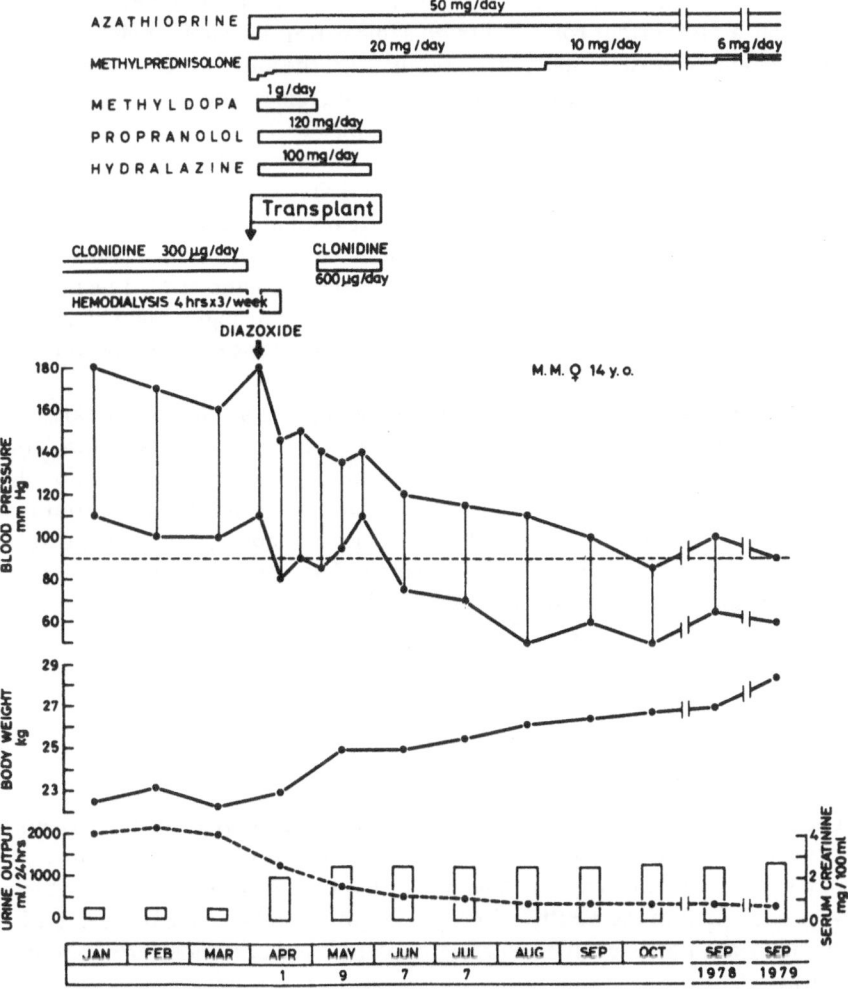

Figure 18 M.M., a 14-year-old female patient on RDT for 3 years, received a cadaver kidney on 3 April 1977. The patient had been hypertensive for many years. After transplantation, severe hypertension during acute rejection required treatment with i.v. diazoxide and then with propranolol, hydralazine, methyldopa and clonidine. Antirejection therapy was successful. As renal function improved, blood pressure fell so that soon all antihypertensive drugs could be withdrawn. The patient is still normotensive with a perfectly functioning graft

The key role of salt and water retention in the pathophysiology of hypertension secondary to CRF is clearly demonstrated by the beneficial effects frequently observed when excess sodium and water are removed by diuretics (Figure 4) or haemodialysis (Figure 3).

In some cases of CRF, neither diuretics nor haemodialysis can normalize blood pressure. It is assumed that in addition to a salt-dependent hypertension so frequently observed in CRF, a salt-independent hypertension may occur in uraemic patients. In these cases the renin–angiotensin system may play an important role. Although some extrarenal sites, such as uterus and splanchnic vessels, may release renin[301,302], the kidney is the main site of renin production. In CRF, renin formation and release does not stop despite the great reduction in renal mass. In fact plasma renin activity in hypertensive uraemic patients varies from low to very high levels[303–311]. The mechanism(s) which elevate plasma renin activity, in some cases despite salt and water retention and ECV expansion, are not known. Alteration in perfusion of severely diseased kidneys and increased activity of the sympathetic nervous system have been proposed as possible mechanisms[283]. The hypertensive effect of the renin–angiotensin system is due to angiotensin II, a very potent vasopressor substance, that also stimulates aldosterone secretion and catecholamine release.

It is well established that, in addition to a vasopressor function, the kidney has a vasodepressor endocrine function. Thus, successful renal transplantation without removal of the host diseased kidneys may frequently normalize severe hypertension that was previously uncontrollable by ultrafiltration haemodialysis (Figure 18). Vasodepressor substances, such as prostaglandins, have been isolated from renal medullary tissue, and the infusion of prostaglandins in experimental animals[312,313], as well as in hypertensive patients with and without CRF, induces a decrease in systemic blood pressure[314–318]. The role played by endogenous prostaglandins in the pathophysiology of hypertension in CRF is not yet known.

Hypertensive retinopathy

The lesions of small blood vessels, which occur in hypertensive patients, may easily be seen by inspecting the optic fundus. Funduscopic examination may show acute and chronic changes of hypertensive retinopathy, which were combined in the Keith–Wagener classification but have been recently classified as 'hypertensive neuroretinopathy' and 'arteriosclerotic retinopathy'[319].

'Hypertensive neuroretinopathy' has been graded from I to IV (Roman numerals), ranging from narrowing of arteriolar lumen (grade I) to arteriovenous nicking (grade II), haemorrhages and exudates (grade III) and papilloedema (grade IV)[319]. Haemorrhages are blotchy or flame-shaped and arise from the optic disc. 'Soft' exudates are areas of white discoloration (due to oedema of the retina) with indefinite margins, sometimes radiating from the macula towards the optic disc in the so-called 'macular star'[22]. Papilloedema, by definition a constant feature of 'malignant' hypertension, may initially be unilateral and may cause blurred vision and lead to blindness.

'Arteriosclerotic retinopathy' has been classified into four groups (Arabic numerals), ranging from focal or general narrowing of the arteriolar lumen (group 1) to arteriovenous nicking with vein still visible (group 2), vein invisible below arteriole (group 3) and venous obstruction combined with arteriolar obliteration (group 4)[319]. Quite characteristic of arteriosclerotic retinopathy is the tortuous and narrow shape of retinal arteries, crossing the veins at right angles (rather than following the usual oblique direction), with retinal veins that appear to be 'compressed' by the arteries (arteriovenous nipping) due to accumulation of connective tissue between the artery and the vein[22]. 'Hard' glistening exudates of a yellowish-white colour may also be seen. They are small in size, with sharply defined margins, sometimes disposed in clusters radiating from the macula[22].

Acute changes of hypertensive neuroretinopathy may appear superimposed on the chronic changes of arteriosclerotic retinopathy, particularly when long-standing hypertension progresses to the 'malignant' phase of hypertension. Frequently retinal lesions do not cause any change in vision. Their evolution is, however, very useful for evaluation of hypertensive patients. To avoid confusion due to different classifications it is better to describe what is observed on funduscopic examination instead of indicating groups or grades[319].

Cardiac complications

Cardiac complications are undoubtedly frequent in CRF. They are mainly due to hypertension, extracellular volume expansion and atherosclerosis. Congestive heart failure frequently occurs in overexpanded patients. In these cases, high-ceiling diuretics or, in advanced uraemia, ultrafiltration dialysis will readily improve cardiac function. Anaemia may precipitate heart failure in these patients. The oxygen supply to the myocardium is reduced, while an increase in cardiac output is required to obtain sufficient oxygen delivery to peripheral tissues[320]. If cardiac failure occurs, renal function deteriorates further.

In patients with long-standing hypertension, left ventricular enlargement may be observed on a chest X-ray. Echocardiogram is particularly useful in defining left ventricular hypertrophy[321] (Figure 19), the signs of which may be clear on electrocardiography.

In advanced uraemia, excessive expansion of extracellular fluid volume may cause pulmonary oedema, even in the absence of raised pulmonary capillary pressure. In this situation, the chest X-ray may show a typical picture of the 'uraemic lung'. This is characterized by dense opacities radiating from the hilum into the body of the lung, while the upper and lower zones and the outer part of the lung remain clear. This picture is usually (but not necessarily) bilateral, assuming a 'butterfly pattern', and is presumably due to increased permeability of pulmonary capillaries, resulting in fibrin exudation in alveoli[322]. Removal of fluid excess by potent diuretics or dialysis will readily reverse the 'uraemic lung'.

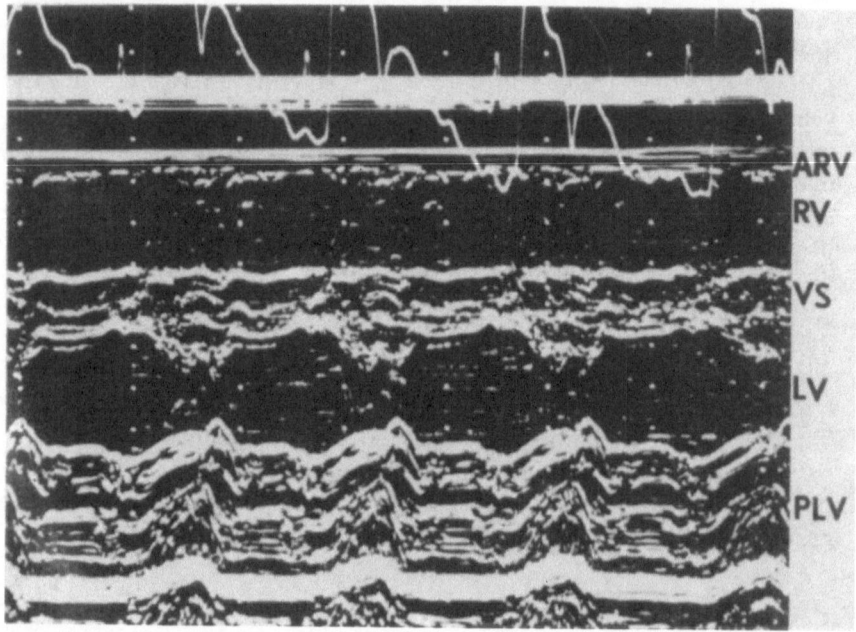

Figure 19 Echocardiogram in a 40-year-old hypertensive patient with left ventricular hypertrophy. The interventricular septum (VS) is 15 mm thick, while the thickness of the posterior wall of the left ventricle (PLV) is 16 mm. (ARV = anterior wall of the right ventricle; RV = cavity of the right ventricle; LV = cavity of the left ventricle)

Uraemic pericarditis is an aseptic fibrino–haemorrhagic pericarditis that may occur in advanced uraemia. Sometimes it appears as a bloody effusion that may cause tamponade. The cause of uraemic pericarditis is not known. Prompt institution of intensive dialysis treatment is usually followed by a dramatic improvement; effusion and pericardial friction rubs may completely disappear after a few dialyses (Figures 20 and 21). In some cases of large bloody effusion, an emergency anterior pericardiectomy may become necessary to avoid tamponade.

Echocardiography is particularly useful in evaluating an enlarged cardiac silhouette, allowing a clear diagnosis of pericardial effusion[323]. The fluid in the pericardial cavity gives a picture of echo-free space between the non-moving parietal pericardium and the moving cardiac walls (Figure 22). This non-invasive procedure may be repeated many times and is highly accurate, allowing diagnosis of pericardial effusions as small as 15 ml[324].

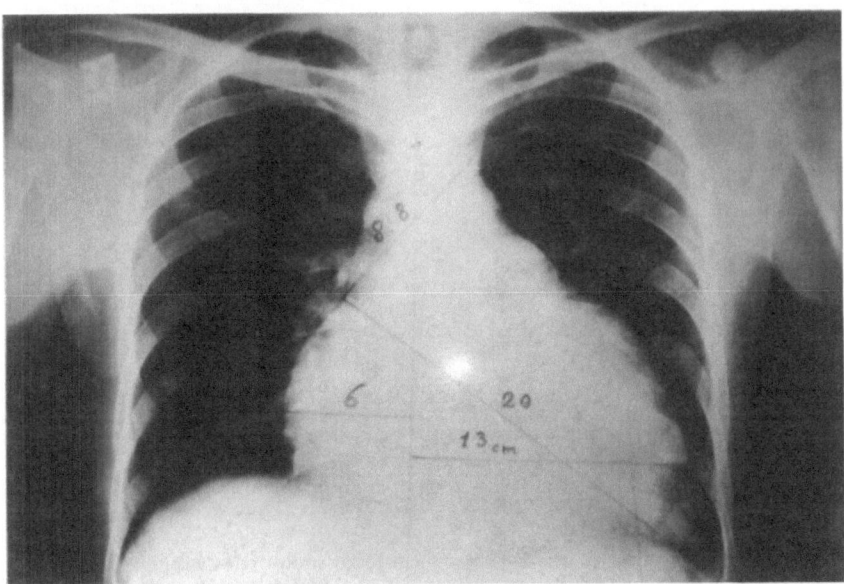

Figure 20   Chest X-ray of a 24-year-old male patient with uraemic pericarditis

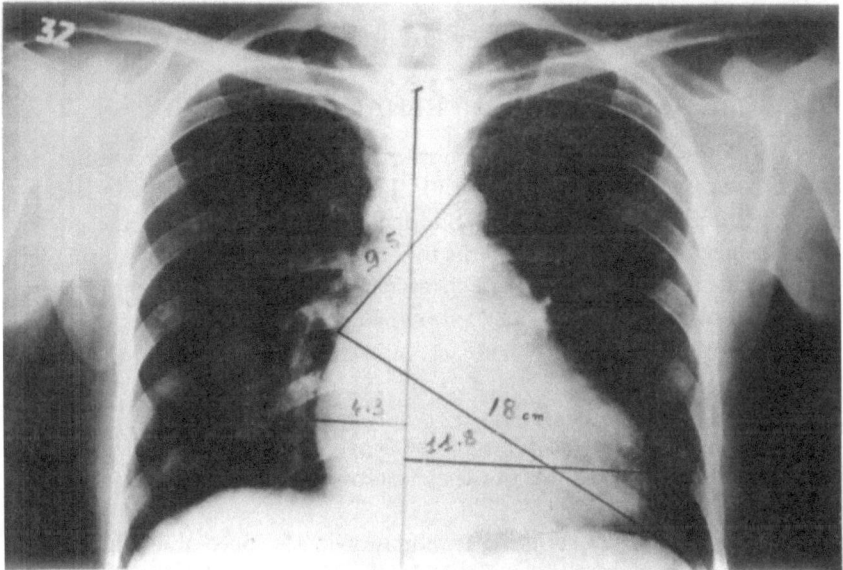

Figure 21   Chest X-ray in the same uraemic patient as in Figure 20 after intensive dialysis treatment. Effusion and pericardial friction rubs completely disappeared with dialysis

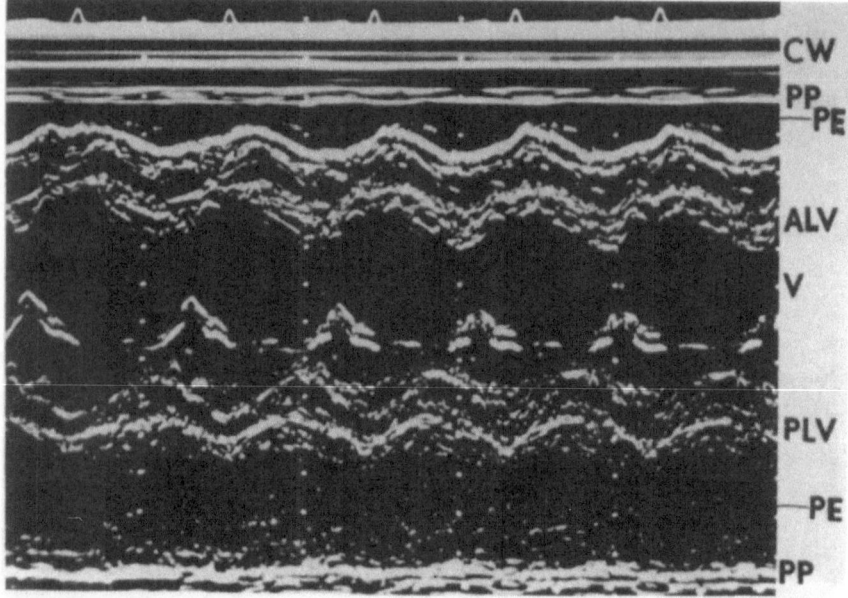

Figure 22 Echocardiogram in a 28-year-old female patient with uraemic pericarditis. Pericardial effusion (PE) is indicated by the presence of echo-free spaces between the non-moving parietal pericardium (PP) and the moving anterior (ALV) and posterior (PLV) walls of the left ventricle. (CW = chest wall; V = cavity of the left ventricle)

CLINICAL ASSESSMENT OF RENAL FUNCTION

It is well known that renal function may be severely impaired without the patient even being aware of being ill. These patients can usually lead an active life and eat a normal diet. Suddenly, anorexia, nausea, retching or vomiting occur, leading the patients to the physician. Laboratory tests then demonstrate an advanced stage of chronic uraemia. In other cases, a routine check-up will bring the patient to seek medical advice.

Uraemic symptoms

It is peculiar of CRF that some of the biochemical abnormalities do not cause symptoms, while most of the symptoms have no known biochemical cause[22].

Anorexia, nausea and vomiting are common in advanced uraemia. Nausea and retching appear initially in the early morning; they then become more frequent and almost continuous, with vomiting occurring two to three times a day.

The tongue is usually dry and the patient complains of a foul taste of ammonia in the mouth, especially on waking in the morning, due to decomposition of urea[22]. The breath smells of urine, hiccoughs are very frequent and constipation or severe diarrhoea may also occur.

Gastrointestinal haemorrhages in the form of haematemesis and melaena, due to peptic ulcer, may appear in the terminal phase of CRF. Other symptoms and signs of uraemia have been described earlier in this chapter, but none of these are pathognomonic of chronic uraemia. Laboratory tests are essential to decide whether or not renal function is impaired and, if so, to evaluate the degree of renal impairment.

Serum creatinine and creatinine clearance

Creatinine is derived from creatine, which comes from creatine phosphate of skeletal muscles. Since the dietary intake of meat is very small in comparison with the total muscle mass of the body, serum concentration of creatinine does not depend on creatine intake with the diet, but mainly on muscle metabolism. Creatinine is excreted only by the kidneys, almost completely by glomerular filtration. Therefore, the filtered load (e.g. 1.2 mg/min if GFR is 120 ml/min and serum creatinine is 1 mg/100 ml) equals the urinary excretion rate (1.2 mg/min in the example) and is identical to the production

Table 5 Effect of GFR on serum concentration of creatinine

Condition	GFR (ml/min)	Serum creatinine (mg/100 ml)	Filtered load of creatinine (mg/min)	Excretion rate of creatinine (mg/min)	Production rate of creatinine (mg/min)	Retention rate of creatinine (mg/min)
A	120	1	1.2	1.2	1.2	0
B I	60	1	0.6	0.6	1.2	0.6
II	60	2	1.2	1.2	1.2	0
C I	40	2	0.8	0.8	1.2	0.4
II	40	3	1.2	1.2	1.2	0
D I	20	3	0.6	0.6	1.2	0.6
II	20	6	1.2	1.2	1.2	0
E I	10	6	0.6	0.6	1.2	0.6
II	10	12	1.2	1.2	1.2	0
F I	5	12	0.6	0.6	1.2	0.6
II	5	24	1.2	1.2	1.2	0

rate (1.2 mg/min, condition A in Table 5). If GFR falls (e.g. to 60 ml/min), and the production rate is not modified (1.2 mg/min in the example), there will be a temporary positive balance for creatinine (condition B I in Table 5) and some creatinine will, in fact, be retained. Thus, serum concentration of creatinine will rise (to 2 mg/100 ml in the example) until the filtered load is restored (condition B II in Table 5) so that the excretion rate of creatinine (1.2 mg/min) again equals the production rate (1.2 mg/min). With a further fall in GFR (conditions C, D, E and F in Table 5), further increases in serum creatinine occur, step by step, until very high values are reached, when the renal function is almost completely lost (condition F II in Table 5). An inverse relationship exists between GFR and serum concentration of creatinine. The normal range for the latter is 0.7–1.2 mg/100 ml*, the wide variation resulting mainly from the influence of age, sex and body size on muscle mass, but also from errors in the measurement. Because of this variation[157], serum concentration of creatinine may not rise above the upper limit of normal range until GFR is reduced by at least 40%. If measurements of serum creatinine were exact, without any variation, a change in serum creatinine from 0.8 mg/100 ml to 1.2 mg/100 ml in an adult man (40 years old, 70 kg body weight) would correspond to a fall in creatinine clearance from 120 ml/min to 80 ml/min.

The problem related to errors in measurement of serum creatinine may, in part, be overcome by repeating two or three times, at intervals of a few days. The effect of changes in muscle mass may be overcome by using endogenous creatinine clearance as a more correct index of GFR. Creatinine clearance is only approximately equal to GFR, since creatinine is partially secreted by renal tubules; but a few ml/min of difference between GFR and creatinine clearance does not make any clinical difference in the evaluation of chronic uraemia. Obviously inulin clearance would be a more accurate measure of GFR, but it is not practicable as a routine renal function test, since inulin has to be infused intravenously and urine collected by bladder catheterization.

For determining creatinine clearance, urine is collected for 24 h after spontaneous voiding, and a blood sample is withdrawn in the morning after fasting. Since the filtered load of creatinine ($P_{Cr} \times Cl_{Cr}$, where P_{Cr} is the plasma or serum concentration of creatinine, identical to the concentration of creatinine in the ultrafiltrate, and Cl_{Cr} is the ultrafiltration rate to be measured) is considered identical to its excretion rate ($U_{Cr} \times V$, where U_{Cr} is the concentration of creatinine in urine and V is the urine volume), the ultrafiltration rate (Cl_{Cr}) may be easily obtained from

$$P_{Cr} \times Cl_{Cr} = U_{Cr} \times V$$

as

$$Cl_{Cr} = \frac{U_{Cr} \times V}{P_{Cr}}$$

Because of collection difficulties, even the determination of creatinine clearance may not be practical. Creatinine clearance, however, may be pre-

---

*Creatinine is the 2-imino-1-methyl-4-imidazolidinone, $C_4H_7B_3O$, with a mol. wt. of 113.12; hence, 100 μmol/1000 = 1.13 mg/100 ml.

dicted from serum creatinine[5]. Several formulas have been suggested for this purpose[325–327]. We prefer the following calculation proposed by Cockcroft and Gault[327].

$$\text{Creatinine clearance (ml/min)} = \frac{(140 - \text{age in years}) \, (\text{kg body weight})}{72 \times \text{serum creatinine (in mg/100 ml)}}$$

For female patients, the value obtained by this calculation should be reduced by 15%.

Plasma urea and blood urea nitrogen (BUN)

Urea is the main end-product of nitrogen metabolism. It is a diamide of carbonic acid (carbamide, $CO(NH_2)_2$, mol. wt. 60) derived from protein catabolism and it is freely diffusible through cellular membranes (RBC and muscle). The distribution of urea is similar to that of water so that blood concentration of urea reflects the concentration of urea in all tissues[328]. Urea concentration in blood is frequently determined by measuring the amount of urea nitrogen (BUN). Since the urea molecule (mol. wt. 60) contains two nitrogen atoms, the weight of which is 28 (atomic wt. of $N = 14$), blood urea concentration may be calculated by multiplying BUN by two (since 28 is approximately half of 60). It should be stressed that, while plasma urea concentration is identical to serum urea concentration, blood urea concentration is slightly (14% according to Goldsmith[329]) lower than plasma or serum urea[328]. Similarly, plasma urea nitrogen (PUN) is identical to serum urea nitrogen (SUN). In clinical practice, however, many doctors use the term BUN when referring to either the serum or plasma urea nitrogen. Thus the values of BUN, PUN and SUN are, in reality, the same and the three symbols (BUN, PUN and SUN) can be used interchangeably.

Urea is excreted almost exclusively by the kidneys. Unlike creatinine, however, urea is not only filtered, but also reabsorbed by the tubules. If GFR falls because of renal disease, the plasma urea must increase much more than the plasma creatinine (which is only filtered) in order to maintain the external nitrogen balance. Furthermore, unlike creatinine, the production of urea depends on dietary protein intake and, should the GFR remain stable whilst protein intake increases, plasma urea would increase significantly. This is evident in the following example (Table 6). From the catabolism of 100 g of protein, 35 g of urea are produced[328] which must be excreted by the kidneys. If we assume that the tubular reabsorption rate of urea is 50% of the filtered load (and we also assume that it remains so both when GFR falls and when dietary protein intake is changed)[157], a male subject with a GFR of 120 ml/min and protein intake of 70 g/day will be in perfect external balance for urea with a plasma concentration of urea of 28 mg/100 ml; the production rate of urea is, in fact, 24.5 g/day (35% of the 70 g of protein introduced with the diet), that is 17 mg/min. Since the filtered load of urea is approximately 34 mg/min (0.28 mg/ml × 120 ml/min) and 50% of the filtered load is reabsorbed, 17 mg/min is also the excretion rate of urea (A in Table 6). Should GFR fall to 60 ml/min (condition B in Table 6), then the filtered load of urea will fall to about 17 mg/min (0.28 mg/ml × 60 ml/min). The consequent decrease in the excretion rate of urea to 8.5 mg/min in a condition of unchanged production rate of 17 mg/min (the dietary protein intake is unchanged) will result in a retention of urea of 8.5 mg/min (B I in Table 6). This positive urea balance will raise the plasma concentration of urea until urea excretion again equals its production, i.e. until a plasma urea concentration of 57 mg/100 ml (B II in Table 6).

Table 6 Effect of GFR and dietary protein intake on plasma concentration of urea

Condition	Dietary protein intake (g/day)	GFR (ml/min)	Plasma urea (mg/100 ml)	Filtered load of urea (mg/min)	Reabsorption rate of urea* (mg/min)	Excretion rate of urea (mg/min)	Production rate of urea†		Retention rate of urea (mg/min)
							(g/day)	(mg/min)	
A	70	120	28	34	17	17	24.5	17	0
B I	70	60	28	17	8.5	8.5	24.5	17	8.5
II	70	60	57	34	17	17	24.5	17	0
C I	100	120	28	34	17	17	35	24	7
II	100	120	40	48	24	24	35	24	0
D I	60	75	28	21	10.5	10.5	21	15	4.5
II	60	75	40	30	15	15	21	15	0
E I	50	60	28	17	8.5	8.5	17.5	12	3.5
II	50	60	40	24	12	12	17.5	12	0
F I	33	40	28	11	5.5	5.5	11.5	8	2.5
II	33	40	40	16	8	8	11.5	8	0

*It is assumed that tubular reabsorption rate of urea is 50% of the filtered load and remains so when GFR falls and when dietary protein intake is changed

†Production rate of urea is calculated from the dietary protein intake considering that 35 g of urea are produced from the catabolism of 100 g of protein

Should the GFR remain unchanged (120 ml/min) but protein intake increase to 100 g/day (condition C), retention of urea of about 7 mg/min will similarly occur because of increased production of urea (about 24 mg/min). In a condition of unchanged filtered load (about 34 mg/min) and excretion (17 mg/min), this retention will raise the plasma concentration until an excretion rate identical to the production rate is reached (24 mg/min), i.e. until a plasma urea concentration of 40 mg/100 ml. Should the GFR fall to 75 ml/min (condition D), 60 ml/min (condition E) and 40 ml/min (condition F) and dietary protein intake decrease to 60 g/day (condition D), 50 g/day (condition E) and 33 g/day (condition F) respectively, similar adjustments would occur in plasma concentration of urea (40 mg/100 ml) in order to eliminate positive urea balance (conditions D II, E II and F II).

It is evident that the same value of plasma urea (40 mg/100 ml) may be observed in normal subjects (GFR of 120 ml/min, condition C II in Table 6) as well as in patients with renal function slightly reduced (GFR of 75 ml/min, condition D II), halved (condition E II) or reduced to one third of normal (condition F II) provided that dietary protein intake is proportionately decreased. Thus, a plasma urea level at the upper limit of the normal range may lull physicians into the wrong impression that renal function is normal even though it is actually reduced to one third of normal. Only the measurement of creatinine clearance will clarify whether renal function is impaired and the extent of this impairment.

The example reported in Table 6 is based on the assumption that tubular reabsorption of urea is 50% of the filtered load and remains constant with increasing impairment of renal function. This assumption is not correct, since urea reabsorption from ultrafiltrate is closely linked to changes in water reabsorption and the fall in fractional reabsorption of water occurring in surviving nephrons in CRF will reduce tubular reabsorption of urea. Furthermore, the example does not take into account the possible reutilization of urea for protein synthesis. These effects, however, will only slightly reduce the extent to which plasma urea must increase in order to restore urea balance[157].

Urine culture

Since it is demonstrated that urinary tract infections may further compromise renal function in chronically diseased kidneys and, since these infections are frequently asymptomatic, it is very important to obtain monthly urine cultures of uraemic patients.

For this purpose, a mid-stream sample is obtained during spontaneous micturition after cleaning the perineum and the labia in women and the urethral meatus in men. Disinfectants should be avoided, since even a small drop of them would sterilize the urine. Urine samples collected by this technique are frequently contaminated by bacteria residing in the urethra and the vulva; hence a quantitative bacterial culture is necessary. If the collected urine is cultured immediately or kept in a refrigerator until it is cultured, a bacterial count greater than 100000/ml gives an 85% probability that a true urinary tract infection exists and this probability rises to 99% when two consecutive cultures with counts greater than 100000/ml are obtained. Bacterial counts less than 10000/ml do not indicate true infection but they are due to contamination. Counts between 10000/ml and 100000/ml must be repeated[22].

A great number of leukocytes in the urinary sediment indicates inflammation in the urinary tract and may suggest (but not prove) the possibility of infection. Infections may, in fact, occur with and without pyuria.

Instrumentation or catheterization of the urinary tract should be avoided, whenever possible, because of the risk of infection.

Excretory urography and renal ultrasonography

Intravenous urography can be used for studying the kidneys of patients with advanced CRF. Usually sufficient visualization of the upper urinary tracts may be obtained by high-dose excretory urography (drip infusion pyelography) with tomography when renal function is as low as 15 ml/min. Poorly functioning kidneys may be visualized by [131I]hippuran ([131I]ortho-iodohippurate) scanning[330–333], but the information obtained by this technique is not comparable with that given by intravenous urography.

Ultrasonic echography is an excellent procedure for visualizing the kidneys and upper urinary tracts of patients with advanced uraemia[334, 335]. It is non-invasive and is the medical application of the same principle employed for detecting submarines by naval 'sonar' (from *SO*und *NA*vigation *R*anging). When electrical energy is applied to a piezoelectric crystal (the transducer), waves of high-frequency sound are generated (ultrasound waves, whose frequency ranges from 1 to 20 MHz, are not audible to the human ear). When these ultrasonic waves are directed into the patients (by applying the vibrating transducer to the skin), they travel in a straight line through body tissues of different physical properties. At each interface between tissues with differing density, some waves are reflected back to the transducer (echoes) and the remainder are transmitted to deeper tissues. For clinical use, therefore, the transducer acts both as transmitter and receiver of ultrasonic waves. After emitting ultrasounds in a few microseconds, it behaves as receiver for several hundred microseconds to detect reflected ultrasonic waves[336]. The echoes returned to the transducer are converted into electric pulses that may be amplified and displayed on an oscilloscope screen as dots of differing brightness (B Mode = Brightness Modulation). If the transducer is moved across the skin surface, a B-scan image (i.e. a two-dimensional cross-sectional display or sonogram) is produced resembling a radiographic tomogram, but with a plane that is parallel to the axis of the ultrasound beam (whereas the plane of the radiograph is perpendicular to the X-ray beam)[336, 337]. The oscilloscope is usually adjusted to store the images as the reflected echoes form them. The images can then be photographed with a Polaroid camera (Figures 23 and 24). They will represent cross-sections of body structures (e.g. longitudinal section of the kidney as in Figure 23a, transverse section of the kidney as in Figure 23b). Echoes appear as white areas while black regions represent absence of echoes. Nephrosonography allows an accurate assessment of the renal size, the contour of the kidneys, their internal architecture and the perirenal structures, even in conditions of impaired renal function[337].

Usually the kidneys are studied by ultrasonography with the patients in the prone position. Longitudinal sections of the organ (Figure 23a) are obtained by moving the transducer across the skin surface along the longitudinal axis of the kidney (i.e. slightly oblique to the vertebral column).

Transverse cross-sectional sonograms (Figure 23b) are obtained by moving the transducer perpendicular to the long axis of the kidney.

The normal kidney appears as an elliptical, ring-shaped structure in longitudinal cross-sectional sonograms (Figure 23a). This appearance is due to better transmission of ultrasound by renal parenchyma (peripheral black area) and to reflection of echoes by the walls of the collecting system and vessels (central echo complex that appears in the sonogram in the form of numerous white areas). In transverse cross-sectional sonograms, the kidney appears more rounded (Figure 23b). Since ultrasound transmission is improved in fluid-filled structures, a renal cyst will appear as a round, sharply outlined, echo-free area in the sonogram (Figure 23c). In case of mild hydronephrosis, echo-free areas (due to dilated urine-filled calyces and pelvis) are surrounded by echoes in the central part of the nephrosonogram (Figure 23d). In severe hydronephrosis, the urine-filled dilated renal pelvis will appear as an echo-free area (i.e. completely black area) in the sonogram[338,339] (Figure 24a), displacing the highly echogenic pelvicalyceal echo complex usually observed in the central part of the normal nephrosonogram[340] (Figure 23a). Polycystic kidneys show, in the nephrosonogram, a

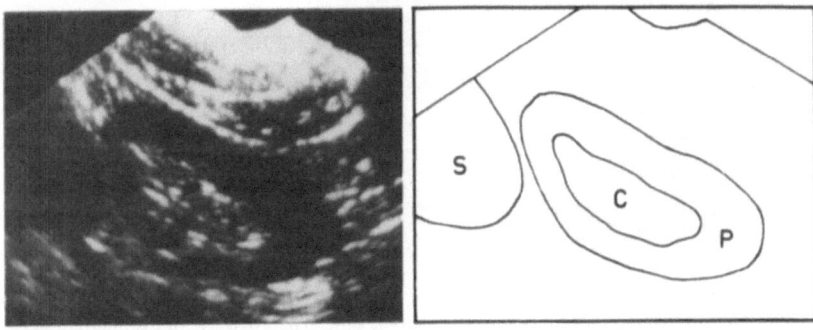

Figure 23a Normal kidney. Longitudinal cross-sectional sonogram of the left kidney in a normal adult subject. The ring-shaped structure is due to better transmission of ultrasounds by renal parenchyma (peripheral black area, P) and to reflection of echoes by the walls of the collecting system and vessels (central area with white spots, C) (S = spleen)

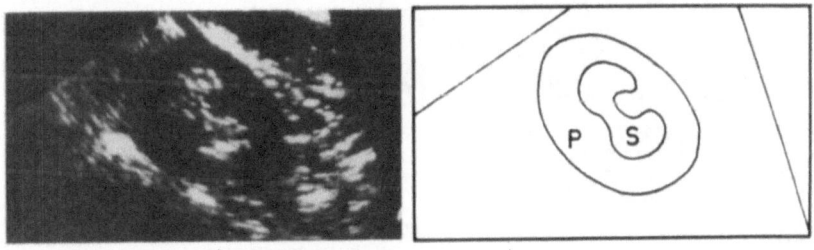

Figure 23b Normal kidney. Transverse cross-sectional sonogram of a normal kidney. (P = renal parenchyma; C = central echo complex)

distortion of the central echo complex that is fragmented by numerous fluid-filled cysts (Figure 24b). Radio-opaque as well as non-radio-opaque renal calculi may also be visualized by ultrasonography; they appear as echogenic foci with typical acoustic shadows obscuring deeper structures[336,341,342] (Figure 24c).

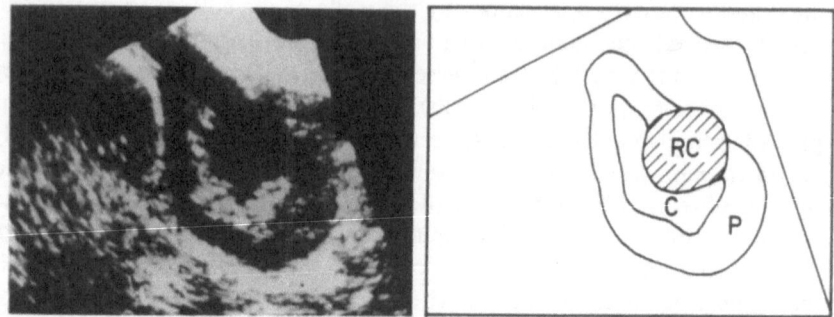

Figure 23c   Renal cyst. The renal cyst appears as a round, sharply outlined, echo-free area (RC) in the dorsal portion of the kidney. (P = renal parenchyma; C = central echo complex)

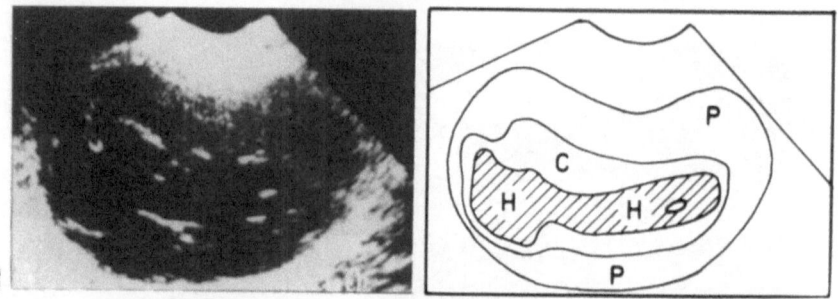

Figure 23d   Hydronephrosis. An echo-free area (H), due to dilated urine-filled calyces and pelvis, is surrounded by echoes (white spots) in the central part of the nephrosonogram in a case of mild hydronephrosis. (P = renal parenchyma; C = central echo complex)

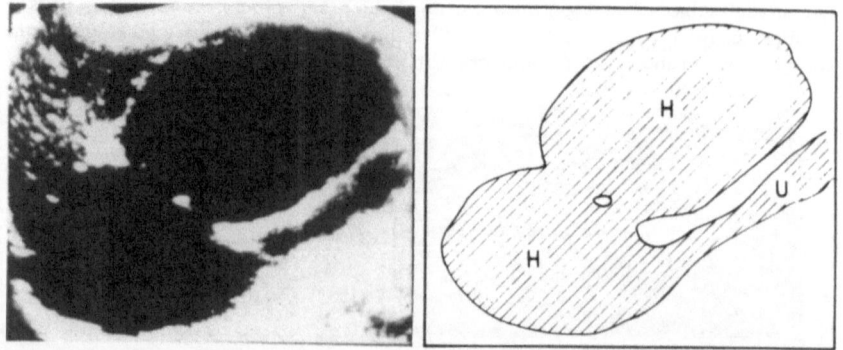

Figure 24a   Hydronephrosis. Two large echo-free areas (H) represent the urine-filled dilated renal pelvis in a case of severe hydronephrosis; the dilated ureter (U) is also visualized

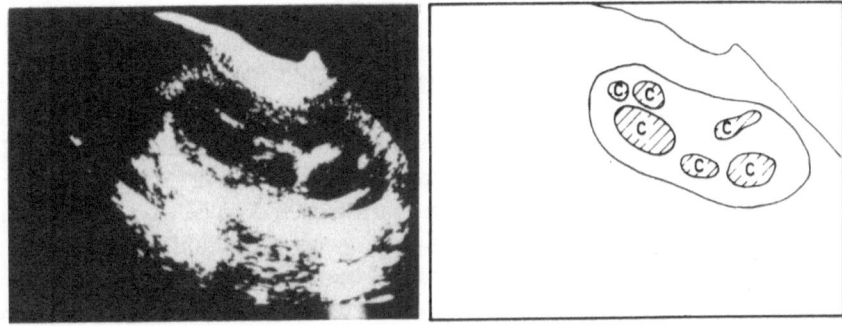

Figure 24b Polycystic kidney. The central echo complex is fragmented by fluid-filled cysts (C)

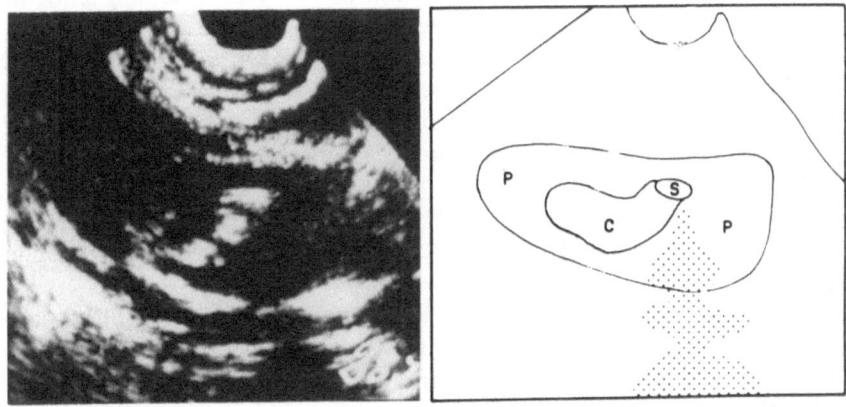

Figure 24c Radio-opaque renal stone (S) in a patient with CRF (creatinine clearance of 15 ml/min). Dense echoes (S), with a marked acoustic shadow on the back, are observed in the central echo complex (C), indicating a renal calculus in the lower part of the renal pelvis. (A radio-opaque stone in the renal pelvis was also demonstrated by a drip infusion pyelography). (P = renal parenchyma)

CONSERVATIVE MANAGEMENT OF CHRONIC RENAL FAILURE

The dietary and pharmacological treatment of CRF, instituted in patients with reduced renal function but before the end-stage CRF requiring dialysis or transplantation, may be termed 'conservative'[110].

The aims of conservative management of CRF are the maintenance of water, electrolyte and acid–base balance, and the reduction of accumulation of waste products of protein metabolism which may be responsible for uraemic toxicity.

Low protein diet

In the early 1960s, Italian investigators demonstrated that the nitrogen balance in uraemic patients could be maintained with diets restricted in nitrogen but containing adequate amounts of essential amino acids[343,344]. It was postulated that a low-protein diet could allow urea nitrogen reutilization for protein synthesis, i.e. ammonia nitrogen derived from urea breakdown could be a nitrogen source for the synthesis of non-essential amino acids[343] and even for the amination of keto-analogues of essential amino acids[345,346]. It has recently been demonstrated that reutilization of urea nitrogen for protein synthesis is quite small and plays no significant role in uraemic patients on dietary treatment[172,347,348].

Dietary treatment remains the key feature of the conservative management of CRF. It has been reported that low-protein diets may slow the progression of CRF[349]. Although this has yet to be confirmed, it is today accepted that the beneficial effect of protein restriction (provided calorie intake is adequate) is not based on reutilization of endogenous nitrogen, as initially proposed, but on reduction of nitrogen load to the gastrointestinal tract and to the whole organism in a condition of reduced capacity for nitrogen excretion[350].

It is a common observation that when anorexia, nausea and vomiting occur in uraemic patients, they respond quite well to protein restriction in the diet.

The aim of low-protein diets in chronic uraemia is to lower blood concentration of nitrogenous compounds to values below those at which uraemic symptoms occur. Furthermore, since hydrogen ions, sulphate, phosphate and potassium derive mainly from exogenous proteins, protein restriction may also be helpful in preventing metabolic acidosis (every 10 g of protein provides 7 mmol of hydrogen ions in the form of sulphated amino acids[110]), hyperphosphataemia and hyperkalaemia. Hence the need for protein restriction in the diet.

An extremely poor dietary intake, however, may be responsible for wasting syndrome. This is a syndrome characterized by decreased body weight, loss of adipose tissue, reduction in muscle mass and in growth in children, a fall in serum concentration of albumin, transferrin and C′3 fraction of complement, and an alteration in plasma and muscle concentration of amino acids[351,352]. Undoubtedly, other concurrent factors may contribute to this syndrome, such as uraemic toxins, endocrine disorders (e.g. hyperparathyroidism) or intercurrent illnesses, but the main causative factor is excessive dietary restriction.

For a correct nutritional management of chronic renal failure, the amount of protein in the diet must be low enough to minimize uraemic toxicity but high enough to prevent malnutrition. Furthermore, a large proportion of these proteins should have a high biological value, i.e. proteins should have most of the nitrogen as essential amino acids and should contain all the essential amino acids in approximately the proportions required by humans[353]. This is obtained mainly from eggs, but also from meat, fowl, fish, milk and milk products[352]. Proteins from vegetables and grains have low biological values and should be limited, although patients usually like this type of food. Very important is an adequate calorie intake, and this should not be less than 35 kcal kg^{-1} day^{-1} in order to prevent protein breakdown for energy purposes.

In a fasting condition, up to 20 g of urea (about 10 g of urea nitrogen) are produced daily by endogenous protein catabolism, i.e. about 60 g of body protein are catabolized each day*. During a nitrogen-free diet with adequate calorie intake, the obligatory protein catabolism is limited to about 15 g of body protein daily, yielding about 5 g of urea daily (about 2.5 g of urea nitrogen per day)[110,328]. Carbohydrates are protein-sparing; they decrease endogenous protein catabolism and the production of nitrogenous waste products provided they are ingested with the dietary protein or taken within 4 h of protein ingestion[353].

In wasted uraemic patients, a larger calorie intake (e.g. 50 kcal/kg body weight) is necessary to allow the limited protein intake to be used for repair of tissue protein deficits[354,355].

Carbohydrates may be given to uraemic patients in the form of sugar, jam, honey, etc. Low-protein wheat-starch products are commercially available as a source of high-calorie food. Low-protein pasta (Aproten, Aglutella) and low-protein wheat-starch flour for making bread and biscuits or pancakes may greatly help in enhancing the palatability of low-protein high-calorie diets. Protein-free carbohydrate supplements are also available as powder to be dissolved in water, milk, juice, etc., in order to increase calorie intake.

Fat is usually provided as butter or oil. Cookbooks, such as the one by Margie et al.[356], may help by providing useful recipes and suggestions. Obviously an expert dietician is of great help to the physician for the dietary management of CRF.

The disappearance, or at least the reduction, of anorexia, nausea and vomiting is usually an expression of adequacy of protein and calorie intake. The relief of uraemic symptoms is secondary to the decrease of endogenous protein catabolism and therefore to reduced accumulation of nitrogenous wastes[110].

In advanced CRF, phenothiazines, such as 0.4 mg kg^{-1} day^{-1} of prochlorperazine in three to four oral doses, may be very helpful in treating uraemic nausea and vomiting[110].

There is still controversy about when protein restriction should be started in patients with CRF. Kopple[352] avoids any restriction if GFR exceeds

---

*Approximately 35 g of urea (about 16 g of urea nitrogen) are produced from the catabolism of 100 g of protein[328].

25 ml/min. Others suggest $20 \, \text{ml min}^{-1} (1.73 \, \text{m}^2)^{-1}$ as the limit below which low-protein diets become necessary[110,353,357,358,359]. In our opinion, protein intake should be restricted when creatinine clearance is lower than 20–25 ml/min and blood urea is greater than 130–150 mg/100 ml (BUN greater than 65–75 mg/100 ml) with a normal unrestricted diet.

According to Kopple[352], when GFR is less than 10–15 ml/min, protein intake should be limited to $0.55–0.60 \, \text{g (kg body weight)}^{-1} \, \text{day}^{-1}$, with a maximum of 40 g/day (70% being high biological value proteins), provided the calorie intake is greater than $35 \, \text{kcal kg}^{-1} \, \text{day}^{-1}$. This protein intake $(0.6 \, \text{g kg}^{-1} \, \text{day}^{-1})$ is higher than that suggested in the Giordano–Giovannetti diet. This is a 20 g protein diet of high biological value proteins containing the minimum requirement of all essential amino acids[343,344]. When adult patients with GRF less than 10 ml/min were randomly assigned to either 20 g protein/day (Giordano–Giovannetti type) or 40 g protein/day of proteins of high biological value, the latter resulted in a slightly greater BUN, but the patients were in positive nitrogen balance (negative with 20 g/day) and they gained in body weight. Additionally, they felt better and

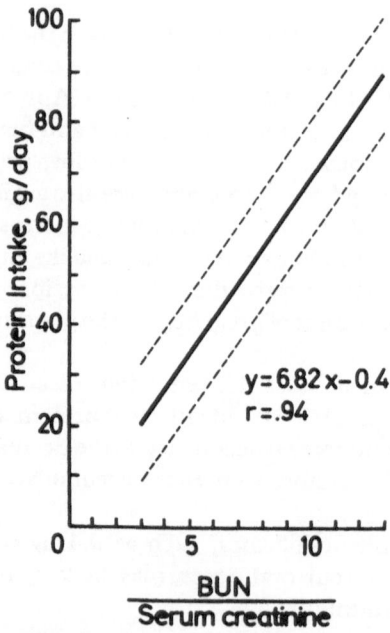

Figure 25 Relationship between dietary protein intake and BUN to serum creatinine ratios in chronically uraemic men not treated with dialysis. The regression line is solid; the interrupted lines represent the 95% confidence limits. Reproduced by kind permission from J. D. Kopple and J. W. Coburn (1974). Evaluation of chronic anemia. *J. Am. Med. Assoc.*, **227**, 41. Copyright 1974 American Medical Association

compliance was higher[360,361]. In fact, patients on more restricted protein intake disliked their diet so much that they frequently consumed 28–30 g rather than 20 g of protein per day[362].

Since uraemic symptoms (anorexia, nausea, vomiting, diarrhoea, twitching and apathy) do not occur until BUN is greater than 90 mg/100 ml, treatment should be aimed at a BUN level of about 60 mg/100 ml (i.e. blood urea 120 mg/100 ml) or less, remembering that it takes 2 to 3 weeks before the BUN level stabilizes after a change in diet[351]. In order to select the optimal dietary protein intake in a single patient, Kopple and Coburn[363] have designed a diagram based on the relationship between the ratios of BUN (or SUN) to serum creatinine and protein intake in chronically uraemic adult men not treated with dialysis (Figure 25). For example, to maintain the BUN of a patient at approximately 60 mg/100 ml, the BUN (60 mg/100 ml) is divided by the serum creatinine (e.g. 8 mg/100 ml) and the resulting ratio (7.5 in this example) corresponds to the protein intake (52 g/day in the example) which will maintain this ratio. Since serum creatinine is affected by renal function and by muscle mass, this diagram cannot be used for small men, women or children. According to Kopple, protein intake in adult men should never be reduced below 40 g/day of high-quality protein, and never below 35 g/day in small men and women[351].

Urinary protein loss is usually not great in CRF. Even when nephrotic syndrome is initially present, urinary proteins usually decrease with the drop in GFR. However, when protein restriction is needed in advanced CRF and there is a significant urinary loss of proteins, it may be necessary to increase protein intake at a rate equivalent (gram for gram) to the urinary loss[352].

When GFR is lower than 4–5 ml/min, RDT should be started[282], since a diet with a protein restriction of 18 to 25 g/day may not control uraemic toxicity and may result in malnutrition[352,364].

Recently, a nutritional regimen involving semisynthetic diets containing essential amino acids and/or their keto and hydroxy analogues (ketoacids and hydroxyacids)* has been suggested as an alternative to dialysis. Some authors suggested the use of only essential amino acids (20–25 g/day)[365], some use a combination of a very low-protein diet (e.g. 20 g protein) and essential amino acids (e.g. 10 g/day)[100,205,366] and others use a mixture of keto analogues of five essential amino acids and the other four essential amino acids (e.g. 16 g/day) plus 20 g protein daily[100,349,367]. When a patient with GFR less than 4–5 ml/min cannot be treated with dialysis or transplantation, a 20 g/day protein diet may be used with supplements of essential amino acids (e.g. 20 g/day in the proportion defined by Rose[368] for daily

---

* Keto acids and hydroxy acids have the same structure in that their respective essential amino acids have a keto or a hydroxy group substituted for the α-amino nitrogen. Since keto acids and hydroxy acids are rapidly converted to their respective amino acids *in vivo*, their use has the same biological effects as amino acids with a lower nitrogen load.

amino acid requirements, but including 1.65 g/day of L-histidine). This dietary treatment will reduce uraemic toxicity and maintain a good nutritional status[369]. Unfortunately such diets are monotonous and unpleasant to take and the substitution of keto acids makes them worse.

Diet in children

Dietary management of chronic uraemia in children and adolescents is more specialized. Uraemic children and adolescents are often malnourished and growth retarded[370,371]. Undoubtedly depletion of minerals, such as potassium or calcium, and hormonal imbalance may play important roles in the failure of children to grow, but the protein/calorie deficiency in the diet is the major cause of poor body growth and reduction in final adult height[370,372,373].

Energy intake in children is usually seriously low and malnutrition is often disguised by fluid retention. On the other hand, the energy requirements of children are much greater than those of adults. Abitrol and Holliday[374] have shown that an energy intake less than $60 \, \text{kcal} \, \text{kg}^{-1} \, \text{day}^{-1}$ causes catabolic loss of body proteins. This energy requirement is undoubtedly far in excess of what children like eating. Kerr et al.[375] have shown that, in order to restore a 7 kg child to the ideal weight of 10 kg, it takes 150 days if the calorie intake is 820 kcal/day and only 19 days with 1180 kcal/day.

Calorie requirements of children depend on age and sex. From 10 to 18 years, $42/64 \, \text{kcal} \, \text{kg}^{-1} \, \text{day}^{-1}$ are required for girls and $50–70 \, \text{kcal} \, \text{kg}^{-1} \, \text{day}^{-1}$ for boys. Calorie requirements increase from 78 to $90 \, \text{kcal} \, \text{kg}^{-1} \, \text{day}^{-1}$ for both girls and boys aged 1 year, while $100–120 \, \text{kcal} \, \text{kg}^{-1} \, \text{day}^{-1}$ is needed by infants under 1 year of age[110,358]. This energy intake should consist of 75% carbohydrate, 20% fat and 5% protein of high biological value or mixture of essential amino acids[110,358].

Protein requirements in childhood also vary in relation to age, sex and degree of renal failure. According to Broyer[358] and Schoenemann[110], a low-protein diet in children should provide the following amounts of protein:

(a) $0.8–1 \, \text{g} \, \text{kg}^{-1} \, \text{day}^{-1}$ (when GFR is $10–20 \, \text{ml} \, \text{min}^{-1} (1.73 \, \text{m}^2)^{-1}$) or $0.7–0.9 \, \text{g} \, \text{kg}^{-1} \, \text{day}^{-1}$ (when GFR is $5–10 \, \text{ml} \, \text{min}^{-1} (1.73 \, \text{m}^2)^{-1}$) in female and male adolescents ranging in age from 18 years to 10 years;

(b) $1.1–1.2 \, \text{g} \, \text{kg}^{-1} \, \text{day}^{-1}$ (when GFR is $10–20 \, \text{ml} \, \text{min}^{-1} (1.73 \, \text{m}^2)^{-1}$) or $0.9–1.0 \, \text{g} \, \text{kg}^{-1} \, \text{day}^{-1}$ (when GFR is $5–10 \, \text{ml} \, \text{min}^{-1} (1.73 \, \text{m}^2)^{-1}$) in 4- to 10-year-old children;

(c) $1.4–1.6 \, \text{g} \, \text{kg}^{-1} \, \text{day}^{-1}$ (GFR $= 10–20 \, \text{ml} \, \text{min}^{-1} (1.73 \, \text{m}^2)^{-1}$) or $1.2–1.4 \, \text{g} \, \text{kg}^{-1} \, \text{day}^{-1}$ (GFR $= 5–10 \, \text{ml} \, \text{min}^{-1} (1.73 \, \text{m}^2)^{-1}$) in children less than 4 years of age (including infants).

It is evident that calorie and protein requirements decrease with increasing age.

The beneficial effects of diets with high biological value proteins and/or essential amino acids in uraemic children and infants are well documented[376,377]. Supplements of essential amino acids to very low protein diets often improve nitrogen balance and weight gain[378] and may stimulate protein synthesis. Indeed, Aronson et al.[359] have reported resumption of growth in a severely uraemic child treated with a low protein diet and essential amino acids (0.5–1 g/100 kcal of essential amino acids).

Synthetic essential amino acids may completely or partially replace protein. The WHO Expert Committee on Energy and Protein Requirements[110] has shown that each gram of dietary protein provides 0.4 g of essential amino acids. It is important, however, that these amino acids are given in the proportions specified by Rose[368]: L-methionine, L-phenylalanine and L-leucine 15.4% each; L-lysine and L-valine 12% each; L-isoleucine 10%; L-tryptophan 3.8%; and L-threonine and L-histidine 7.5% each. The L-histidine should be added to the accepted eight essential amino acids as it has been shown to be essential in infancy and severe uraemia[379–381].

Recently, keto analogues of essential amino acids have been used in conjunction with a restricted protein diet. Preliminary experience with both essential amino acid and keto analogue supplements to low-protein diets seems to support the hope of deferring dialysis in end-stage CRF[348,382]. Uraemic patients receiving such treatment have clearly shown an initial improvement in their renal function[100,349]. Furthermore, in patients already on RDT, but with some residual renal function, nutritional therapy with analogues could replace dialysis for prolonged periods[382]. These observations support the view that uraemia is nephrotoxic and that factors such as protein malnutrition, hyperuricaemia and elevated Ca × P product in the blood may contribute to progression of renal failure[382]. In favour of this hypothesis are the observations of improved renal function when hyperuricaemia was corrected (Figure 13) and the preliminary results of the beneficial effect of low-phosphorus diet plus phosphate binders on the progression of CRF[383].

Some investigators claim that nitrogen balance is more positive, both in adults and in children, and growth of infants is better when dietary supplements contain only amino acids rather than a mixture of amino acids and some keto analogues[377]. Further studies are therefore necessary before deciding what is the ideal diet in respect to protein metabolism and particularly the value of keto analogues.

Vitamin supplements

Low-protein diets may induce water-soluble vitamin deficiency, since restriction of both protein of low biological value and potassium limits the intake of leafy vegetables and fruits. Furthermore, boiling vegetables to reduce their potassium content lowers their water-soluble vitamins[110].

Administration of one multivitamin tablet will usually correct or prevent any water-soluble vitamin deficiency in non-dialysed uraemic patients. Alternatively, supplements of at least the following vitamins should be given: folic acid[110,384,385], 1 mg/day; vitamin C[352], 70–100 mg/day; and pyridoxine[110] (vitamin B_6, the deficiency of which is mainly due to reduced synthesis[385]), 25–50 mg/day. According to Kopple[352], non-dialysed uraemic patients should receive the following supplements: thiamine (B_1), 1.5 mg/day; riboflavin (B_2), 1.8 mg/day; pantothenic acid (B_5), 5 mg/day; niacin, 20 mg/day; pyridoxine hydrochloride (B_6), 5 mg/day; vitamin B_{12}, 3 µg/day; vitamin C, 70–100 mg/day; and folic acid, 1 mg/day.

Hypertriglyceridaemia, diet and lipid-lowering drugs

There is evidence that a defect in triglyceride removal is an important factor in the development of hypertriglyceridaemia in uraemic patients[221,386–388], but diet is also an important factor influencing plasma triglyceride levels. A direct correlation has been shown to exist between triglyceride production and plasma concentration in uraemic subjects[388].

However, patients with CRF are usually placed on low-protein diets in which wheat-starch foodstuffs and high carbohydrate and fat desserts represent the main sources of calories. Fats are therefore used to provide energy, to give essential fatty acids and, last but not least, to enhance the palatability of the diet[110], although fat is considered less effective than carbohydrates in minimizing endogenous protein catabolism[328]. Hence, carbohydrates remain the major source of calories, and even a moderate increase in carbohydrate intake has been shown to raise plasma triglycerides (at least in subjects with normal renal function)[389].

Recently promising results have been obtained in treatment of uraemic hypertriglyceridaemia from a slight reduction in carbohydrate intake and better selection of lipids in the diet. When non-nephrotic uraemic subjects with hypertriglyceridaemia (256 ± 57 mg/100 ml) on 'conventional' diets (i.e. 10% of total calories as protein, 50% as carbohydrates and 40% as fat, with a polyunsaturated to saturated fat ratio of 0.2) were switched to a 'low carbohydrate' diet in which calories (35 kcal (kg body weight)$^{-1}$ day^{-1} were supplied by 35% as carbohydrates, 55% as fat with polyunsaturated to saturated fat ratio of 2, and 10% as protein, serum triglyceride level fell from a mean value of 256 to 160 mg/100 ml over an 11-day period[388]. These results show that reduction in carbohydrate intake and substitution of polyunsaturated fat for saturated fat lowers triglycerides in uraemic hypertriglyceridaemia, as well as in non-uraemic type IV hyperlipidaemia[390,391]. Further studies are necessary to elucidate which one of these two factors, the lower carbohydrate intake or greater substitution of polyunsaturated for saturated fat, is more important in reducing the high blood levels of triglyceride in chronic uraemia.

On the basis of these observations, we advise uraemic patients to avoid cooked fat, fried food and baked fatty meat, to use corn oil and sunflower oil (both rich in polyunsaturated fatty acids) in preference to olive oil, and margarine in preference to butter, and to absolutely avoid alcohol.

Clofibrate is capable of reducing plasma concentrations of both low density and very low density lipoproteins. It has been used for treating uraemic hyperlipidaemia (type IV hyperlipidaemia); but the dosage should be low (not exceeding 1.5 g/week) to prevent accumulation and consequent severe and painful myositis with elevated CPK levels[214,392,393]. Some authors advocate the use of clofibrate in uraemic hypertriglyceridaemia[394-396], but others are opposed to its use[392].

Recently a large and long clinical trial of the effects of clofibrate (1.6 g/day) on the incidence of coronary heart disease in apparently normal men with high serum cholesterol has raised some concern about its use as a lipid-lowering drug. A randomized double-blind study[397] was carried out under the auspices of WHO in three European centres (Edinburgh, Budapest and Prague). In 15 745 males, aged 30–59 years with an average follow-up of 5.3 years, clofibrate appeared to be effective in reducing the incidence of major ischaemic heart disease. This effect was attributed to a fall in serum cholesterol averaging 9%. But the study also showed a significant increase in deaths due to non-cardiovascular diseases, such as liver disease, cholelithiasis and neoplasms at all levels of the alimentary tract[397,398]. These results may represent a fortuitous association or direct toxic effects of clofibrate[398], but it was concluded that clofibrate should not be recommended for community-wide prevention of ischaemic heart disease[397,398].

Furthermore, some countries (e.g. Federal Republic of Germany) have withdrawn drugs containing clofibrate and many nephrologists no longer use clofibrate for treating uraemic hyperlipidaemia.

Whether lipid-lowering regimens (including dietary modification in fat intake) share the same problems is still an unanswered question[399]. It should, however, be stressed that nicotinic acid, another potent hypolipidaemic drug, also increases biliary neutral sterol excretion[400].

Salt intake

The 'floor' and 'ceiling' for sodium excretion can be determined in uraemic patients by external balance study at different salt intakes. Thus, if the patient has a 'salt-free' diet (a diet with the lowest known salt content will usually provide less than 1 g of NaCl/day) for 4 days, the 24-hour urinary sodium excretion on the fourth day will give the 'floor' value in that patient. Similarly, if the patient is maintained for 4 days on the same 'salt-free' diet but with the addition of 10 or 12 g (exactly weighed) of NaCl per day, the 24-hour urinary sodium excretion on the fourth day will give the 'ceiling'[14].

Usually there is no need to establish 'floor' and 'ceiling' values for sodium excretion in all chronic uraemic patients. If the patient has no oedema and his blood pressure is normal, his usual salt intake can be maintained. In uraemic patients without hypertension, but with anorexia, salt leaks should be suspected and investigated, and salt replacement given as soon as possible.

In cases of hypertension, congestive heart failure, nephrotic syndrome or advanced liver disease, sodium restriction becomes mandatory and sometimes potent diuretics should be used in high doses. Usually, when sodium balance is controlled, thirst is adequate to control water balance, but, when GFR is lower than 5 ml/min, water restriction becomes necessary, independently of sodium, to prevent overhydration[352].

Treatment of hypertension in CRF

In adults, treatment of hypertension may be considered successful when diastolic blood pressure falls to 90 mmHg or below (systolic blood pressure not greater than 130 mmHg in men under 45, 140 mmHg in men over 45, and 160 mmHg in women)[319] all day long.

Since treatment with antihypertensive drugs is long-term, care should be taken to avoid too many pills at different hours of the day, since patient compliance is inversely related to the difficulty of dosage schedules.

As salt and water retention plays a key role in the pathophysiology of the hypertension secondary to CRF, the treatment of uraemic hypertension must rely on the correction of salt retention (item (a) in Figure 17). The first step in the management of uraemic hypertension is therefore dietary restriction of salt. Scribner and co-workers introduced the concept of 'basal sodium excretion', i.e. the highest 24-hour urinary sodium excretion that is compatible with normotension in each patient with CRF[284,401]. Blood pressure in uraemic patients may be normalized if dietary sodium intake is reduced to the level of their basal sodium excretion. Some uraemic patients (less than 20%) have very high basal sodium excretion (greater than 200 mmol/24 h) so that they remain normotensive whatever their sodium intake is[294]. In most uraemic patients, however, basal sodium excretion is below 70–80 mmol/24 h, so that salt restriction with the diet is usually not sufficient to reduce sodium intake to the level of urinary sodium output. In such cases we can still correct salt retention (item (a) in Figure 17), and hence hypertension, by using diuretic agents to increase basal sodium excretion. Thiazides are the most commonly used diuretics when GFR is greater than 40 ml/min. With further loss of renal function, more powerful diuretics, such as ethacrynic acid or furosemide, should be used. We have recently shown that muzolimine is the best high-ceiling diuretic because of its long-acting saluretic effect and its effectiveness in patients with very low renal function[21]. We have frequently obtained normalization of systemic blood pressure in hypertensive patients with advanced uraemia (creatinine clearance as low as 7–8 ml/min) by increasing salt excretion with muzolimine (Figure 4).

While on treatment with diuretic agents, serum uric acid must be monitored, since most diuretics cause hyperuricaemia. Promising results have recently been obtained with ticrynafen, or tienilic acid (2,3-dichloro-4(2-thienylcarbonyl) phenoxyacetic acid), a new non-sulphonamide diuretic with antihypertensive effects, similar to those of thiazides, but with associated uricosuric activity sufficient to prevent hyperuricaemia[402–406]. As the site of action of this diuretic is the same as for thiazides[407], presumably it is effective only when GFR is greater than 40 ml/min.

The uricosuric effect of ticrynafen may cause problems such as stone formation due to uric acid precipitation or nucleation of calcium oxalate by monosodium urate crystals[408]. More significant, acute renal failure has recently been described in hypertensive patients treated with ticrynafen[409–411], but it has been claimed that this may be prevented by adequate hydration[412].

Spironolactone should sometimes be used in association with diuretics in order to prevent hypokalaemia. However, it should be stressed that:

(a) It takes 3 to 5 days before the effects of spironolactone on potassium excretion become detectable;
(b) Excessive spironolactone administration may cause hyperkalaemia; and
(c) Spironolactone may cause gynaecomastia in some patients.

If salt restriction and diuretics fail to normalize systemic blood pressure, antihypertensive drugs must be used. Firstly, in order to influence cardiac output (item (b) in Figure 17) we use β-adrenergic blockers, such as propranolol. We start with a very low dosage (e.g. 20 mg of propranolol daily) to test the sensitivity of the patient to the drug, and then slowly increase the dosage in two, three or even four divided doses (e.g. 20 mg × 4 daily of propranolol). It should be remembered that:

(a) β-Adrenergic blockers are contraindicated in patients with bronchial asthma or with cardiac A-V block;
(b) They may cause congestive heart failure in patients with heart disease (sometimes secondary to long-standing severe hypertension);
(c) They cause bradycardia which will limit their dosage.

Better results in blocking β-adrenergic receptors have been claimed with the use of the so-called cardioselective β-blockers. After the demonstration of two types of adrenergic receptors, α- and β-receptors[413], it was subsequently shown that β-receptors could be divided into two types, termed β_1-receptors (cardiostimulation and lipolysis) and β_2-receptors (bronchodilatation and vasodilatation). This led to the development of drugs acting selectively at either β_1- or β_2-receptors[414]. Propranolol blocks both β_1- and β_2-receptors; other cardioselective β-blockers, such as metoprolol and atenolol, only antagonize the action of sympathomimetic amines on β_1-receptors[415-418]. This property of cardioselective β-blocking drugs makes them particularly suitable for patients with acute or chronic obstructive pulmonary disease[416] for the β_2-receptors remain available for adrenergic bronchodilatation. They may also be preferable for treating hypertension, since the β_2-receptors in peripheral arterioles are not blocked[414]. Unfortunately, this selectivity for β_1-receptors is limited to low doses and β_2-receptor blockade occurs in most patients when the dose of metoprolol or atenolol exceeds 100 mg/day[414].

Clinical trials have shown that the antihypertensive effects of propranolol, metoprolol and atenolol are quantitatively similar[419-422] and that they are effective both in standing and supine positions. Their antihypertensive action[414] results from:

(a) Reduction in cardiac output,
(b) A fall in plasma renin activity, and, possibly
(c) Their action on the central nervous system which reduces sympathetic outflow.

Atenolol is long-acting so that the usual dosage is 100 mg once daily in patients with normal renal function[421,423]. This property makes atenolol a useful drug to improve compliance. Because it is excreted through the kidneys, the dose interval may need to be prolonged (e.g. 100 mg every other day, or even 3 or 4 days) in patients with moderate to severe renal failure[418].

β-Blockers may increase atherogenesis because of their effects on lipid and carbohydrate metabolism. Such effects are probably less important with cardioselective β-blocking drugs[414].

Labetalol has recently been suggested as the ideal agent for replacing β-adrenergic blockers. It is a combined α- and β-adrenoceptor antagonist. The α-adrenoceptor-blocking effect of labetalol can lower systemic blood pressure by reducing total peripheral resistance (item (c) in Figure 17), while the reflex tachycardia that usually follows α-adrenergic blockade is not observed because of its β-blocking effect. Labetalol is not contraindicated in patients with bronchial asthma because of its α-adrenergic blocking activity. However, congestive heart failure and cardiac A-V blocks are contraindications for the use of this drug. Labetalol is an efficient antihypertensive agent in uraemic patients either alone (Figure 26) or in association with diuretics.

Peripheral vasodilator drugs are the antihypertensive agents of third choice, i.e. they are used when diuretics and β-adrenergic blockers are not sufficient to control hypertension. They include hydralazine, minoxidil and prazosin.

Hydralazine and minoxidil are direct-acting vasodilators, since they reduce the tone of the arterioles by a direct relaxant effect on vascular smooth muscle. A fall in total peripheral resistance (item (c) in Figure 17)

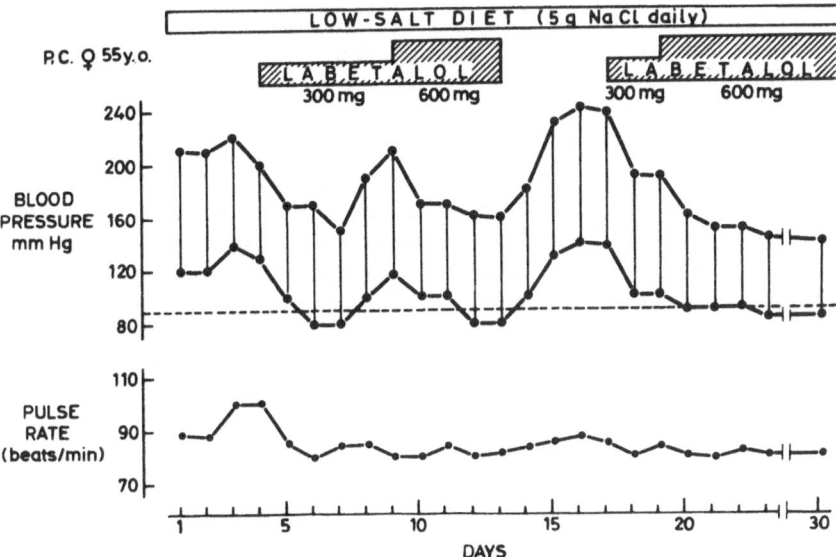

Figure 26 P.C. is a 55-year-old female with hypertension in chronic renal failure (creatinine clearance of 40 ml/min). After a low-salt diet, blood pressure was still 205/120 mmHg or greater. 300 mg daily of labetalol were given in three divided doses, increasing to 600 mg daily after a few days. With the drug, blood pressure fell to 160/80 mmHg. Withdrawal of labetalol was followed by a rise in blood pressure to the pretreatment values. Further treatment with labetalol was again successful, especially when the dosage was maintained at 600 mg daily; pulse rate was stabilized at 80 beats/min

will result, with a consequent fall in systemic blood pressure. The hyperdynamic state of the circulation induced by these drugs may cause anginal pain in patients with coronary artery insufficiency (not infrequent in longstanding hypertension). The association of a β-adrenergic blocker will control the reflex tachycardia secondary to peripheral vasodilatation. Untoward effects of hydralazine include headache and nasal congestion. Sometimes the headache is so severe as to require a change in antihypertensive therapy.

At present minoxidil is the most powerful antihypertensive agent and is effective in treating life-threatening 'malignant' hypertension[424–426]. It must be used with a β-adrenergic blocker to control reflex tachycardia, and with a diuretic (a high-ceiling diuretic in advanced CRF) to prevent salt retention. It may be given in two daily doses, since its effect, which begins within 2 h, usually lasts at least 17 h (Figure 27). The side-effect of this drug, which limits its use in females and children, is hypertrichosis, which appears within 2–3 weeks of treatment[426]. The use of minoxidil should be limited to cases of severe hypertension refractory to high doses of conventional anti-hypertensive drugs. We have also used it in dialysis patients and in transplanted patients during rejection episodes associated with severe hypertension[427].

Prazosin is an antihypertensive drug that reduces peripheral vascular resistance (item (c) in Figure 17) by blocking vascular α-adrenergic receptors. This mechanism of action is different from that of hydralazine and minoxidil, both of which have a direct effect on vascular smooth muscle[428]. Prazosin may be used as a single agent in the treatment of hypertension, especially in patients who cannot tolerate β-adrenergic blockers because of bronchial asthma or congestive heart failure. It does not cause reflex tachycardia, presumably because of its combined action of reducing vascular tone in both the resistance bed (arterioles) and capacitance bed (veins), so that increases in venous return and cardiac output are avoided[428,429]. These effects make the drug particularly suitable for treating hypertensive patients with congestive heart failure. An important and troublesome side-effect of prazosin is transitory postural hypotension, with faintness, dizziness and

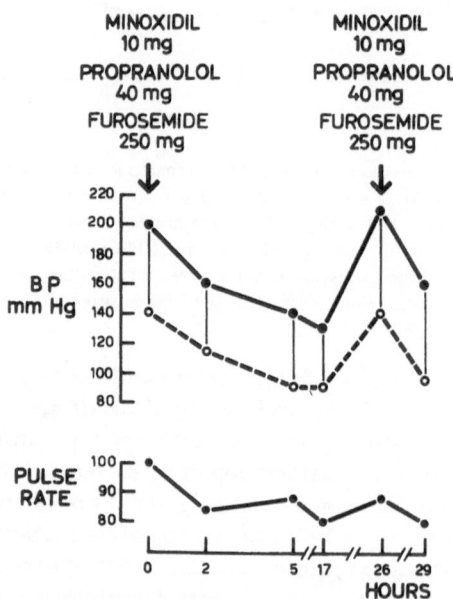

Figure 27   S.V., a 24-year-old male patient with advanced chronic renal failure (creatinine clearance of 18 ml/min), had severe hypertension, uncontrolled by conventional antihypertensive medications. Oral administration of 10 mg of minoxidil, associated with 40 mg of propranolol (to control reflex tachycardia) and 250 mg of furosemide (to prevent salt retention), caused a significant fall in arterial pressure from 200/140 to 160/115 mmHg within 2 h. After 5 h, BP was 140/90 mmHg and remained unchanged until 17 h. The BP then rose again to 208/140 so that another dose of minoxidil + propranolol + furosemide was given

palpitation, that occurs soon after the first dose of the drug ('first-dose phenomenon')[430]. This seems to be related to the lack of compensatory increase in catecholamine release after a rapid fall in blood pressure[428]. This phenomenon is exaggerated by sodium depletion[430], and, in order to avoid it, we advise the patient to take the initial dose (only 1 mg) of prazosin late in the evening before going to bed. The dosage may then be increased, in divided daily doses, up to 30 mg/day, until the desired reduction in blood pressure is obtained. Prazosin is well tolerated, even at high doses, in hypertensive patients with CRF[431]. We frequently combine it with diuretics and β-adrenergic blockers. This combination may prevent the increase in severity and frequency of pre-existing angina described by others after prazosin[432].

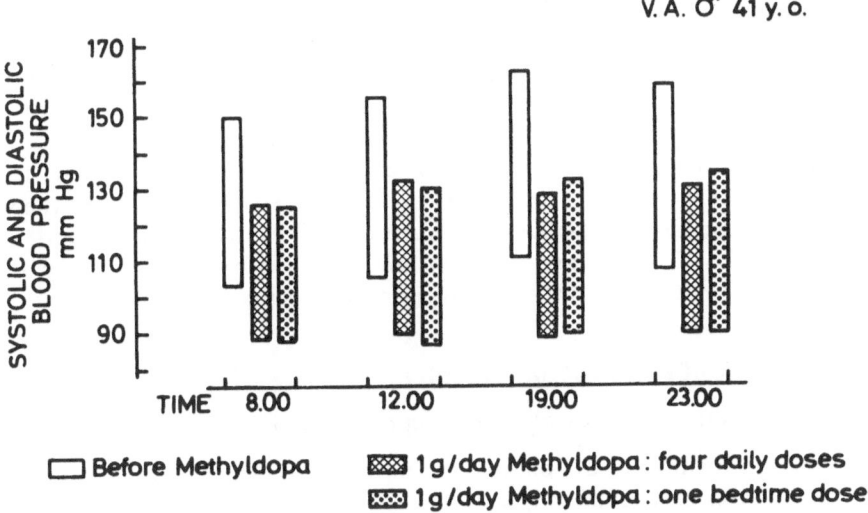

Figure 28   V.A., a 41-year-old male patient with hypertension ranging between 150/103 and 162/110 mmHg, was treated for 3 months with 1 g methyldopa daily, in four divided doses, and then for the next 3 months with 1 g methyldopa daily as a single bedtime dose. Systolic and diastolic blood pressure fell to the same extent with the two regimens

Methyldopa and clonidine are other antihypertensive agents which are also widely used in chronic uraemia. They belong to the class of antihypertensive drugs which act via the central nervous system. Both methyldopa (by forming methylnoradrenalin) and clonidine have their main effect on the catecholamine receptors, probably the α-receptors in the CNS. The activation of these receptors will reduce the efferent sympathetic activity on heart, blood vessels and adrenal glands, and it will increase efferent vagal activity leading to bradycardia. The consequent re-adjustment of sympathetic and vagal activity will lower the systemic blood pressure[433]. The central action of these drugs accounts for the sedation and sleepiness that represent their main side-effect. A dry mouth, due to inhibition of salivation, is also frequent, especially with clonidine. Because of vagal bradycardia, clonidine cannot be used as a single antihypertensive agent at high doses. The combination of clonidine and hydralazine is, however, quite satisfactory in this respect. A severe 'rebound' hypertension has been described after rapid withdrawal of clonidine therapy[434]. It should be administered in divided daily doses, e.g. 75 µg × 4 daily, as the initial dose, which may be then slowly increased up to 300 µg × 4 daily.

Evidence suggests that the antihypertensive effect of methyldopa persists much longer than its plasma half-life so that the total daily dosage may be given as a single dose at night[435, 436]. We have observed identical results with single doses and four daily doses (Figure 28). The administration of a single dose at night may minimize the sedative side-effects and also improve compliance.

Guanethidine is another antihypertensive drug which may be useful for treating uraemic patients with hypertension not adequately controlled by other agents. Its action results from the depression of postganglionic adrenergic nerves. Guanethidine can almost completely inhibit sympathetic vasomotor tone and may therefore cause postural hypotension. It is necessary to start treatment with very low doses (e.g. 10 or even 5 mg daily) and then gradually increase the dosage, at intervals of not less than 4–5 days, until a standing diastolic blood pressure of 90 mmHg or less is achieved. It may be used in association with other antihypertensive agents.

Treatment of renal osteodystrophy

There are four objectives when treating renal osteodystrophy:

(1) The maintenance of plasma concentration of calcium and phosphorus within the normal range,
(2) The suppression and prevention of secondary hyperparathyroidism,
(3) The restoration of the skeleton to normal, and
(4) The prevention or correction of metastatic calcification[74].

These objectives may be achieved by adequate control of phosphate and calcium intake, by treatment with vitamin D and other vitamins and, in some cases, by total or subtotal parathyroidectomy.

Phosphate and calcium intake

Consideration of phosphate metabolism in CRF ('trade-off' hypothesis of Bricker)[437] suggests that a reduction in phosphate intake proportional to the fall in overall GFR should prevent adaptive hyperphosphaturia in residual nephrons and consequent secondary hyperparathyroidism. This has been demonstrated in uraemic dogs where PTH levels were maintained at normal for 1 year and only slightly elevated after 2 years by proportional reduction of phosphate intake. (This slight rise in PTH was counteracted[39] by addition of $25\text{-}OHD_3$.) Similar results have been obtained in uraemic patients[14, 74]. In the conservative management of CRF, a low-phosphate diet may be used when plasma phosphate is normal[438]. It is essential when plasma phosphate is increased above 5 mg/100 ml in order to prevent metastatic calcification and the reciprocal fall in ionized calcium which would lead to a rise in parathyroid gland activity. The ideal is to maintain plasma phosphate in the range of 3–4 mg/100 ml.

Reduction in dietary phosphate is not easy, since phosphorus is a ubiquitous substance present in almost all foodstuffs, particularly meat and dairy products. The best approach is therefore reduction of the enteric absorption of ingested phosphorus with phosphate-binding gels, such as aluminium hydroxide and/or magnesium hydroxide. These antacids minimize the amount of ingested phosphorus available for absorption, increasing the content of phosphate with faeces. Since reduction in protein intake implies a fall in phosphate intake, phosphate-binding gels are not usually necessary, while uraemic patients are on low-protein diets, until a creatinine clearance of 10 ml/min or less.

In hyperphosphataemia, up to 6 g/day of aluminium hydroxide gel may be given either in the form of a suspension or tablets (of 0.3 g, 0.5 g or 0.6 g each; Alucol and Amphojel) starting with two or three tablets with each meal. The association of aluminium hydroxide with magnesium hydroxide (Maalox and Aludrox tablets or suspension) is effective and especially useful in patients with a tendency to constipation if treated with aluminium hydroxide alone. Calcium carbonate (5–10 g/day orally) may also be used, since it binds phosphate in the gut. However, the rise in plasma calcium which follows calcium carbonate administration may be dangerous (because of the consequent rise in plasma calcium × plasma phosphorus product) in cases of severe hyperphosphataemia. The use of calcium carbonate is restricted to prolonged maintenance treatment once plasma phosphate has been lowered by other means.

Hypophosphataemia must be avoided. Excessive reduction in phosphate intake may cause a hypophosphataemic syndrome characterized by haemolytic anaemia, myopathy and osteomalacia[439–441].

Lowering of plasma phosphate is usually associated with a rise in plasma concentration of calcium and a fall in blood levels of PTH[442]. Sometimes, however, normalization of phosphataemia is insufficient to adequately control secondary hyperparathyroidism because of persistent low levels of plasma calcium and supplements of calcium therefore become necessary.

Because of impaired intestinal absorption, calcium intake in chronic uraemia should range between 1 and 1.5 g/day. However, dietary intake is often insufficient, since the diets of uraemic patients are usually low in dairy products. In these circumstances, dietary calcium may be supplemented with calcium salts, such as calcium gluconate (containing 8% elemental calcium), calcium lactate (12% elemental calcium) or calcium carbonate (40% elemental calcium), up to a total daily intake of 1–1.5 g elemental calcium. As mentioned, calcium carbonate is also phosphate binding and calcium chloride should be avoided because of its acidifying properties[74]. In patients with advanced CRF and coexistent osteomalacia and elevated alkaline phosphatase, calcium intake may be slowly increased up to 4 g/day of elemental calcium, but this should only be done after normalization of plasma phosphate[74].

Treatment with vitamin D

Uraemic patients with osteomalacia, and children with renal rickets, may respond to small doses of vitamin D, such as 0.10–0.45 mg of vitamin D_2 daily[57]. The vitamin D requirement in normal men is 0.0025–0.01 mg daily[443,444]. According to Massry and Coburn[74], however, the starting dose of vitamin D_2 (or D_3) in uraemic patients should be 0.625–1.25 mg/day. Generalized bone pain and muscle weakness may disappear with the progressive rise in plasma calcium and fall in plasma alkaline phosphatase. If clinical, biochemical and radiological improvement is not evident after 6–12 weeks of treatment, the dosage of vitamin D may be increased, but only gradually and by no more than 1.25 mg/day every 4–8 weeks[50,74]. It has been reported that doses as high as 5 mg/day are sometimes necessary for beneficial effects on bone lesions in chronic uraemia[445].

Calcium supplements may be given as calcium salts, but not in milk, since milk raises the plasma phosphate, predisposing to soft tissue calcification. Plasma concentration of calcium and phosphate must be monitored at least once a week during treatment in order to prevent hypercalcaemia and hyperphosphataemia.

Patients resistant to vitamin D_2 (or D_3) at doses in the range 1.25–2.50 mg/day may respond beneficially to dihydrotachysterol (AT10*)[446] at doses[74] of 125–250 µg/day, which may then be increased[447] up to 375 µg/day.

To be active, dihydrotachysterol requires hepatic hydroxylation in position 25. More recently, 25-hydroxydihydrotachysterol has been synthesized and has shown[50,62] an affinity for intestinal and bone receptor sites greater than that of vitamin D or AT10, and equal to that of 1,25-$(OH)_2D_3$. 1,25-$(OH)_2D_3$ has proved quite successful in improving bone mass and calcium absorption and in decreasing circulating PTH and alkaline phosphatase at doses of 0.25–2.5 µg/day in limited long-term therapeutic trials in uraemic patients with vitamin D-resistant renal osteodystrophy[188,448–450]. Promising preliminary results have also been obtained with 5,6-trans-25-OHD₃. Similarly, the most recent synthetic analogue of vitamin D_3, which is 1-α-hydroxycholecalciferol (1-α-OHD₃), has been shown to be as successful as 1,25-$(OH)_2D_3$ in treating vitamin D-resistant renal osteodystrophy[451–453]. 1-α-OHD₃ may be used in daily doses of 1–2 µg for long periods and 9–10 weeks of treatment results in progressive improvement in enteric absorption

---

* AT10 is a mixture of irradiation products of ergosterol containing dihydrotachysterol as the primary active form[74].

of calcium and in skeletal mineral content[50]. While hydroxylation in position 25 seems to be necessary for activity, its biological effect has been demonstrated in anephric patients[453].

Fournier et al.[454] have recently shown that, in end-stage renal disease, large doses of 25-OHD$_3$ (50–100 µg/day) are more effective in bone mineralization than 'physiological' doses (1–2 µg/day) of 1-α-OHD$_3$, despite finding a smaller increase in PCa × PPO$_4$ product. This suggests that 25-OHD$_3$ may be a better vitamin D metabolite for treating renal osteomalacia. However, a negative correlation has been observed between histological changes in the mineralization in bone biopsies and changes in PCa × PPO$_4$ product and this suggests a direct action of 25-OHD$_3$ on bone. The decrease in the PCa × PPO$_4$ product can be accounted for by the deposition of calcium and phosphate in bone. Similar exciting effects of 25-OHD$_3$ in treating uraemic bone disease have been also reported by others[455,456]. The more rapid reversal of hypercalcaemia induced by 1-α-OHD$_3$, however, makes it less hazardous than 25-OHD$_3$ in treating renal osteodystrophy[454].

Concentration of plasma calcium and alkaline phosphatase should be monitored during treatment with vitamin D. Excess vitamin D will cause hypercalcaemia, whereas insufficient dosages will maintain high levels of alkaline phosphatase.

Other vitamins

In uraemic patients, plasma concentrations of vitamin C and pyridoxine are low, especially when on low-protein diets. Since these vitamins are important cofactors in the formation of the collagen molecule and its maturation[457,458], supplements of them should be given[62]. Multivitamin preparations containing vitamin A should be avoided, since vitamin A stimulates the resorption of bone and cartilage[459–461], possibly through increased secretion of PTH[462]. Furthermore, plasma concentration of this vitamin is already elevated in chronic uraemia[62].

Parathyroidectomy

Secondary hyperparathyroidism may not be controlled by low phosphorus intake, nor by supplements of calcium salts and/or administration of vitamin D. In these cases, soft tissue calcification, pruritus, severe renal osteodystrophy and/or persistent excessive secretion of PTH despite normalization of plasma calcium and phosphate will be indications for subtotal parathyroidectomy[62,75]. Some authors prefer total parathyroidectomy to prevent future growth of the remaining parathyroid tissue and need for another operation. The beneficial effect of surgical intervention is usually striking: pruritus may disappear in 1 week[73,95,97–99], soft tissue calcification will be greatly reduced[62] and mineralization of skeletal defects may often occur[62,73]. The number of chronic uraemic patients undergoing para-thyroidectomy[99] varies from 2 to 20%.

Treatment of itching

Itching is one of the most frequent complaints of patients with advanced chronic renal failure. Lowering the plasma calcium × plasma phosphorus product is sometimes helpful in treating it. It has also been reported that parathyroidectomy is frequently followed by dramatic relief of itch-ing[73,95,97–99], but this operation is usually undertaken only when other manifestations of severe hyperparathyroidism are present[95,99].

Symptomatic treatment is frequently necessary. Patients should be advised to avoid those factors that are known to exacerbate pruritus, such as overheating (heavy physical exercise and hot baths should be avoided), rubbing or scratching, clothes which are made of nylon or wool or are tightly fitting[97]. Topical emollients, such as greasy creams or ointments, applied just after a bath may be helpful in reducing dryness of the skin which is so frequently observed in uraemic patients and is known to exacerbate pruritus. Menthol and phenol applied locally may be useful, but alcohol, which causes dryness, and topical corticosteroid creams or ointments, which induce skin atrophy, bruising and bacterial superinfection, are contra-indicated[97]. Oral antihistamines and tranquillizers may be of some temporary help but they cause drowsiness. Ultraviolet phototherapy (twice weekly for 4 weeks) has been shown by Gilchrest[97] to be particularly effective and safe in the management of uraemic pruritus. Patients treated this way may remain free of itching for many months and may be treated successfully again when pruritus recurs.

Treatment of hyperkalaemia

In chronic uraemia, serum potassium is stabilized within, or slightly above, the upper limit of normal (i.e. 5–5.5 mmol/l). This level of serum potassium does not require any treatment. Sometimes, however, hypoaldosteronism may complicate CRF leading to hyperkalaemia[109]. In these cases, serum potassium concentration may be normalized following mineralocorticoid hormone administration[463]. Similarly, hyperkalaemia may follow long-term treatment with spironolactone; serum potassium normalizes as soon as the drug is withdrawn.

Excessive potassium intake with food (meat, fruits, fruit juices, green vegetables, etc.) may result in very high levels of serum potassium. When chronic hyperkalaemia occurs in uraemic patients, dietary restriction of potassium becomes necessary, since potassium (as well as hydrogen ions, sulphate and phosphate) derives mainly from exogenous proteins. A low-protein diet is useful for treating mild (less than 6 mmol/l) persistent hyperkalaemia, as well as metabolic acidosis and hyperphosphataemia. If dietary restriction of potassium is not sufficient to lower serum potassium to 5 mmol/l, oral administration of potassium exchange resins, in addition to a low-protein diet, is required. It should be remembered that hyperkalaemia may be secondary to chronic metabolic acidosis. In these cases, it is readily improved by correction of the acidosis with alkali.

Severe hyperkalaemia may occur in chronic uraemic patients because of hypercatabolic states or during exacerbations of renal failure (e.g. following extracellular volume depletion). Emergency treatment may be necessary and this includes:

(a) Slow intravenous infusion of calcium salts (1–2 ml/min of 10% calcium gluconate).

(b) Intravenous infusion of sodium bicarbonate (calcium salts *cannot* be added to the solution of sodium bicarbonate) or sodium lactate (calcium salts *can* be added to the solution of sodium lactate) even if acidosis is not present.

(c) Intravenous infusion of glucose (e.g. 500 ml of a 10% solution). Glucose will reduce serum potassium in 15–20 min (K^+ will move into the cells with glucose) and this effect will last 2–4 h. Insulin is not usually necessary but, if used, it should be limited to a very small amount to avoid late hypoglycaemia (e.g. five units of regular insulin subcutaneously or in the infusion).

(d) Administration of potassium exchange resins (such as sodium polystyrene sulphonate or Kayexalate) orally or by enema. Kayexalate may be given orally, in doses of 20 g, three or four times daily, together with 20 ml of 70% sorbitol with each dose of resin to prevent faecal impaction. Alternatively, 50 g of resin in 50 ml of 70% sorbitol and 100 ml of tap water may be given as a retention enema. Beneficial effects will be evident ½–1 h after an enema and 1–2 h after oral administration.

(e) Dialysis: whenever possible haemodialysis should be used as it lowers serum potassium in 30 min. If not available, peritoneal dialysis will suffice[464]. It should be stressed, however, that dialysis must be associated with the other emergency treatments (i.e. items (a), (b) and (c)).

Treatment of metabolic acidosis

Mild metabolic acidosis is a constant feature of advanced CRF and frequently requires no treatment. It is a stable acidosis with a plasma bicarbonate concentration of approximately 20 mmol/l. This reduction in bicarbonate concentration makes uraemic patients particularly prone to pH changes. Should acidosis progress and the arterial pH fall lower than 7.35, or plasma bicarbonate fall to less than 20 mmol/l, treatment is essential. It may be based on restriction of H^+ generation from metabolism by using a low-protein diet* together with oral alkali, such as sodium bicarbonate. The amount of sodium bicarbonate to be used as a daily oral supplement is decided in an empirical manner on the basis of the response of arterial pH and plasma bicarbonate. We usually start with 2 g/day and increase the dose appropriately. Five g/day are usually sufficient for the correction of mild acidosis, although sometimes 8–9 g/day are necessary. If sodium restriction is necessary, sodium bicarbonate may be used to partly or completely replace dietary salt. Some patients may dislike the gas formation that follows ingestion of bicarbonate as it causes abdominal bloating and belching. They may prefer sodium citrate, but one mole of citrate, when completely oxidized, yields three moles of bicarbonate. Calcium carbonate (6–10 g/day) may also be used for alkalinization in hypocalcaemic patients, provided plasma phosphate is not too high. It is particularly useful in those patients requiring sodium restriction because of heart failure or severe hypertension.

Severe metabolic acidosis (e.g. pH of 7.1 and $[HCO_3^-]_P$ less than 10 mmol/l) requires intravenous infusion of sodium bicarbonate. The amount of bicarbonate to be infused may be roughly estimated from the body weight of the patient and his initial plasma bicarbonate concentration, assuming that 50% of body weight is total body water and that this approximates to the 'bicarbonate space'[129]. Thus, if patient's weight is 66 kg, total body water will be 33 l (66 × 0.5). If plasma $[HCO_3^-]$ is 16 mmol/l and we wish to bring it to 26 mmol/l, it is necessary to infuse 10 mmol of HCO_3^- for each litre of total body water, i.e. 330 mmol. This may be accomplished by i.v. infusion of 330 mmol of sodium bicarbonate in the form of isotonic solution (1/6 mol/l or 1.4 g/100 ml). Since $NaHCO_3$ 1/6 mol/l (1.4 g/100 ml) solution contains 167 mmol/l of HCO_3^-, the i.v. infusion of 2 l (i.e. 334 mmol of HCO_3^-) is sufficient to normalize the plasma bicarbonate concentration of the patient. A slow correction of the acidosis is, however, preferable. We suggest the i.v. infusion of 500 ml of $NaHCO_3$ 1/6 mol/l (83.5 mmol of HCO_3^-) daily for 4 days. The expected rise in plasma bicarbonate concentration is 2.5 mmol/day, and this correction occurs 2–4 h after finishing the i.v. infusion when an equilibrium state has been reached and after partitioning of buffering between intracellular and extracellular spaces has occurred[129]. Obviously, arterial pH, P_{CO_2} and bicarbonate concentration must be closely monitored during replacement therapy. Garella et al.[465] have shown that the bicarbonate requirement for correcting extreme metabolic acidosis is much greater than the amount calculated, since the apparent 'bicarbonate space' in this situation is as great as 200% of body weight.

Isotonic sodium lactate ($NaC_3H_5O_3$ 1/6 mol/l solution is a 1.87 g/100 ml solution with 167 mmol of lactate ion) may replace the isotonic sodium bicarbonate ($NaHCO_3$ 1/6 mol/l solution is a 1.4 g/100 ml solution with

---

*Every 10 g of protein[110] provides 7 mmol of H^+.

167 mmol of bicarbonate ion), since lactate ions are metabolized by the liver to bicarbonate. 167 mmol of lactate is converted by the liver to 167 mmol of bicarbonate. Sodium lactate, however, cannot be used in patients with liver disease because of difficulties in the conversion of lactate to bicarbonate. Similarly, sodium lactate should not be used in lactic acidosis as there is already an excess of lactate ion to be metabolized[466].

Rapid correction of severe metabolic acidosis must always be avoided. The equilibration of bicarbonate concentration between blood and cerebro-spinal fluid is slow, so that a rapid rise in plasma bicarbonate is not necessarily associated with a simultaneous rise in brain bicarbonate. The increase in blood pH, however, is responsible for a reduction in ventilation and consequent rise in blood P_{CO_2}. Since CO_2 is readily diffusible, the higher blood P_{CO_2} is quickly transmitted to the cerebrospinal fluid and brain where the increased P_{CO_2}, in the presence of a continuing low bicarbonate concentration, will result in a further drop in the already low pH[467]. This sharp fall in the pH of the cerebrospinal fluid may cause nausea, vomiting, giddiness and disturbances of consciousness[22].

In some patients, it is difficult to bring the blood level of bicarbonate to normal because they have type II renal tubular acidosis. This is usually detectable when plasma bicarbonate concentration is raised to within the normal range[147].

As previously mentioned, changes in acid–base balance may modify the serum concentration of potassium by a redistribution of K^+ between intra- and extracellular fluid. Thus metabolic acidosis will increase serum potass-ium concentration by 0.6 mmol/l for every 0.1 unit change in arterial pH[113,116]. This phenomenon should be remembered when correcting meta-bolic acidosis, for a patient with normal serum concentration of potassium and severe metabolic acidosis has a 'potassium deficiency' and will experi-ence dangerous hypokalaemia when the metabolic acidosis is corrected unless potassium supplements are given.

Correction of metabolic acidosis in chronic uraemia may precipitate tetany and even seizures. Many uraemic patients have hypocalcaemia, and the metabolic acidosis protects them against tetany from hypocalcaemia. Once the acidosis is corrected, this protection is lost. Oral administration of several grams of calcium gluconate or intravenous infusion of at least 10 ml of a 10% solution of calcium gluconate prior to alkali therapy may prevent this complication.

It is a common opinion that the mild metabolic acidosis seen in chronic uraemia should not be corrected and that it is not necessary to raise the plasma level of bicarbonate above 20 mmol/l. If the dangerous effect of acidosis on bones is confirmed as an important factor in the development of uraemic osteodystrophy, we believe that this view should be reconsidered and abnormalities of acid–base balance completely corrected by constant oral administration of bicarbonate supplements.

Treatment of anaemia in CRF

The anaemia of CRF is usually asymptomatic, presumably because of the slow adaptation of the patients.

Transport of oxygen to peripheral tissues normally depends on four factors[468]:

(1) Pulmonary gas exchange,
(2) Cardiac output,
(3) Haemoglobin concentration, and
(4) Affinity of the haemoglobin for oxygen.

When haemoglobin concentration falls in CRF, compensatory adjustments may occur in cardiac output and the affinity of the haemoglobin for oxygen but not in pulmonary gas exchange[187]. Cardiac output presumably increases because of peripheral vasodilatation[469,470]. The major compensatory adjustment, however, is the decrease in haemoglobin affinity for oxygen which allows increased oxygen release to peripheral tissues. It results from metabolic acidosis[471] and from hyperphosphataemia[472] through an increase in intracellular concentration of 2,3-diphosphoglycerate (2,3-DPG)* and ATP.

Anaemia in CRF should not be treated until it becomes symptomatic. Administration of erythropoietin may be the ideal form of therapy, but erythropoietin is not yet available for therapy. Oral or parenteral iron is useless and may even be dangerous (it may cause haemosiderosis) unless depletion of iron stores has been demonstrated. The determination of serum iron concentration or total iron-binding capacity[227] is of little help in this respect. Depletion of iron is best demonstrated by staining bone marrow smears for iron or by evaluating the serum level of ferritin, as the latter seems to be an accurate index of iron stores[473].

Attempts have been made to stimulate the endogenous production of erythropoietin in uraemic patients. Cobalt and androgens are both efficient in this respect. Cobalt stimulates the renal production of erythropoietin by causing cellular hypoxia[474,475], but the administration of cobalt chloride may cause nausea, vomiting and thyroid enlargement, and this makes cobalt unsuitable for treating uraemic anaemia[228].

Oral of parenteral androgens have two effects:

(a) They stimulate endogenous production of erythropoietin, both by the kidneys[476] and at extrarenal sites[187,477,478];
(b) They have a direct stimulating effect on bone marrow stem cells[228].

Unfortunately, androgens may cause hypertriglyceridaemia[479,480], fluid retention, growth retardation, hepatic injury, hirsutism and masculinization

---

*Unfortunately the intracellular production of 2,3-DPG that is increased by hyperphosphataemia is instead impaired by acidosis[228].

in women and priapism in men[187,228]. Their use should be restricted to essential cases for short periods.

When uraemic anaemia becomes symptomatic, transfusion of whole blood or packed erythrocytes becomes necessary. The possibility of transmitting hepatitis by blood transfusion remains an unsolved problem, although careful screening minimizes the risks. Fortunately, recent studies have shown that transfusion therapy does not jeopardize a future transplant. Indeed, it may be beneficial[481-488].

Other conservative therapeutic regimens

Oral sorbents

Oral sorbents have been used in recent years for conservative treatment of chronic uraemia. Polyaldehydes in the form of oxystarch or oxycellulose have been proposed by Giordano and his co-workers for adsorbing urea and ammonia in the gastrointestinal tract of uraemic patients[489-491]. By using 40 g/day of wet oxystarch by mouth, 1.5 g of nitrogen have been removed[490] in 24 h; the administration of 100 g/day of moistened oxycellulose resulted[491] in the removal of more than 4 g of nitrogen in 24 h.

More recently, Yatzidis and co-workers[492,493] have proposed the use of a new sorbent, locust bean gum, which is a non-digested polymer of mannose derived from the seeds of the *Ceratonia siliqua* tree (carob). The administration of 25 g/day of locust bean gum in hypertensive uraemic patients resulted in the normalization of blood pressure within 3 weeks of treatment and in a significant drop in serum urea, creatinine and phosphorus[493]. Further studies with these substances are necessary.

Soil bacterial enzymes

The management of chronic uraemia by bacterial enzymes, proposed by Setälä[494,495], is very interesting.

The rationale of this therapeutic method is the utilization of non-protein-nitrogen waste products in the gastrointestinal tract of the uraemic patients by using specifically adapted lyophilized enzymes obtained from selected non-pathogenic soil micro-organisms. The patient swallows enterosoluble capsules containing these enzymes which are pre-adapted to decompose urea, creatinine, uric acid, guanidino butyric acid, guanidino succinic acid and even the so-called 'middle molecules'. Other substances, such as ammonia, potassium, phosphorus and presumably vasoconstrictive peptides, are also used by these enzymes.

For removal of water, Setälä suggests non-toxic water-adsorbing agents, such as sodium alginate. These can be safely administered by mouth but should be packed in enterocoated gelatin capsules[495]. Clinical studies have shown that even renoparenchymal hypertension is normalized by this treat-ment[494], but more extensive trials are necessary before accepting this thera-peutic regimen as standard management of chronic uraemia.

USE OF DRUGS IN PATIENTS WITH CHRONIC RENAL FAILURE

The excretory function of the kidneys is not limited to elimination of waste products and excess salt and water, but it extends to the excretion of a large number of common drugs. Some of these drugs are excreted entirely by the kidneys (group A), others only partially by the renal route (group B), a third group are completely eliminated by non-renal routes (group C). Obviously, for drugs that are eliminated by non-renal routes, any impairment of renal function does not effect their elimination (Figure 29). For all other drugs, the excretion is reduced in proportion to the fall in renal function but more steeply for drugs that are excreted solely by the kidneys (Figure 29). When these drugs are given in the normal dosage schedule to patients with CRF, the reduction in renal excretion may lead to toxic levels in the blood which may further deteriorate renal function and/or cause damage to other organs. When renal function is impaired, adequately adjusted dosage schedules are needed to ensure blood levels that are sufficient for the therapeutic effect without toxic accumulation. This is obtained either by reducing the dose administered to uraemic patients or by giving the usual dose but less often, or both. This adjustment in the dosage schedule is based on the removal rate of each drug from the body. The usual means of expressing this is the 'halflife' (or 'halftime' or $t_{1/2}$). It may be defined as the time required for the blood concentration of the drug to decrease to one-half its initial value[496]. During each $t_{1/2}$, the blood concentration will decline by one half, so that after two halflives blood concentration will be 25%, after three halflives 12.5%, after four halflives 6.25% and so on. This means that 97% of the drug is eliminated by five halflives[497,498].

For drugs that are excreted wholly or largely unchanged by the kidneys, the halflife is directly proportional to the volume of distribution of the drug and inversely proportional to its renal clearance. This accounts for differ-ences in $t_{1/2}$ between drugs when renal function is normal. A drug with a large volume of distribution and low renal clearance has a long halflife while a drug with a small volume of distribution and high renal clearance has a short halflife. It also explains the increase in $t_{1/2}$ when renal function is impaired[496].

For many drugs, dosage schedules for different degrees of renal impair-ment have been described and these will be listed later in this chapter. For any other drug, the change in dose or dose interval may be calculated for each uraemic patient in relation to the creatinine clearance using the follow-ing formulae suggested by Anderson et al.[497]:

$$\text{Dose for uraemic patient} = \text{Normal dose} \times \frac{f(K_f - 1) + 1}{1}$$

$$\text{Dose interval for uraemic patient} = \text{Normal dose interval} \times \frac{1}{f(K_f - 1) + 1}$$

where f is the fraction of the drug normally excreted in the urine and K_f is the ratio of the patient's creatinine clearance/normal creatinine clearance.

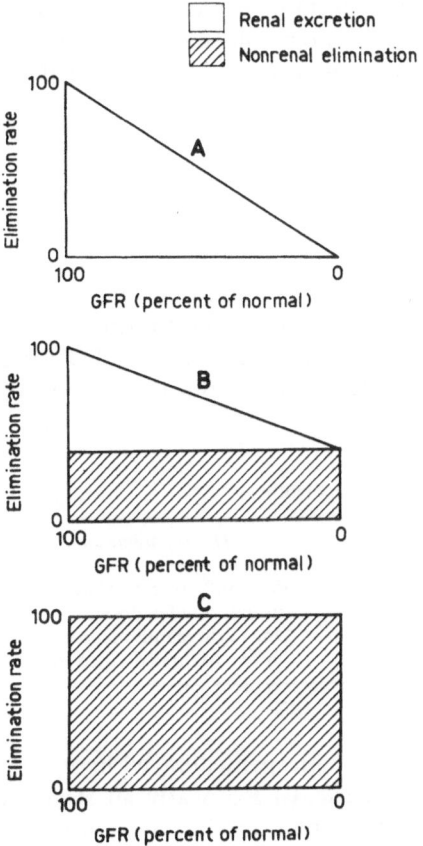

Figure 29 Relationship between elimination rate and GFR for drugs eliminated only by the kidneys (A), by both renal and non-renal routes (B) and entirely by non-renal routes (C)

Antibacterial drugs

Penicillins

Penicillin G. Penicillin G is highly effective against many species of Gram-positive and Gram-negative cocci (strains of *Staphylococcus aureus*,

Pneumococcus, Streptococcus, Gonococcus and *Meningococcus*), strains of *Corynebacterium diphtheriae*, the *Treponema pallidum* and many species of Gram-negative bacilli[499]. It is administered by intramuscular or intravenous injections. When renal function is normal, as much as 60–90% of the injected dose is rapidly excreted by the kidneys, mainly by proximal tubular secretion, whilst a small amount is eliminated in bile[497,499]. The normal halflife of penicillin G is 30–40 min[500]. In anuric patients, the halflife is 7–20 h, and, in anuric patients with hepatic dysfunction[497], it is prolonged to 16–31 h. Possible toxic effects of penicillin G include allergic reactions, nephropathy in the form of glomerulonephritis or interstitial nephritis[501,502], and neuroencephalopathy with hyperirritability, hallucinations, seizures, myoclonic jerks and coma[498,503,504].

Penicillin G is available as a sodium salt or potassium salt. Since each million units of penicillin G contains 1.7 mmol of sodium or potassium[497,498], the use of massive doses in CRF may cause excessive sodium load or hyperkalaemia[504].

Penicillin G may be used in normal doses[504] (e.g. one million units every 6 h) in uraemic patients with creatinine clearance greater than 10 ml/min. With creatinine clearance lower than this, the dosage should not exceed one to three million units per day in two to three divided doses[497,505]. No further modification of dosage is necessary during haemodialysis or peritoneal dialysis[504].

Schedule 1   Penicillin G

GFR	Dose (parenteral use)
> 10 ml/min	Four million units or more daily (in four divided doses)
< 10 ml/min	One to three million units daily (in two to three divided doses)

Methicillin. This semisynthetic penicillin, without any effect on Gram-negative bacteria, is bactericidal for nearly all strains of *Staphylococcus aureus*, especially for penicillinase-producing strains[499]. It may be administered only by the parenteral route. More than 65% of a parenteral dose is eliminated in the urine within 4 h by both glomerular filtration and tubular secretion[506]; part of it is also metabolized by the liver.

The halflife of methicillin is 0.5–1 h when renal function is normal and becomes 4 or more hours when creatinine clearance is less than 10 ml/min[496–498]. Toxic effects of methicillin are similar to those of penicillin, including interstitial nephritis[497]. The dosage of methicillin may remain normal until a creatinine clearance of 10 ml/min; the following schedules have been suggested[497]:

Schedule 2 Methicillin

GFR	Dose (parenteral use)
>10 ml/min	1–2 g every 4 h
<10 ml/min	1–2 g every 8–12 h
RDT	1–2 g every 8–12 h

In cases of hepatic dysfunction in CRF with GFR less than 10 ml/min, a further reduction in dosage is necessary[497].

Ampicillin. Ampicillin is a broad-spectrum semisynthetic penicillin, effective on both Gram-positive and Gram-negative bacteria. It is well absorbed after oral administration and is available both for oral and parenteral use. When renal function is normal, 50–90% of the drug is excreted in the urine[507,508], the remainder being metabolized/excreted by the liver[497]. The normal halflife is 1–2 h and becomes 6–20 h in anuric patients[496–498,507,508].

Toxic effects of ampicillin are similar to those of penicillin G, including generalized seizures[497]. Interstitial nephritis has been described after ampicillin therapy[509] with deterioration of renal function[497]. Febrile and skin reactions to ampicillin seem more frequent in patients with CRF unless the dosage is reduced in proportion to the fall in renal function[496].

With GFR greater than 75 ml/min, no modification in standard dose (i.e. 50 mg kg^{-1} day^{-1}) is necessary, but, with values less than 75 ml/min, dosage of the drug should be reduced as follows[497]:

Schedule 3 Ampicillin

GFR	Dose (oral and parenteral use)
>75 ml/min	50 mg kg^{-1} day^{-1}
50–75 ml/min	30–40 mg kg^{-1} day^{-1}
10–50 ml/min	10–20 mg kg^{-1} day^{-1}
<10 ml/min	5–10 mg kg^{-1} day^{-1}

Significant amounts of the drug (30% of more) are removed with haemodialysis but not with peritoneal dialysis[496–498].

Carbenicillin. Carbenicillin is a broad-spectrum semisynthetic antibiotic, active against Gram-positive and Gram-negative bacteria, including *Pseudomonas aeruginosa*. Its renal excretion is about 60% when renal function is normal; the halflife is 1 h and increases to 16 h in anephric patients[496,498].

Each gram of carbenicillin contains 4.7 mmol of sodium[497]; this must be considered when sodium restriction is needed. High doses of carbenicillin may cause metabolic acidosis[510].

The following dosage schedules have been proposed in relation to renal function[497,504]:

Schedule 4   Carbenicillin i.v.

GFR	Dose (intravenous use)
> 30 ml/min	4–5 g every 4 h
10–30 ml/min	2–4 g every 6–12 h
< 10 ml/min	2 g every 12 h
< 10 ml/min + hepatic dysfunction	2 g every 24 h
RDT	2 g every 24 h + 2 g after each dialysis section
Peritoneal dialysis	2 g every 6–12 h

An oral carbenicillin preparation is available and is now commonly used for treating urinary tract infections. Effective urinary concentration[511,512] can only be obtained with creatinine clearance greater than 20–30 ml/min.

Schedule 5   Carbenicillin oral

GFR	Dose (oral use)
> 20–30 ml/min	2–4 g/day
< 20–30 ml/min	—

Oxacillin, cloxacillin, flucloxacillin, dicloxacillin and nafcillin. These semi-synthetic penicillins are very active against *Staphylococcus aureus* and other Gram-positive cocci. Their renal elimination is about 40–45% for oxacillin and nafcillin and 60–70% for cloxacillin and dicloxacillin. Since their half-life (normally $\frac{1}{2}$ h) is only slightly increased in anephric patients, the non-renal elimination (through the liver) must be increased with the fall of renal function[496,497].

Toxic effects of these antibiotics are similar to those occurring with other penicillins[497]. Alterations in dosage are not necessary in chronic uraemia, nor in patients undergoing haemodialysis or peritoneal dialysis[496,497]. Therefore:

Schedule 6   Oxacillin, cloxacillin, flucloxacillin, dicloxacillin, nafcillin

GFR	Dose (oral or parenteral use)
120–0 ml/min	250–500 mg every 6 h (in children, 25–50 mg (kg body weight)$^{-1}$ day^{-1} in four divided doses)

Cephalosporins

These antibiotics are effective against Gram-positive and Gram-negative micro-organisms. They are highly nephrotoxic (especially cephaloridine), producing proximal tubular damage and renal failure[513–518]. Their nephrotoxicity is enhanced by simultaneous administration of furosemide[515,516,519–521] and other nephrotoxic drugs, such as gentamicin[522,523].

The renal toxicity of these antibiotics and their renal excretion (50–90%) makes it necessary to reduce their dosage with the fall in glomerular filtration rate in order to prevent further deterioration of renal function.

Cephaloridine. Cephaloridine should never be used in renal patients.

Cephalothin. Cephalothin is effective only after parenteral administration: 50–70% is excreted in the urine, while 30% is metabolized by the liver to desacetylcephalothin. Its halflife is 0.5 h when renal function is normal and is increased up to 12–20 h in end-stage renal failure[496–498]. The following dosage schedules, based on the suggestions of different authors[496,497,524], may be used in relation to the renal function:

Schedule 7 Cephalothin

GFR	Dose (parenteral use)
> 30 ml/min	15–35 mg/kg body weight every 4–6 h
5–30 ml/min	20 mg/kg body weight every 6–12 h
< 5 ml/min	20 mg (kg body weight)$^{-1}$ day^{-1}
RDT	2–4 g as loading dose, then 1 g every 12–24 h as maintenance dose (1 g should be repeated at the end of each dialysis section)
Peritoneal dialysis	1 g every 6 h

Cephalexin. Cephalexin is well absorbed when taken orally and is excreted mainly (80–100%) by the kidneys. Its halflife is 0.9–1 h when renal function is normal and is increased up to 25–30 h in end-stage renal failure[496,497]. The following schedules are suggested[497,504]:

Schedule 8 Cephalexin

GFR	Dose (oral use)
> 75 ml/min	500 mg every 6 h
50–75 ml/min	500 mg every 8 h
20–50 ml/min	500 mg every 12 h
< 20 ml/min	500 mg every 24 h
RDT	500 mg daily + 500 mg at the end of each dialysis section

Cefazolin. Cefazolin is effective only after parenteral administration: 60–90% is excreted unchanged in the urine. Its halflife is 1.9–2 h when renal function is normal and is increased up to 40–57 h in end-stage renal failure[496,497]. The following dosage schedules have been suggested[525]:

Cefoxitin

This is a new β-lactam antibiotic (a semisynthetic cephamycin, closely related to the cephalosporins), effective in the therapy of infections due to both Gram-positive and Gram-negative micro-organisms, including many that are resistant to penicillins and cephalosporins[526-528]. It is particularly useful in treating anaerobic infections[529,530]. Many strains of *Pseudomonas*, *Enterobacter cloacae* and methicillin-resistant *Staphylococci* are resistant to cefoxitin. Each gram of cefoxitin contains 2.3 mmol of sodium.

Cefoxitin is excreted in the urine in a bacteriologically active form[531]. Dosage of the drug should be reduced in proportion to the fall in renal function. Concurrent treatment with potent diuretics does not prolong the serum halflife of cefoxitin or induce nephrotoxicity[532].

Schedule 9　Cefazolin

GFR	Dose (parenteral use)
>60 ml/min	500 mg every 6 h
30–60 ml/min	500 mg as loading dose; then 250 mg every 6 h
5–30 ml/min	500 mg as loading dose; then 250 mg every 12 h
<5 ml/min	500 mg as loading dose; then 250 mg every 48 h
RDT	500 mg as loading dose; then 250 mg every 48 h + 250 mg at the end of each dialysis section

Schedule 10　Cefoxitin

GFR	Dose (parenteral use)
>50 ml/min	1–2 g every 6–8 h
30–50 ml/min	1–2 g every 8–12 h
10–30 ml/min	1–2 g every 12–24 h
5–10 ml/min	0.5–1 g every 12–24 h
<5 ml/min	0.5–1 g every 24–48 h
RDT	1–2 g after each dialysis section

Aminoglycosides

These broad-spectrum antibiotics, active against Gram-positive and Gram-negative bacteria, are effective after parenteral administration. Unfortunately, they are both highly ototoxic, causing deafness and damage to the vestibular part of the inner ear, and nephrotoxic. At a dosage of 4 mg (kg body weight)$^{-1}$ day^{-1} they cause damage of the proximal tubules and a fall in glomerular ultrafiltration in normal animals[533]. Acute neuromuscular blockade with respiratory paralysis[534] has also been described after amino-glycosides.

The nephrotoxicity of these antibiotics is enhanced by salt depletion and by the association with cephalosporins, especially cephaloridine, or furosemide. They are excreted mainly in the urine so that their halflife of about 2–3 h is increased to 60–70 h in oliguric–anuric patients[496]. It is essential to reduce the dosage of these drugs in proportion to the fall in the glomerular filtration rate. Serum creatinine should be carefully monitored during treatment with aminoglycosides.

Gentamicin, tobramicin and sisomicin. These are very useful antibiotics, especially against Gram-negative bacteria, including *Pseudomonas* and *Proteus*. However, renal function may be significantly impaired in normal subjects even by standard doses[535,536]. Further deterioration of renal function may occur in uraemic patients unless adequate adjustments in dosage are made[497,504]. The following dosage schedules are suggested for these antibiotics:

Schedule 11 Gentamicin, tobramicin, sisomicin

GFR	Dose (parenteral use)
>70 ml/min	1 mg/kg body weight every 8–12 h
50–70 ml/min	1 mg/kg body weight every 12–16 h
30–50 ml/min	1 mg/kg body weight every 24 h
10–30 ml/min	0.5 mg/kg body weight every 24 h
5–10 ml/min	0.5 mg/kg body weight every 48 h
RDT	1 mg/kg body weight after each dialysis section

For adult patients, it has been suggested that the interval in hours between normal doses (1 mg/kg body weight) can be calculated by multiplying serum creatinine mg/100 ml by eight.

Amikacin. This is an aminoglycoside, active against Gram-positive and Gram-negative bacteria. The normal dose is 7.5 mg/kg body weight. The interval in hours between normal doses can be calculated, in adult patients, by multiplying serum creatinine (mg/100 ml) by nine.

Kanamicin. This is an extremely toxic antibiotic which is only rarely used. Toxic effects include neurotoxicity (acute neuromuscular blockade), nephrotoxicity (renal impairment or acute renal failure) and non-reversible auditory damage which is related to both height and duration of drug blood levels[497,504]. Since most of this drug is excreted in the urine, the dosage should be reduced with decreased renal function. Thus, the standard dose of 7 mg/kg body weight may be given every third halflife[504,537] when the half-life is calculated as follows[504]:

$$\text{halflife (h)} = \frac{3.6 \times \text{body weight (kg)}}{\text{creatinine clearance (ml/min)}}$$

Schedule 12 Kanamicin

GFR	Dose
>70 ml/min	7 mg/kg body weight every 8–10 h
70–75 ml/min	7 mg/kg body weight every third halflife (calculated as stated above)
RDT	4.5 mg/kg body weight after each dialysis section

Streptomycin. This very toxic aminoglycoside antibiotic is commonly used for treating tuberculosis; 30–80% is excreted in the urine, so that its halflife, normally 2–3 h, is increased to 70–110 h when renal function is severely impaired[496,497]. It is potentially nephrotoxic, but its main toxic effects are vestibular toxicity and nerve deafness. The use of streptomycin in uraemic patients should be avoided, rifampicin being the drug of choice for treating tuberculosis in chronic uraemia[497,504]. If used, blood levels should be measured repeatedly. The next dose should be given only when the blood concentration[504] falls below 4 μg/ml. The following dosage schedules have been suggested as a rough guideline for adult patients with CRF[498,504]:

Schedule 13 Streptomycin

GFR	Dose (parenteral use)
>70 ml/min	1 g/day
30–50 ml/min	0.5 g/day
10–20 ml/min	0.25 g/day
<10 ml/min	0.25 g twice a week
RDT	0.25 g after each dialysis section

Colistimethate or colistin (colomycin)

Colistin is a very toxic antibiotic, effective against Gram-negative bacteria including *Pseudomonas*: 75% is excreted in the urine so that its normal half-life of 3–8 h increases to 10–20 h with the fall in renal function[496,497]. Toxic effects of colistin include renal impairment and neurological reactions (paraesthesias; acute neuromuscular blockade with respiratory paralysis)[497,504]. The following dosage schedules have been proposed[498,504]:

Schedule 14 Colistin

GFR	Dose (parenteral use)
>80 ml/min	2.5 mg/kg body weight every 12 h
40–80 ml/min	1.5 mg/kg body weight every 12 h
5–40 ml/min	1.5 mg/kg body weight every 18–36 h
Anuria	2 mg/kg body weight once only
RDT	2 mg/kg body weight every 12 h

Tetracyclines

These antibiotics have a wide range of antimicrobial activity against both Gram-positive and Gram-negative bacteria. They may be given orally but their intestinal absorption is reduced by meals and antacids. Urinary excretion ranges from 15–35% for doxycycline to 70% for oxytetracycline[497]. The halflife is normally 8–13 h for tetracycline, oxytetracycline, demethyl-chlortetracycline, methacycline and minocycline, and is significantly increased with the fall in renal function. Impaired renal function has only slight effects on the halflife of chlortetracycline (normal halflife 6 h) and none on doxycycline[497] (normal halflife 15–25 h). It has been demonstrated that, with the possible exception of doxycycline, the urinary or renal tissue concentration of tetracyclines is too low in chronic uraemia to have inhibitory effects on Gram-negative bacteria[497].

With the exception of doxycycline[538], all tetracyclines are contraindicated in CRF because of their toxic effects[496–498, 504]. These include an antianabolic effect (with the consequent increase in blood urea concentration), the aggravation of uraemic symptoms in patients with CRF and deterioration of renal function[539]. Furthermore, demethylchlortetracycline may impair the renal concentrating ability and cause reversible nephrogenic diabetes insipidus[540]. Outdated or improperly stored tetracyclines may cause a reversible Fanconi-like syndrome[541].

Doxycycline. Doxycycline is non-toxic so that it may be given in normal doses even in patients with CRF[497, 504, 538]:

Schedule 15   Doxycycline

GFR	Dose (oral or parenteral use)
120–0 ml/min and RDT	200 mg as a loading dose; then 100 mg/day as a maintenance dose

Chloramphenicol

Because of its toxic effects (particularly bone marrow depression), chloramphenicol is now used only for treating typhoid fever. It is well absorbed when taken orally, conjugated in the liver with glucuronides and excreted in urine in the inactive form. Its halflife is normally 3 h and is increased up to 7 h in renal failure[496, 497]. Because of this relatively short halflife in severe uraemia, it is not necessary to make any change in its normal dosage in CRF[504].

Schedule 16   Chloramphenicol

GFR	Dose (oral use)
120–0 ml/min and RDT	500 mg every 6 h

Lincomycin

This relatively non-toxic antibiotic, available for oral and parenteral use, is effective against some Gram-positive bacteria and some anaerobic organisms. Only 5–25% is excreted in the urine the remainder being metabolized by the liver. The halflife is normally 4–5 h and becomes 10 h in end-stage renal failure[496,497]. The following dosage schedules have been suggested[496–498,504]:

Schedule 17   Lincomycin

GFR	Dose (oral and parenteral use)
>70 ml/min	500 mg every 6–8 h
10–70 ml/min	500 mg every 12 h
<10 ml/min	500 mg every 24–36 h
RDT	250–500 mg every 12 h

Erythromycin

This relatively non-toxic antibiotic is effective against Gram-positive and some Gram-negative bacteria. Its urinary excretion is less than 15%, the remainder being metabolized and excreted by the liver. The halflife is normally 1–2 h and is increased to 4–6 h in end-stage renal failure[496,497]. Because of the relatively short halflife, even in severe uraemia, it has been stated that no changes in dosage are necessary in CRF[496–498,504]. More recently, however, several cases of reversible deafness, especially in elderly patients, have been reported in advanced uraemia following treatment with erythromycin in normal doses[542,543]. Thus, a total dosage not exceeding 1.5 g/day has been suggested for patients with end-stage renal failure, with frequent testing of hearing acuity and avoiding any association with other potentially ototoxic drugs[543].

Schedule 18   Erythromycin

GFR	Dose (oral use)
120–10 ml/min	500 mg every 6 h
<10 ml/min	500 mg every 8 h
RDT	500 mg every 8 h

Fosfomycin

This antibiotic is effective against Gram-positive and Gram-negative bacteria, including *Pseudomonas*: 90% is excreted unchanged in the urine so that a reduction in dosage is required in CRF. Each gram of the drug contains 14.5 mmol of sodium and this must be considered when sodium restriction is needed. In normal subjects, the usual dosage is 3–4 g/day, but this may be increased up to 20 g in severe infections. The following dosage schedules have been suggested in CRF[544,545]:

Schedule 19   Fosfomycin

GFR	Dose (oral and parenteral use)
>40 ml/min	1 g every 6 h
20–40 ml/min	1 g every 8 h
10–20 ml/min	1 g every 12 h
<10 ml/min	1 g every 24 h
RDT	1 g/day (after dialysis on day of haemodialysis)

Rifampicin

Rifampicin is a relatively non-toxic antibiotic. It is the drug of choice for treating tuberculosis in uraemic patients[504]. It is well absorbed after oral administration, even if taken with meals, and is mostly metabolized and excreted by the liver, only 3–30% being excreted in the urine. The halflife is 2–5 h in normal subjects and is not increased in uraemic patients[496,497]. No dosage changes are necessary in CRF until very low renal function unless concomitant hepatic dysfunction is present[497,504] and removal by dialysis is probably insignificant[496].

Schedule 20   Rifampicin

GFR	Dose (oral use)
120–10 ml/min	450–600 mg/day
<10 ml/min	300–450 mg/day
RDT	300–450 mg/day

Sulphamethoxazole–trimethoprim (co-trimoxazole = Bactrim)

This mixture of sulphonamides is available in tablets containing 400 mg of sulphamethoxazole and 80 mg of trimethoprim, the normal dose being two tablets twice daily: 60–80% is excreted in urine. Its normal halflife is 10–15 h, but this is increased to 24–30 h in advanced renal failure[496,497,504]. Toxic effects of co-trimoxazole include bone-marrow suppression with neutropenia, thrombocytopenia and aplastic anaemia, folic acid deficiency and deterioration of renal function[546]. Dosage must be reduced with the fall in renal function[496,497,504].

Schedule 21   Sulphamethoxazole–trimethoprim

GFR	Dose (oral use)
>50 ml/min	1–2 tablets × 2/day
10–50 ml/min	1 tablet × 2/day
<10 ml/min	1 tablet/day
RDT	1 tablet/day (after dialysis)

Nitrofurantoin

Nitrofurantoin is a toxic drug commonly used for treating urinary tract infections[496,497,504], but its urinary concentration is inadequate to have an antibacterial effect when creatinine clearance is less than 50 ml/min.

Toxic effects of nitrofurantoin include gastrointestinal disturbances, haemolytic anaemia, pulmonary infiltrates and peripheral neuropathy, especially in patients with renal impairment[497]. It is contraindicated in patients with renal failure.

Schedule 22   Nitrofurantoin

GFR	Dose (oral use)
> 50 ml/min	50 mg × 4/day
< 50 ml/min	—

Nalidixic acid

Nalidixic acid is commonly used for treating urinary tract infections due to Gram-negative bacteria. Its halflife is 1–2 h in normal subjects and is increased up to 20 h in advanced CRF. Significant urinary concentration of active drug may be obtained[497] until a creatinine clearance as low as 20 ml/min. Resistance of bacteria to the drug may occur during treatment. Toxic effects include phototoxic reactions in the skin of patients with CRF, hepatic toxicity, gastrointestinal and neurological disturbances[497,504].

Schedule 23   Nalidixic acid

GFR	Dose (oral use)
> 20 ml/min	500 mg × 4/day (in children: 50 mg (kg body weight)$^{-1}$ day^{-1} in four divided doses)
< 20 ml/min	—

Oxolinic acid

Oxolinic acid is a chemotherapeutic agent, used in the treatment of urinary tract infections, with a structure and antibacterial spectrum similar to those of nalidixic acid. Its effect is, however, more prolonged, since urine concentrations are adequate up to 12 h after a single dose[547]. Furthermore, some strains of bacteria that are resistant to nalidixic acid may be sensitive to oxolinic acid[548]. As with nalidixic acid, resistance of bacteria to oxolinic acid may occur during treatment[549].

Urine concentrations of oxolinic acid remain adequate with decreasing renal function until a creatinine clearance as low as 10 ml/min (serum creatinine of 10 mg/100 ml in an adult patient)[550]. Side-effects, which include insomnia and gastrointestinal symptoms, are not frequent and do not increase with depression of renal function[550, 551].

Schedule 24   Oxolinic acid

GFR	Dose (oral use)
> 10 ml/min	500–750 mg × 2/day
< 10 ml/min	—

Pipemidic acid

Pipemidic acid is used for treating urinary tract infections due to Gram-negative bacteria (including *Pseudomonas aeruginosa*). It is well absorbed after oral administration and excreted mainly in the urine in a bacteriologically active form. Significant urinary concentration of active drug is obtained[552, 553] until a creatinine clearance as low as 30 ml/min. Toxic effects may be phototoxic reactions in the skin and gastrointestinal disturbances.

Schedule 25   Pipemidic acid

GFR	Dose (oral use)
> 30 ml/min	400 mg every 12 h
< 30 ml/min	—

Other drugs

Isoniazid (isonicotinic acid hydrazide, INAH)

Isoniazid is used in the treatment of tuberculosis, usually associated with ethambutol, streptomycin or rifampicin. It is mostly metabolized by the liver with less than 25% excreted unchanged in urine. Its halflife is 1–4 h and is not increased in renal failure[496, 497]. Toxic effects include gastrointestinal symptoms, hepatic toxicity, peripheral neuropathy, optic neuritis, seizures and pyridoxine-responsive anaemia (vitamin B_6 supplements are therefore necessary)[497, 504].

Schedule 26   Isoniazid

GFR	Dose (oral use)
> 50 ml/min	100 mg × 3/day
< 50 ml/min	100 mg × 2/day
RDT	100 mg × 2/day

Ethambutol

Ethambutol is used in the treatment of tuberculosis. It is well absorbed after oral administration and excreted mostly in urine. Its halflife is 2–4 h in normal subjects and is increased to 10 h in advanced uraemia[496,497]. Toxic effects include optic neuritis with decrease in visual acuity and loss of ability to perceive the colour green. Usually, recovery occurs when the drug is withdrawn, but we have seen at least one case of irreversible blindness following long-standing treatment with high doses of ethambutol. Visual abnormalities seem to be dose-related and dosage should be reduced with the fall in renal function[497,504].

Schedule 27 Ethambutol

GFR	Dose (oral use in a single dose daily)
> 50 ml/min	25 mg (kg body weight)$^{-1}$ day^{-1}
25–50 ml/min	15–25 mg (kg body weight)$^{-1}$ day^{-1}
10–25 ml/min	7.5–15 mg (kg body weight)$^{-1}$ day^{-1}
< 10 ml/min	5 mg (kg body weight)$^{-1}$ day^{-1}
RDT	18 mg (kg body weight)$^{-1}$ day^{-1} (after dialysis on day of haemodialysis)
Peritoneal dialysis	18 mg (kg body weight)$^{-1}$ day^{-1}

It is important to test the visual acuity and the ability to perceive the colours monthly during treatment with ethambutol.

Digoxin

The halflife of digoxin is normally 30–40 h and is increased to 4–5 days in advanced CRF. Reduction in dosage is therefore necessary in CRF in order to avoid digitalis intoxication. If possible, serum digoxin levels should be measured in uraemic patients under treatment; the normal therapeutic range[504] is between 1 and 2 ng/ml.

Schedule 28 Digoxin

GFR	Dose (oral use)
< 50 ml/min	0.1–0.25 mg/day

Cyclophosphamide

Cyclophosphamide is an alkylating agent used both for its antitumour effects and its immunosuppressive properties. After oral or intravenous administration, it undergoes biotransformation in the liver into an aldehyde derivative, aldophosphamide, which is the active form of the drug: 50–60%

of the total administered dose is excreted in the urine. The normal halflife is 5–6 h and this is increased in CRF or by the administration of allopurinol[497].

Toxic effects of cyclophosphamide include gastrointestinal disturbances, hepatic toxicity, alopecia, haemorrhagic cystitis, sterility (testicular atrophy with azoospermia and ovarian destruction) and bone marrow depression with leukopenia and thrombocytopenia[5,497,554]. Because of its toxic effects, especially on bone marrow, and its excretion in the urine, cyclophosphamide should be used in lower dosage with the fall in renal function[497].

Schedule 29 Cyclophosphamide

GFR	Dose (oral or i.v. use)
> 80 ml/min	3–5 mg (kg body weight)$^{-1}$ day^{-1}
< 80 ml/min	1–3 mg (kg body weight)$^{-1}$ day^{-1}
RDT	1–2 mg (kg body weight)$^{-1}$ day^{-1} (after dialysis on day of haemodialysis)

Therapy with cyclophosphamide must be guided by keeping the total leukocyte count[5] above 3000/mm^3.

Azathioprine

Azathioprine is used as an immunosuppressive drug. It is well absorbed when taken orally and metabolized by the liver. Its metabolites are excreted in the urine, but there is also some urinary excretion of unchanged azathioprine[497]. Toxic effects include hepatic toxicity and bone marrow suppression with leukopenia and thrombocytopenia[554]. In advanced CRF, reduction in dosage is necessary to prevent severe leukopenia and/or thrombocytopenia.

Schedule 30 Azathioprine

GFR	Dose (oral use)
> 80 ml/min	2–5 mg (kg body weight)$^{-1}$ day^{-1}
80–10 ml/min	1.5–3 mg (kg body weight)$^{-1}$ day^{-1}
< 10 ml/min	1–1.5 mg (kg body weight)$^{-1}$ day^{-1}

Therapy with azathioprine must be controlled by keeping the total leukocyte count above 3000/mm^3, lymphocyte count above 500/mm^3 and platelet count above 100000/mm^3. Associated treatment with allopurinol will increase the immunosuppressive and toxic effects of azathioprine, since allopurinol decreases the degradation of the drug and a reduction of dosage of azathioprine becomes necessary[5,554].

Glucocorticosteroids

Since the halflife of glucocorticosteroids is not modified by the fall in renal function, no reduction in dosage is necessary in CRF[497].

Phenacetin

CRF may occur after prolonged ingestion of phenacetin and possibly of other analgesic compounds. It has been shown that interstitial nephritis and papillary necrosis are frequent in patients who ingest phenacetin[496]. Furthermore, aspirin (acetylsalicyclic acid) should be used with caution and only for short periods in patients with CRF[497].

Insulin and oral hypoglycaemic agents

Insulin. With the impairment of renal function, insulin requirement by diabetic patients is decreased and uraemic patients are prone to hypoglycaemia; this usually requires lower dosage of insulin.

Tolbutamide. This is the best oral hypoglycaemia agent in CRF. Its halflife is not increased with the fall in renal function and it may be used in normal dosage in uraemic patients[497].

Chlorpropamide. The long halflife (35 h) which is further increased in CRF (the drug is excreted in the urine) excludes the use of chlorpropamide in uraemic patients[496,497,504].

Phenformin. The urinary excretion of this drug (which is reduced with the fall in renal function) and the induction of lactic acidosis in patients with impaired renal function preclude its use in uraemic patients[496,497,504].

Tricyclic antidepressants

These drugs (imipramine, amitriptyline, nortriptyline, etc.) are used to treat depression. No reduction in dosage is necessary in uraemic patients[497].

Phenothiazines

These drugs (chlorpromazine, promazine, etc.), used in the treatment of psychiatric disorders, do not require reduction in dosage in uraemic patients[497].

Diazepam and other benzodiazepines

These drugs, used as sedatives, require lower dosages in CRF (especially at the beginning of treatment) in order to avoid excessive sedation.

References

1 Kluthe, R., Oeschlen, D., Quirin, H. and Jedinsky, H. J. (1971). Six years experience with a special low-protein diet. In Kluthe, R., Berlyne, G. and Burton, B. (eds.) *Uremia: International Conference on Pathogenesis, Diagnosis and Therapy*, p. 250. (Stuttgart: Georg Thieme Verlag)

2 Johnson, W. J., O'Kane, H., Woods, J. E. and Elveback, L. R. (1973). Survival of patients with end-stage renal disease. *Mayo Clin. Proc.*, **48**, 18

3 Alfrey, A. C. (1976). Chronic renal failure: manifestations and pathogenesis. In Schrier, R. W. (ed.) *Renal and Electrolyte Disorders*, pp. 319–347. (Boston: Little, Brown and Company)

4 Brunner, F. P., Brynger, H., Chantler, C., Donckerwolcke, R. A., Hathway, R. A., Jacobs, C., Selwood, N. H. and Wing, A. J. (1979). Combined report on regular dialysis and transplantation in Europe, IX, 1978. *Proc. Eur. Dial. Transplant. Assoc.*, **16**, 1

5 Andreucci, V. E. (1977). *Le Glomerulonefriti*, p. 275. (Naples, Italy: Idelson Publisher)

6 Walker, W. G. and Solez, K. (1979). Renal involvement in disorders of connective tissue. In Earley, L. E. and Gottschalk, C. W. (eds.) *Strauss and Welt's Diseases of the Kidney*. 3rd Edn., pp. 1259–1288. (Boston: Little, Brown and Company)

7 Fine, L. G., Schlondorff, D., Trizna, W., Gilbert, R. M. and Bricker, N. S. (1978). Functional profile of the isolated uremic nephron. *J. Clin. Invest.*, **61**, 1519

8 Platt, R. (1952). Structural and functional adaptations in renal failure. *Br. Med. J.*, **1**, 1313 and 1372

9 Dorhout-Mees, E. J. (1959). Role of osmotic diuresis in impairment of concentrating ability in renal disease. *Br. Med. J.*, **1**, 1156

10 Dorhout-Mees, E. J. (1959). Relation between maximal urine concentration, maximal water reabsorption capacity and mannitol clearance in patients with renal disease. *Br. Med. J.*, **1**, 1159

11 Gilbert, R. M., Weber, H., Turchin, L., Fine, L. G., Bourgoignie, J. J. and Bricker, N. S. (1976). A study of the intrarenal recycling of urea in the rat with chronic experimental pyelonephritis. *J. Clin. Invest.*, **58**, 1348

12 Kokko, J. P. and Rector, F. C. Jr. (1972). Countercurrent multiplication system without active transport in inner medulla. *Kidney Int.*, **2**, 214

13 Brickner, N. S., Klahr, S. and Lubowitz, H. (1972). The kidney in chronic renal disease. In Maxwell, M. H. and Kleeman, C. R. (eds.) *Clinical Disorders of Fluid and Electrolyte Metabolism*. 2nd Edn., pp. 697–725. (New York: McGraw-Hill)

14 Bricker, N. S., Bourgoignie, J. J. and Weber, H. (1976). The renal response to progressive nephron loss. In Brenner, B. M. and Rector, F. C. Jr. (eds.) *The Kidney*, pp. 703–736. (Philadelphia: W. B. Saunders Company)

15 Epstein, F. H. (1977). Disturbances in renal concentrating ability. In Andreoli, T. E., Grantham, J. J. and Rector, F. C. Jr. (eds.) *Disturbances in Body Fluid Osmolality*, pp. 251–265. (Bethesda: American Physiological Society)

16 Kleeman, C. R., Adams, D. A. and Maxwell, M. H. (1961). An evaluation of maximal water diuresis in chronic renal disease. I. Normal solute intake. *J. Lab. Clin. Med.*, **58**, 169

17 Andreucci, V. E. (1978). *Manual of Renal Micropuncture*, p. 514. (Naples, Italy: Idelson Publisher)

18 Bricker, N. S., Fine, L. G., Kaplan, M., Epstein, M., Bourgoignie, J. J. and Light, A. (1978). 'Magnification phenomenon' in chronic renal disease. *N. Engl. J. Med.*, **299**, 1287

19 Slatopolsky, E., Elkan, I., Weerts, C. and Bricker, N. S. (1968). Studies on the characteristics of the control system governing sodium excretion in uremic man. *J. Clin. Invest.*, **47**, 521

20 Coleman, A. J., Arias, M., Carter, N. W., Rector, F. C. Jr. and Seldin, D. W. (1966). The mechanism of salt wastage in chronic renal disease. *J. Clin. Invest.*, **45**, 1116

21 Dal Canton, A., Russo, D., Gallo, R. and Andreucci, V. E. (1981). Muzolimine: a new high-ceiling diuretic suitable for patients with advanced renal disease. *Br. Med. J.*, **282**, 595

22 de Wardener, H. E. (1973). *The Kidney. An Outline of Normal and Abnormal Structure and Function*, p. 432. (Edinburgh: Churchill Livingstone)

23 Morgan, D. B. and Thomas, T. H. (1979). Water balance and hyponatraemia. *Clin. Sci.*, **56**, 517

24 Sherwood, L. M., Mayer, G. P., Ramberg, C. F., Kronberg, D. S., Aurbach, G. D. and Potts, J. T. (1968). Regulation of parathyroid hormone secretion; proportional control by calcium. Lack of effect of phosphate. *Endocrinology*, **83**, 1043

25 Reiss, E., Canterbury, J. M., Bercovitz, M. A. and Kaplan, E. L. (1970). The role of phosphate in the secretion of parathyroid hormone in man. *J. Clin. Invest.*, **49**, 2146

26 Bricker, N. S., Slatopolsky, E., Reiss, E. and Avioli, L. V. (1969). Calcium, phosphorus and bone in renal disease and transplantation. *Arch. Intern. Med.*, **123**, 543

27 Slatopolsky, E., Caglar, S., Pennell, J. P., Taggart, D. D., Canterbury, J. M., Reiss, E. and Bricker, N. S. (1971). On the pathogenesis of hyperparathyroidism in chronic renal disease. *J. Clin. Invest.*, **50**, 492

28 Slatopolsky, E., Caglar, S., Gradowska, L., Canterbury, J., Reiss, E. and Bricker, N. S. (1972). On the prevention of secondary hyperparathyroidism in experimental chronic renal disease using 'proportional reduction' of dietary phosphorus intake. *Kidney Int.*, **2**, 147

29 Slatopolsky, E. and Bricker, N. S. (1973). The role of phosphorus restriction in the prevention of secondary hyperparathyroidism in chronic renal disease. *Kidney Int.*, **2**, 141

30 Avioli, L. V., Birge, S., Lee, S. W. and Slatopolsky, E. (1968). The metabolic fate of vitamin D_3-^{3}H in chronic renal failure. *J. Clin. Invest.*, **47**, 2239

31 Avioli, L. V., Scott, S., Lee, S. W. and De Luca, H. F. (1969). The nature of the defect in intestinal Ca absorption in chronic renal disease. *Science*, **166**, 1159

32 Coburn, J. W., Koppel, M. H., Brickman, A. S. and Massry, S. G. (1973). Study of intestinal absorption of calcium in patients with renal failure. *Kidney Int.*, **3**, 264

33 Slatopolsky, F., Hruska, K. and Rutherford, W. E. (1975). Current concepts of parathyroid hormone and vitamin D metabolism: perturbations in chronic renal disease. *Kidney Int.*, **7**, S-90

34 Reiss, E., Canterbury, J. M. and Kanter, A. (1969). Circulating parathyroid hormone concentration in chronic renal insufficiency. *Arch. Intern. Med.*, **124**, 417

35 Arnaud, C. D. (1973). Hyperparathyroidism and renal failure. *Kidney Int.*, **4**, 89

36 Arnaud, C. D., Goldsmith, R. S., Bordier, P. J. and Sizemore, G. W. (1974). Influence of immunoheterogeneity of circulating parathyroid hormone on results of radioimmunoassays of serum in man. *Am. J. Med.*, **56**, 785

37 Reiss, E. and Canterbury, J. M. (1974). Spectrum of hyperparathyroidism. *Am. J. Med.*, **56**, 794

38 Kaplan, M. A., Canterbury, J. M., Bourgoignie, J. J., Veliz, G., Gavellas, G., Reiss, E. and Bricker, N. S. (1979). Reversal of hyperparathyroidism in response to dietary phosphorus restriction in the uremic dog. *Kidney Int.*, **15**, 43

39 Rutherford, W. E., Bordier, P., Marie, P., Hruska, K., Harter, H., Greenwalt, A., Blondin, J., Haddad, J., Bricker, N. and Slatopolsky, E. (1977). Phosphate control and 25-hydroxycholecalciferol administration in preventing experimental renal osteodystrophy in the dog. *J. Clin. Invest.*, **60**, 332

40 Goldman, R. and Bassett, S. (1954). Phosphorus excretion in renal failure. *J. Clin. Invest.*, **33**, 1623

41 Slatopolsky, E., Robson, A. M., Elkan, I. and Bricker, N. S. (1968). Control of phosphate excretion in uremic man. *J. Clin. Invest.*, **47**, 1865

42 Massry, S. G., Friedler, R. M. and Coburn, J. W. (1973). Excretion of phosphate and calcium. Physiology of their renal handling and relation to clinical medicine. *Arch. Intern. Med.*, **131**, 828

43 Popovtzer, M. M., Schainuck, L. I., Massry, S. G. and Kleeman, C. R. (1970). Divalent ion excretion in chronic kidney disease. Relation to degree of renal insufficiency. *Clin. Sci.*, **38**, 297

44 Stanbury, S. W. (1971). Calcium and phosphorus metabolism in renal failure. In Strauss, M. B. and Welt, L. G. (eds.) *Diseases of the Kidney*. 2nd Edn., pp. 305–333. (Boston: Little, Brown and Company)

45 Brickman, A. S., Coburn, J. W., Rowe, P. H., Massry, S. G. and Norman, A. W. (1974). Impaired calcium absorption in uremic man: evidence for defective absorption in the proximal small intestine. *J. Lab. Clin. Med.*, **84**, 791

46 Parker, R. F., Vergne-Marini, P., Hull, A. R., Pak, C. Y. C. and Fortran, J. S. (1974). Jejunal absorption and secretion of calcium in patients with chronic renal disease on hemodialysis. *J. Clin. Invest.*, **54**, 358

47 Clarkson, E. M., McDonald, S. J. and de Wardener, H. E. (1966). The effect of a high intake of calcium carbonate in normal subjects and patients with chronic renal failure. *Clin. Sci.*, **30**, 425

48 Clarkson, E. M., Eastwood, J. B., Koutsaimanis, K. G. and de Wardener, H. E. (1973). Net intestinal absorption of calcium in patients with chronic renal failure. *Kidney Int.*, **3**, 258

49 Avioli, L. V. (1972). Intestinal absorption of calcium. *Arch. Intern. Med.*, **129**, 345

50 Avioli, L. V. (1978). Renal osteodystrophy and vitamin D. *Dial. Transplant.*, **7**, 244

51 Avioli, L. V. (1978). Controversies regarding uremia and acquired defects in vitamin D_3 metabolism. *Kidney Int.*, **13** (suppl. 8), S-36

52 Counts, S. J., Baylink, D. J., Shen, F. H., Scherrard, D. J. and Hickman, R. O. (1975). Vitamin D intoxication in an anephric child. *Ann. Intern. Med.*, **82**, 196

53 Stern, P., De Luca, H. F. and Ikekawa, N. (1975). Bone-resorbing activities of 24-hydroxy stereoisomers of 24-hydroxyvitamin D_3 and 24,25-dihydroxyvitamin D_3. *Biochem. Biophys. Res. Commun.*, **67**, 965

54 Atkins, D. (1976). A possible role of 24,25-dihydroxycholecalciferol in bone resorption. *J. Endocrinol.*, **69**, 28P

55 Lee, S. W., Russell, J. and Avioli, L. V. (1977). 25-Hydroxycholecalciferol to 1,25-dihydroxycholecalciferol: conversion impaired by systemic metabolic acidosis. *Science*, **195**, 994

56 Gray, R. W., Wilz, D. R., Calda, A. E. and Lemann, J. Jr. (1977). The importance of phosphate in regulating plasma 1,25(OH)$_2$ vitamin D levels in humans: studies in healthy subjects, in calcium-stone formers and in patients with primary hyperparathyroidism. *J. Clin. Endocrinol. Metab.*, **45**, 299

57 Lumb, G. A., Mawer, E. B. and Stanbury, S. W. (1971). The apparent vitamin D resistance of chronic renal failure. *Am. J. Med.*, **50**, 421

58 Brancaccio, D., Graziani, G., Galmozzi, C. and Ponticelli, C. (1977). 25-Hydroxyvitamin deficiency and osteomalacia in chronic renal failure. *Lancet*, **1**, 199

59 Kanis, J. A., Oliver, D., Ledingham, J. G. G. and Russell, R. G. G. (1976). Evidence that endogenous calcitonin protects against renal bone disease. *Lancet*, **2**, 1322

60 Martin, B. F. and Jacoby, F. (1949). Diffusion phenomenon complicating the histochemical reaction for alkaline phosphatase. *J. Anat.*, **83**, 351

61 Tanzer, F. S. and Navia, J. M. (1973). Calcitonin inhibition of intestinal phosphate absorption. *Nature (London)*, **242**, 221

62 Avioli, L. V. and Teitelbaum, S. L. (1979). Renal osteodystrophy. In Earley, L. E. and Gottschalk, C. W. (eds.) *Strauss and Welt's Diseases of the Kidney*. 3rd Edn., pp. 307–370. (Boston: Little, Brown and Company)

63 Haussler, M. R. and McCain, T. H. (1977). Basic and clinical concepts related to vitamin D metabolism and action. *N. Engl. J. Med.*, **297**, 974

64 Habener, J. F. and Potts, J. T. (1978). Biosynthesis of parathyroid hormone. *N. Engl. J. Med.*, **299**, 635

65 Stanbury, S. W. (1966). The treatment of renal osteodystrophy. *Ann. Intern. Med.*, **65**, 1133

66 Vosik, W. M., Anderson, C. F., Steffee, W. P., Johnson, W. J., Arnaud, C. D. and Goldsmith, R. S. (1972). Successful medical management of osteitis fibrosa due to 'tertiary' hyperparathyroidism. *Mayo Clin. Proc.*, **47**, 110

67 Buckle, R. M. (1970). Hyperparathyroidism in chronic renal failure: assessment of autonomy by plasma-parathyroid hormone response to alterations in calcium. *Lancet*, **2**, 234

68 O'Riordan, J. L. H., Page, J., Kerr, D. N. S., Walls, J., Moorhead, J., Crockett, R. E., Franz, H. and Ritz, E. (1970). Hyperparathyroidism in chronic renal failure and dialysis osteodystrophy. *Q. J. Med.*, **39**, 359

69 Eastwood, J. B., Bordier, Ph. J. and de Wardener, H. E. (1973). Some biochemical, histological, radiological and clinical features of renal osteodystrophy. *Kidney Int.*, **4**, 128

70 Stanbury, S. W. (1968). Bone disease in uremia. *Am. J. Med.*, **44**, 714

71 Stanbury, S. W., Lumb, G. A. and Mawer, E. B. (1969). Osteodystrophy developing spontaneously in the course of chronic renal failure. *Arch. Intern. Med.*, **124**, 274

72 Massry, S. G. and Coburn, J. W. (1972). Renal osteodystrophy. In Maxwell, M. H. and Kleeman, C. R. (eds.) *Clinical Disorders of Fluid and Electrolyte Metabolism*. 2nd Edn., pp. 505–539. (New York: McGraw-Hill)

73 Katz, A. I., Hampers, C. L., Wilson, R. E., Bernstein, D. S., Washman, A. and Merrill, J. P. (1968). The place of subtotal parathyroidectomy in the management of patients with chronic renal failure. *Trans. Am. Artif. Intern. Organs*, **14**, 376

74 Massry, S. G. and Coburn, J. W. (1976). Divalent ion metabolism and renal osteodystrophy. In Massry, S. G. and Sellers, A. (eds.) *Clinical Aspects of Uremia and Dialysis*. pp. 304–387. (Springfield, Ill.: C. C. Thomas)

75 Katz, A. I., Hampers, C. L. and Merrill, J. P. (1969). Secondary hyperparathyroidism and renal osteodystrophy in chronic renal failure. *Medicine*, **48**, 333

76 Haust, M. D., Landing, B. H., Holmstrand, K., Currarino, G. and Smith, B. S. (1964). Osteosclerosis of renal disease in children: comparative pathologic and radiographic studies. *Am. J. Pathol.*, **44**, 141

77 Mehls, O., Ritz, E., Krempien, B., Willich, E., Bommer, J. and Schärer, K. (1973). Roentgenological signs in the skeleton of uremic children: an analysis of the anatomical principles underlying the roentgenological changes. *Pediatr. Radiol.*, **1**, 183

78 Campos, C., Arata, R. O. and Mautalen, C. A. (1976). Parathyroid hormone and vertebral osteosclerosis in uremic patients. *Metabolism*, **25**, 495

79 Kaln, D. N., Doyle, F. H., Pennock, J. and Foster, G. V. (1970). Parathyroid hormone and experimental osteosclerosis. *Lancet*, **1**, 1363

80 Jaworski, Z. F. G., Lok, E. and Wellington, J. L. (1975). Impaired osteoclastic function and linear bone erosion rate in secondary hyperparathyroidism associated with chronic renal failure. *Clin. Orthop.*, **107**, 298

81 Parsons, V., Davies, C., Goode, C., Ogg, C. and Siddiqui, J. (1971). Aluminium in bone from patients with renal failure. *Br. Med. J.*, **4**, 73

82 Conger, J. D., Hammond, W. S., Alfrey, A. C., Contiguglia, S. R., Stanford, R. E. and Huffer, W. E. (1975). Pulmonary calcification in chronic dialysis patients. *Ann. Intern. Med.*, **83**, 330

83 Oreopoulos, D. G., Pitel, S. and Husdan, H. (1974). Contrasting effect of haemodialysis and peritoneal dialysis on the inhibition of *in vivo* calcifications by uremic serum. *Can. Med. Assoc. J.*, **110**, 43

84 Velentzas, C. and Oreopoulos, D. G. (1979). Soft tissue calcification in chronic renal failure. *Int. J. Artif. Organs*, **2**, 6

85 Berkow, J. W., Fine, B. S. and Zimmerman, L. E. (1964). Unusual ocular calcification in hyperparathyroidism. *Am. J. Ophthalmol.*, **66**, 814

86 Berlyne, C. M. and Shaw, A. G. (1967). Red eyes in renal failure. *Lancet*, **1**, 4

87 Berlyne, C. M. (1968). Microcrystalline conjunctival calcification in renal failure: a useful clinical sign. *Lancet*, **2**, 366

88 Caner, J. E. and Decker, J. L. (1964). Recurrent acute (? gouty) arthritis in chronic renal failure treated with periodic hemodialysis. *Am J. Med.*, **36**, 571

89 Continguglia, S. R., Alfrey, A. C., Miller, N. L., Runnels, D. E. and Le Geros, R. Z. (1973). Nature of soft tissue calcification in uremia. *Kidney Int.*, **4**, 229

90 Boner, G., Jacob, E. T., Perzner, S. and Jungmann, A. (1971). Diffuse calcification of lungs in a patient on maintenance hemodialysis. *Isr. J. Med. Sci.*, **7**, 1182

91 Terman, D. S., Alfrey, A. C., Hammond, W. S., Donndelinger, T., Ogden, D. A. and Holmes, J. H. (1971). Cardiac calcification in uremia. *Am. J. Med.*, **50**, 744

92 Carlström, D., Engfeldt, B., Engström, A. and Ringertz, N. (1953). Studies on the chemical composition of normal and abnormal blood vessel walls. I. Chemical nature of calcified deposits. *Lab. Invest.*, **2**, 325

93 Bernstein, D. S., Pletka, P., Hartner, R. S., Hampers, C. L. and Merrill, J. P. (1971). Effect of total parathyroidectomy and uremia on the chemical composition of bone, skin, and aorta in rats. *Isr. J. Med. Sci.*, **7**, 513

94 Arieff, A. I. and Massry, S. G. (1974). Calcium metabolism of brain in acute renal failure. *J. Clin. Invest.*, **53**, 387

95 Massry, S. G., Popovtzer, M. M., Coburn, J. W., Makoff, D. L., Maxwell, M. H. and Kleeman, C. R. (1968). Intractable pruritus as a manifestation of secondary hyperparathyroidism in uremia. *N. Engl. J. Med.*, **279**, 697

96 Massry, S. G., Coburn, J. W., Hartenbower, D. L., Shinaberger, J. H., de Palma, J. R., Chapman, E. and Kleeman, C. R. (1970). Mineral contents of the human skin in uremia: effect of secondary hyperparathyroidism and hemodialysis. *Proc. Eur. Dial. Transplant. Assoc.*, **7**, 146

97 Gilchrest, B. (1978). Uremic pruritus. Management and possible pathogenesis. *Dial. Transplant.*, **7**, 1021

98 Massry, S. G., Coburn, J. W., Hortenbower, D., Shinaberger, J. H., de Palma, G. R., Chapman, E. and Kleeman, C. R. (1971). The effect of calcemic disorders and uremia on the mineral content of skin. *Isr. J. Med. Sci.*, **7**, 514

99 Hampers, C. L., Katz, A. J., Wilson, R. E. and Merrill, J. P. (1968). Disappearance of 'uremic' itching after subtotal parathyroidectomy. *N. Engl. J. Med.*, **279**, 695

100 Walser, M., Mitch, W. E. and Collier, V. U. (1979). The effect of nutritional therapy on the course of chronic renal failure. *Clin. Nephrol.*, **11**, 66

101 Legros, R. Z., Contiguglia, S. R. and Alfrey, A. C. (1973). Pathological calcifications associated with uremia. Two types of calcium phosphate deposits. *Calc. Tiss. Res.*, **13**, 173

102 Alfrey, A. C., Solomons, C. C., Ciricilla, J. and Miller, N. L. (1976). Extraosseous calcification: evidence for abnormal pyrophosphate metabolism in uremia. *J. Clin. Invest.*, **57**, 692

103 Whittier, F. and Freeman, R. (1971). Potentiation of metastatic calcification in vitamin-D-treated rats by magnesium. *Am. J. Physiol.*, **220**, 209

104 Platt, R. (1950). Sodium and potassium excretion in chronic renal failure. *Clin. Sci.*, **9**, 367

105 van Ypersele de Strihou, C. (1977). Potassium homeostasis in renal failure. *Kidney Int.*, **11**, 496

106 Silva, P., Hayslett, J. P. and Epstein, F. H. (1973). The role of Na–K-activated adenosine triphosphatase in potassium adaptation. *J. Clin. Invest.*, **52**, 2665

107 Schon, D. A., Silva, P. and Hayslett, J. P. (1974). Mechanism of potassium excretion in renal insufficiency. *Am. J. Physiol.*, **227**, 1323

108 Schrier, R. W. and Regal, E. M. (1972). Influence of aldosterone on sodium, water and potassium metabolism in chronic renal disease. *Kidney Int.*, **1**, 156

109 Gerstein, A. R., Kleeman, C. R., Gold, E. M., Franklin, S. S., Maxwell, M. H., Gonick, H. C., Feffer, M. L. and Steninman, T. I. (1968). Aldosterone deficiency in chronic renal failure. *Nephron*, **5**, 90

110 Schoeneman, M. (1978). Dietary and pharmacologic treatment of chronic renal failure. In Edelmann, C. M. Jr. (ed.) *Pediatric Kidney Disease*, pp. 475–487. (Boston: Little, Brown and Company)

111 Hayes, C. P., McLeod, M. E., Robinson, R. R. and Stread, E. A. (1967). An extrarenal mechanism for the maintenance of potassium balance in severe chronic renal failure. *Trans. Assoc. Am. Physicians*, **80**, 207

112 Berlyne, G. M., van Laethem, L. and Ben Ari, J. (1971). Exchangeable potassium and renal potassium handling in advanced chronic renal failure in man. *Nephron*, **8**, 264

113 Scribner, B. H. and Burnell, J. M. (1956). Interpretation of the serum potassium concentration. *Metabolism*, **5**, 468

114 Bilbrey, G. L., Carter, N. W., White, M. G., Schilling, J. F. and Knochel, J. P. (1973). Potassium deficiency in chronic renal failure. *Kidney Int.*, **4**, 423

115 Patrick, J. (1977). The assessment of body potassium stores. *Kidney Int.*, **11**, 476

116 Burnell, J. M., Villamil, M. F., Nyeno, B. T. and Scribner, B. H. (1956). Effect in humans of extracellular pH change on relationship between serum potassium concentration and intracellular potassium. *J. Clin. Invest.*, **35**, 935

117 Dickerman, H. W. and Walker, W. G. (1964). Effect of cationic amino acid infusion on potassium metabolism *in vivo*. *Am. J. Physiol.*, **206**, 403

118 Hertz, P. and Richardson, J. A. (1972). Arginine-induced hyperkalemia in renal failure patients. *Arch. Intern. Med.*, **130**, 778

119 Goldfarb, S., Cox, M., Singer, I. and Goldberg, M. (1976). Acute hyperkalemia induced by hyperglycemia: hormonal mechanisms. *Ann. Intern. Med.*, **84**, 426

120 Perez, G., Siegel, L. and Schreiner, G. E. (1972). Selective hypoaldosteronism with hyperkalemia. *Ann. Intern. Med.*, **76**, 757

121 Schambelan, M., Stockigt, J. R. and Biglieri, E. G. (1972). Isolated hypoaldosteronism in adults: a renin-deficiency syndrome. *N. Engl. J. Med.*, **287**, 573

122 Weidmann, P., Reinhart, R., Maxwell, M. H., Rowe, P., Coburn, J. W. and Massry, S. G. (1973). Syndrome of hyporeninemic hypoaldosteronism and hyperkalemia in renal disease. *J. Clin. Endocrinol. Metab.*, **36**, 965

123 Weidmann, P., Maxwell, M. H., Rowe, P., Winer, R. and Massry, S. G. (1975). Role of the renin–angiotensin–aldosterone system in the regulation of plasma potassium in chronic renal disease. *Nephron*, **15**, 35

124 De Leiva, A., Christlieb, A. R., Melby, J. C., Graham, C. A., Day, R. P., Luetscher, J. A. and Zager, P. G. (1976). Big renin and biosynthetic defect of aldosterone in diabetes mellitus. *N. Engl. J. Med.*, **295**, 639

125 Luke, R. G., Allison, M. and Davidson, J. (1969). Hyperkalemia and renal tubular acidosis due to renal amyloidosis. *Ann. Intern. Med.*, **70**, 1211

126 Popovtzer, M. M., Katz, F. H., Pinggera, W. F., Robinette, J., Halgrimson, C. G. and Butkus, D. E. (1973). Hyperkalemia in salt-wasting nephropathy. *Arch. Intern. Med.*, **132**, 203

127 Maxwell, M. H. and Kleeman, C. R. (1972). *Clinical Disorders of Fluid and Electrolyte Metabolism*. 2nd Edn., p. 1164. (New York: McGraw-Hill)

128 Makoff, D. L. and de Palma, J. R. (1976). Electrolyte and acid–base abnormalities. In Massry, S. G. and Sellers, A. L. (eds.) *Clinical Aspects of Uremia and Dialysis*, pp. 284–303. (Springfield, Ill.: C. C. Thomas)

129 Makoff, D. L. (1972). Acid–base metabolism. In Maxwell, M. H. and Kleeman, C. R. (eds.) *Clinical Disorders of Fluid and Electrolyte Metabolism*. 2nd Edn., pp. 297–346. (New York: McGraw-Hill)

130 Relman, A. S., Lennon, E. J. and Lemann, J. Jr. (1961). Endogenous production of fixed acid and the measurement of the net balance of acid in normal subjects. *J. Clin. Invest.*, **40**, 1621

131 Albert, M. S. and Winters, R. W. (1966). Acid–base equilibrium of blood in normal infants. *Pediatrics*, **37**, 728

132 Kildeberg, P., Engel, K. and Winters, R. W. (1969). Balance of net acid in growing infants. *Acta Paediatr. Scand.*, **58**, 321

133 Salcedo, J. R., Jackson, M. L., Coleman, T. N., Rao, D. D. and Chan. J. M. (1976). Endogenous net acid production in infants, children and adults. *Pediatr. Res.*, **10**, 443

134 Welt, L. G. and Burnett, C. H. (1966). Acidosis and alkalosis. In Harrison, T. R. (ed.) *Principles of Internal Medicine*. 5th Edn., pp. 321–333. (New York: McGraw-Hill)

135 Swan, R. C. and Pitts, R. F. (1955). Neutralization of infused acid by nephrectomized dogs. *J. Clin. Invest.*, **34**, 205

136 Singer, R. B., Clark, J. K., Barker, E. S., Crosley, A. P. Jr. and Elkinton, R. (1955). The acute effects in man of rapid intravenous infusion of hypertonic bicarbonate solution. I. Changes in acid–base balance and distribution of the excess buffer base. *Medicine*, **34**, 51

137 Rector, F. C., Jr., Carter, N. W. and Seldin, D. W. (1965). The mechanism of bicarbonate reabsorption in the proximal and distal tubule of the kidney. *J. Clin. Invest.*, **44**, 278

138 McCance, R. A. and von Finck, M. A. (1947). Titratable acidity pH, ammonia and phosphate in urines of very young infants. *Arch. Dis. Child.*, **22**, 200

139 McCance, R. A. and Widdowson, E. M. (1960). Renal aspects of acid–base control in the newly born. *Acta Paediatr. Scand.*, **49**, 409

140 Wrong, O. and Davies, H. E. F. (1959). The excretion of acid in renal disease. *Q. J. Med.*, **28**, 259

141 Madison, L. L. and Seldin, D. W. (1955). Adaptation of ammonia-producing enzymes in the human kidney during chronic acidosis as revealed by the administration of precursor amino acids. *Clin. Res. Proc.*, **3**, 136

142 Bricker, N. S., Klahr, S. and Rieselbach, R. E. (1964). The functional adaptation of the diseased kidney. I. Glomerular filtration rate. *J. Clin. Invest.*, **43**, 1915

143 Dorhout-Mees, E. J., Machado, M., Slatopolsky, E., Klahr, S. and Bricker, N. S. (1966). The functional adaptation of the diseased kidney. III. Ammonium excretion. *J. Clin. Invest.*, **45**, 289

144 Simpson, D. P. (1971). Control of hydrogen in homeostasis and renal acidosis. *Medicine*, **50**, 503

145 Davies, H. E. F. and Wrong, O. (1957). Acidity of urine and excretion of ammonium in renal disease. *Lancet*, **2**, 625

146 Schwartz, W. B. and Polak, A. (1960). Electrolyte disorders in chronic renal disease. *J. Chronic Dis.*, **11**, 319

147 Schwartz, W. B., Hall, P. W., Hays, R. M. and Relman, A. S. (1959). On the mechanism of acidosis in chronic renal disease. *J. Clin. Invest.*, **38**, 39

148 Lubowitz, H., Purkerson, M. L., Rolf, D., Weisser, F. and Bricker, N. S. (1971). The effect of nephron loss on proximal tubular bicarbonate reabsorption in the rat. *Am. J. Physiol.*, **220**, 457

149 Espines, C. H. (1975). The influence of salt intake on the metabolic acidosis of chronic renal failure. *J. Clin. Invest.*, **56**, 286

150 Raisz, L. G. (1972). Calcium, phosphate, magnesium and trace elements. In Maxwell, M. H. and Kleeman, C. R. (eds.) *Clinical Disorders of Fluid and Electrolite Metabolism*. 2nd Edn., pp. 347–399. (New York: McGraw-Hill)

151 Muldowney, F. P., Donohue, J. F., Carroll, D. W., Powell, D. and Freaney, R. (1972). Parathyroid acidosis in uremia. *Q. J. Med.*, **41**, 321

152 Coe, F. L. (1974). Magnitude of metabolic acidosis in primary hyperparathyroidism. *Arch. Intern. Med.*, **134**, 262

153 Arruda, J. A. L., Carrasquillo, T., Cubria, A., Rademacher, D. R. and Kartzman, N. A. (1976). Bicarbonate reabsorption in chronic renal failure. *Kidney Int.*, **9**, 481

154 Goodman, A. D., Lemann, J. Jr., Lennon, E. J. and Relman, A. S. (1965). Production, excretion and net balance of fixed acid in patients with renal acidosis. *J. Clin. Invest.*, **44**, 495

155 Lemann, J. Jr., Litzow, J. R. and Lennon, E. J. (1966). The effects of chronic acid loads in normal man: further evidence for the participation of bone mineral in the defense against chronic metabolic acidosis. *J. Clin. Invest.*, **45**, 1608

156 Litzow, J. R., Lemann, J. Jr. and Lennon, E. J. (1967). The effect of treatment of acidosis on calcium balance in patients with chronic azotemic renal disease. *J. Clin. Invest.*, **46**, 280

157 Valtin, H. (1979). *Renal Dysfunction: Mechanisms Involved in Fluid and Solute Imbalance*, p. 499. (Boston: Little, Brown and Company)

158 Astrup, P., Jorgensen, K., Siggaard Anderson, O. and Engel, K. (1960). Acid–base metabolism: new approach. *Lancet*, **1**, 1035

159 Brackett, N. C. Jr., Cohen, J. and Schwartz, W. B. (1965). Carbon dioxide titration curve of normal man. *N. Engl. J. Med.*, **272**, 6

160 West, C. D. and Smith, W. C. (1956). An attempt to elucidate the cause of growth retardation in renal disease. *Am J. Dis. Child.*, **91**, 460

161 Cooke, R. E., Boyden, D. G. and Haller, E. (1960). The relationship of acidosis and growth retardation. *J. Pediatr.*, **57**, 326

162 Pellegrino, E. D. and Biltz, R. M. (1965). The composition of human bone in uremia. *Medicine*, **44**, 397

163 Kopple, J. D. (1976). Nitrogen metabolism. In Massry, S. G. and Sellers, A. L. (eds.) *Clinical Aspects of Uremia and Dialysis*. 2nd Edn., pp. 241–273. (Springfield, Ill.: C. C. Thomas)

164 Bergstrom, J. and Furst, P. (1978). Uremic toxins. In *Proceedings VII International Congress of Nephrology* (Montreal, June 18–23, 1978), pp. 669–675. (Basel: S. Karger)

165 Hewlett, A. W., Gilbert, Q. O. and Wickett, A. D. (1916). The toxic effects of urea on normal individuals. *Arch. Intern. Med.*, **18**, 636

166 Javid, M. (1958). Symposium on surgery of the head and neck: urea—new use of an old agent. *Surg. Clin. N. Am.*, **38**, 907

167 Merrill, J. P., Legrain, M. and Hoigne, R. (1953). Observations on the role of urea in uremia. *Am. J. Med.*, **14**, 519

168 Memoli, B., Calderaro, V., Terracciano, V., Caputo, A., Santoro, L., Perretti, A., Caruso, G. and Andreucci, V. E. (1980). L'emofiltrazione come alternativa all'emodialisi nel trattamento dell'uremia terminale. Risultati preliminari. *La Riforma Medica*, **95**, 535

169 Johnson, W. J., Hagge, W. W., Wagoner, R. D., Dinapoli, R. P. and Rosevear, J. W. (1972). Effects of urea loading in patients with far-advanced renal failure. *Mayo Clin. Proc.*, **47**, 21

170 Johnson, W. J., Hagge, W. W., Wagoner, R. D., Dinapoli, R. P. and Rosevear, J. W. (1975). Toxicity arising from urea. *Kidney Int.*, 7 (Suppl. 3), S-288

171 Walser, M. and Bodenlos, L. J. (1959). Urea metabolism in man. *J. Clin. Invest.*, **38**, 1617

172 Mitch, W. E., Lietman, P. S. and Walser, M. (1977). Effects of oral neomycin and kanamycin in chronic uremic patients. I. Urea metabolism. *Kidney Int.*, **11**, 116

173 Walser, M. (1974). Urea metabolism in chronic renal failure. *J. Clin. Invest.*, **53**, 1385

174 Preuss, H. G., Davis, B. B., Maher, J. F., Bise, B. W. and Schreiner, G. E. (1966). Ammonia metabolism in renal failure. *Ann. Intern. Med.*, **65**, 54

175 Sorensen, L. B. (1959). Degradation of uric acid in man. *Metabolism*, **8**, 687

176 Steele, T. H. and Rieselbach, R. E. (1967). The contribution of residual nephrons within the chronically diseased kidney to urate homeostasis in man. *Am. J. Med.*, **43**, 876

177 Steele, T. H. and Rieselbach, R. E. (1976). The renal handling of urate and other organic anions. In Brenner, B. M. and Rector, F. C. Jr. (eds.) *The Kidney*, pp. 442–476. (Philadelphia: W. B. Saunders Company)

178 Verger, D., Leroux, R. C., Ganter, P. and Richet, G. (1967). Les tophus gotteux de la médullaire rénale des urémiques chroniques: étude de 17 cas découvert au cours de 62 autopsies. *Nephron*, **4**, 356

179 Rieselbach, R. E., Bentzel, C. J., Cotlove, E., Frei, E. and Freireich, E. J. (1964). Uric acid excretion and renal function in the acute hyperuricemia of leukemia: pathogenesis and therapy of uric acid nephropathy. *Am. J. Med.*, **37**, 872

180 Massry, S. G. (1977). Is parathyroid hormone a uremic toxin? *Nephron*, **19**, 125

181 Massry, S. G. and Goldstein, D. A. (1978). Role of parathyroid hormone in uremic toxicity. *Kidney Int.*, **13** (Suppl. 8), 39

182 Massry, S. G. and Goldstein, D. A. (1979). The search for uremic toxin(s) "X". "X" = PTH. *Clin. Nephrol.*, **11**, 181

183 Bailey, G. L., Griffith, H. J. L. and Merrill, J. P. (1972). Avascular necrosis of the femoral head in patients on chronic hemodialysis. *Trans. Am. Soc. Artif. Intern. Organs*, **48**, 401

184 Chatterjee, S. N., Friedler, R. M., Berne, T. V., Oldham, S. G., Singer, F. R. and Massry, S. G. (1976). Persistent hypercalcemia after successful renal transplantation. *Nephron*, **17**, 1

185 Massry, S. G., Gordon, A., Coburn, J. W., Kaplan, L., Franklin, S. G., Maxwell, M. H. and Kleeman, C. R. (1970). Vascular calcification and peripheral necrosis in a renal transplant recipient: reversal of lesions following subtotal parathyroidectomy. *Am. J. Med.*, **49**, 416

186 Gibstein, R. H., Coburn, J. W., Adams, D. A., Lee, D. B. N., Parsa, K. P., Sellers, A., Suki, W. N. and Massry, S. G. (1976). Calciphylaxis in man: a syndrome of tissue necrosis and vascular calcification in 11 patients with chronic renal disease. *Arch. Intern. Med.*, **136**, 1273

187 Eschbach, J. W. (1976). Anemia. In Massry, S. G. and Sellers, A. L. (eds.) *Clinical Aspects of Uremia and Dialysis*. 2nd Edn., pp. 146–178. (Springfield, Ill.: C. C. Thomas)

188 Brickman, A. S., Sherrard, D. J., Jowsey, J., Singer, F. R., Baylink, D. J., Maloney, N., Massry, S. G., Norman, A. W. and Coburn, J. W. (1974). Effect of 1,25-dihydroxy-cholecalciferol on skeletal lesions and plasma parathyroid hormone in uremic osteo-distrophy. *Arch. Intern. Med.*, **134**, 883

189 Better, P. S., Shasha, S. M., Windver, J. and Chaimovitz, C. (1976). Improvement in the anemia of hemodialysis patients following parathyroidectomy. *Proc. Am. Soc. Nephrol.*, **9**, 1

190 Cantin, M. (1965). Kidney, parathyroid and lipemia. *Lab. Invest.*, **14**, 1691

191 Loew, H., Schultz, H. and Busch, G. (1975). Klinische Aspekte der Impotenz mannlicher Dauerdialysepatienten. *Med. Welt.*, **26**, 1651

192 Massry, S. G., Goldstein, D. A., Procci, W. R. and Kletsky, O. A. (1977). Impotence in patients with uremia: a possible role for parathyroid hormone. *Nephron*, **19**, 305

193 Alfrey, A. C., Mishell, J. M., Burks, J., Contiguglia, S. R., Rudolph, H., Lewin, E. and Holmes, J. H. (1972). Syndrome of dyspraxia and multifocal seizures associated with chronic hemodialysis. *Trans. Am. Soc. Artif. Intern. Organs*, **18**, 257

194 Guisado, R., Arieff, A. I. and Massry, S. G. (1975). Changes in the electroencephalogram in acute uremia. *J. Clin. Invest.*, **55**, 738

195 Goldstein, D. A. and Massry, S. G. (1978). Effects of parathyroid hormone administration and its withdrawal on brain calcium and electroencephalogram. *Miner. Elect. Metab.*, **1**, 84

196 Goldstein, D. A., Chui, L. A. and Massry, S. G. (1978). Effect of parathyroid hormone and uremia on peripheral nerve calcium and motor nerve conduction velocity. *J. Clin. Invest.*, **62**, 88

197 Avram, M. M., Iancu, M., Morrow, P., Feinfeld, D. and Huatuco, A. (1979). Uremic syndrome in man: new evidence for parathormone as a multisystem neurotoxin. *Clin. Nephrol.*, **11**, 59

198 Simenoff, M. L., Saukonen, J. J., Burke, J. F., Schaedler, R. W., Vogel, W. H., Boree, K. and Lasker, N. (1978). Importance of aliphatic amines in uremia. *Kidney Int.*, **12** (Suppl. 8), S-16

199 Wathen, R., Smith, M., Keshaviah, P., Conty, C. and Shapiro, F. (1975). Depressed *in vitro* aggregation of platelets of chronic hemodialysis patients: a role for cyclic AMP. *Trans. Am. Soc. Artif. Intern. Organs*, **21**, 320

200 Babb, A. L., Popovich, R. P. and Christopher, T. G. (1971). The genesis of the square meter-hour hypothesis. *Trans. Am. Soc. Artif. Intern. Organs*, **17**, 81

201 Bergstrom, J., Asaba, H., Furst, P., Gordon, A., Quadracci, L. and Zimmerman, L. (1976). Middle molecules in uremia. In *Proceedings VI International Congress of Nephrology* (Firenze, June 8–12, 1975), pp. 600–611. (Basel: S. Karger)

202 Bergstrom, J. and Furst, P. (1976). Uremic middle molecules. *Clin. Nephrol.*, **5**, 143

203 Migone, L., Dall'Aglio, P. and Buzio, C. (1975). Middle molecules in uremic serum, urine and dialysis fluid. *Clin. Nephrol.*, **3**, 82

204 Bergstrom, J., Furst, P., Asaba, H. and Oules, R. (1978). Dialysis and middle molecules. *Dial. Transplant.*, **7**, 344

205 Bergstrom, J., Furst, P. and Noree, L. O. (1975). Treatment of chronic uremic patients with protein-poor diet and oral supply of essential amino acids. I. Nitrogen balance studies. *Clin. Nephrol.*, **3**, 187

206 Bergstrom, J. and Furst, P. (1978). Uremic toxins. *Kidney Int.*, **13** (Suppl. 8), S-9

207 Bergstrom, J., Furst, P. and Zimmerman, L. (1979). Uremic middle molecules exist and are biologically active. *Clin. Nephrol.*, **11**, 229

208 Perkoff, G. T., Clayton, L. T. and Newton, J. D. (1958). Mechanism of impaired glucose intolerance in uremia. *Diabetes*, **7**, 375

209 Westervelt, F. B. Jr. and Shreiner, G. E. (1962). The carbohydrate intolerance of uremic patients. *Ann. Intern. Med.*, **57**, 266

210 Bierman, E. L. (1970). Abnormalities of carbohydrate and lipid metabolism in uremia. *Arch. Intern. Med.*, **126**, 790

211 Fichman, M. P. (1976). Effect of uremia and dialysis on carbohydrate and lipid metabolism. *Dial. Transplant.*, **5**, 12

212 Rabbin, R., Simon, N. M. and Steiner, S. (1970). Effect of renal disease on renal uptake and excretion of insulin in man. *N. Engl. J. Med.*, **282**, 182

213 Hampers, C. L., Lowrie, E. G., Soeldner, J. S. and Merrill, J. P. (1970). The effect of uremia upon glucose metabolism. *Arch. Intern. Med.*, **126**, 870

214 Bagdade, J. D. (1976). Hyperlipidemia. In Massry, S. G. and Sellers, A. L. (eds.) *Clinical Aspects of Uremia and Dialysis*, pp. 230–240. (Springfield, Ill.: C. C. Thomas)

215 Fredrickson, D. S., Levy, R. I. and Lees, R. S. (1967). Fat transport in lipoproteins—an integrated approach to mechanisms and disorders. *N. Engl. J. Med.*, **276**, 34

216 Albrink, M. J. and Man, E. B. (1959). Serum triglycerides in coronary artery disease. *Arch. Intern. Med.*, **103**, 4

217 Losowsky, M. and Kenward, D. H. (1968). Lipid metabolism in acute and chronic renal failure. *J. Lab. Clin. Med.*, **71**, 736

218 Carlson, L. A. and Bottinger, L. E. (1972). Ischemic heart disease in relation to fasting values of plasma triglycerides and cholesterol: Stockholm prospective study. *Lancet*, **1**, 865

219 Salel, A. F., Riggs, K., Mason, D. T., Amsterdam, E. A. and Zelis, R. (1974). The importance of type IV hyperlipoproteinemia as a predisposing factor in coronary artery disease. *Am. J. Med.*, **57**, 897

220 Bagdade, J. D., Porte, D. Jr. and Biermann, E. L. (1968). Hypertriglyceridemia: a metabolic consequence of chronic renal failure. *N. Engl. J. Med.*, **279**, 181

221 Bagdade, J. D. (1970). Uremic lipemia. *Arch. Intern. Med.*, **126**, 875

222 Bagdade, J. D. (1975). Atherosclerosis in patients undergoing maintenance hemodialysis. *Kidney Int.*, **7** (Suppl. 3), S-370

223 Erslev, A. J. (1970). Anemia of chronic renal disease. *Arch. Intern. Med.*, **126**, 774

224 Kasanen, A. and Kalliomaki, J. L. (1957). Correlation of some kidney function tests with hemoglobin in chronic nephropathies. *Acta Med. Scand.*, **158**, 213

225 Desforges, J. F. and Dawson, J. P. (1958). The anemia of renal failure. *Arch. Intern. Med.*, **101**, 326

226 Joske, R. A., McAlister, J. M. and Prankerd, T. A. J. (1956). Isotope investigation of red cell production and destruction in chronic renal disease. *Clin. Sci.*, **15**, 511

227 Loge, J. P., Lange, R. D. and Moore, C. V. (1958). Characterization of the anemia associated with chronic renal insufficiency. *Am. J. Med.*, **24**, 4

228 Erslev, A. J. and Shapiro, S. S. (1979). Hematologic aspects of renal failure. In Earley, L. E. and Gottschalk, C. W. (eds.) *Strauss and Welt's Diseases of the Kidney*. 3rd Edn., pp. 227–306. (Boston: Little, Brown and Company)

229 O'Brien, R. T. and Pearson, H. A. (1978). Hematologic disturbances in uremia. In Edelman, C. M. (ed.) *Pediatric Kidney Disease*, pp. 401–407. (Boston: Little, Brown and Company)

230 Callen, I. R. and Limarzi, L. R. (1950). Blood and bone marrow studies in renal disease. *Am. J. Clin. Pathol.*, **20**, 3

231 Magid, E. and Hilden, M. (1967). Ferrokinetics in patients suffering from chronic renal disease and anemia. *Scand. J. Haematol.*, **4**, 33

232 Erslev, A. J. (1955). Physiologic control of red cell production. *Blood*, **10**, 954

233 Jacobson, L. O., Goldwasser, E., Gumey, C. W., Fried, W. and Plzak, L. (1959). Studies on erythropoietin: the hormone regulating red cell production. *Ann. NY Acad. Sci.*, **77**, 551

234 Erslev, A. J. (1959). The effect of anemic anoxia on the cellular development of nucleated red cells. *Blood*, **14**, 386

235 Erslev, A. J. (1964). Erythropoietin *in vitro*. II. Effect on 'stem cells'. *Blood*, **24**, 331

236 Glass, J., Lavidor, L. M. and Robinson, S. H. (1975). Use of cell separation and short-time culture techniques to study erythroid cell development. *Blood*, **46**, 705

237 Erslev, A. J. (1975). Renal biogenesis of erythropoietin. *Am J. Med.*, **58**, 25

238 Fisher, J. W., Busuttil, R., Rodgers, G. M., Mujovic, V., Paulo, L., Fink, G. and George, W. J. (1975). The kidney and erythropoietin production: a review. In Nakao, K., Fisher, J. W. and Takaku, F. (eds.) *Erythropoiesis*, p. 315. (Tokyo: University Tokyo Press)

239 Hirashima, K. and Takaku, F. (1962). Experimental studies on erythropoietin. II. The relationship between juxtaglomerular cells and erythropoietin. *Blood*, **20**, 1

240 Goldfarb, B. and Tobian, L. (1963). Relationship of erythropoietin to renal juxtaglomerular cells. *Proc. Soc. Exp. Biol. Med.*, **112**, 65

241 Demopoulos, H. B., Highman, B., Altland, P. D., Gerving, M. A. and Kaley, G. (1965). Effects of high altitude on granular juxtaglomerular cells and their possible role in erythropoietin production. *Am. J. Pathol.*, **46**, 497

242 Busuttil, R. W., Roh, B. L. and Fisher, J. W. (1971). Cytological localization of erythropoietin in the human kidney using the fluorescent antibody technique. *Proc. Soc. Exp. Biol. Med.*, **137**, 327

243 Busuttil, R. W., Roh, B. L. and Fisher, J. W. (1972). Further evidence of a site of production of erythropoietin in the hypoxic dog kidney. *Acta Haematol.*, **47**, 238

244 Gordon, A. S., Cooper, G. W. and Zanjani, E. D. (1967). The kidney and erythropoiesis. *Semin. Hematol.*, **4**, 337

245 Peschle, C., Marone, G., Genovese, A., Quattrin, S. and Condorelli, M. (1975). Studies on the erythrogenin–erythropoietin system. In Nakao, K., Fisher, J. W. and Takaku, F. (eds.) *Erythropoiesis*, p. 241. (Tokyo: University Tokyo Press)

246 Erslev, A. J. (1974). *In vitro* production of erythropoietin by kidneys perfused with a serum-free solution. *Blood*, **44**, 77

247 Bozzini, C. E., Devoto, F. C. H. and Tonio, J. M. (1966). Decreased responsiveness of hematopoietic tissue to erythropoietin in acutely uremic rats. *J. Lab. Clin. Med.*, **68**, 411

248 Van Dyke, D., Keighley, G. and Lawrence, J. (1963). Decreased responsiveness to erythropoietin in a patient with anemia secondary to chronic uremia. *Blood*, **22**, 838

249 Fisher, J. W., Hatch, F. E., Roh, B. L., Allen, R. C. and Kelley, B. J. (1968). Erythropoietin inhibitors in kidney extracts and plasma from anemic uremic human subjects. *Blood*, **31**, 440

250 Erslev, A. J. (1975). The effect of uremic toxins on the production and metabolism of erythropoietin. *Kidney Int.*, Suppl. 2, S-129

251 Zucker, S., Lysik, R. M. and Mohammad, G. (1976). Erythropoiesis in chronic renal disease. *J. Lab. Clin. Med.*, **88**, 528

252 Fried, W. (1972). The liver as a source of extrarenal erythropoietin production. *Blood*, **40**, 671

253 Peschle, C., Marone, G., Genovese, A., Rappaport, J. A. and Condorelli, M. (1976). Increased erythropoietin production in anephric rats with hyperplasia of the reticuloendothelial system induced by colloidal carbon or zymosan. *Blood*, **47**, 325

254 Tyler, H. R. (1968). Neurologic disorders in renal failure. *Am. J. Med.*, **44**, 734

255 Tyler, H. R. (1971). Neurologic complications of uremia. In Strauss, M. B. and Welt, L. G. (eds.) *Diseases of the Kidney*. 2nd Edn., pp. 335–342. (Boston: Little, Brown and Company)

256 Teschan, P. E. and Ginn, H. E. (1976). The nervous system. In Massry, S. G. and Sellers, A. (eds.) *Clinical Aspects of Uremia and Dialysis*, pp. 3–33. (Springfield, Ill.: C. C. Thomas)

257 Martinez, W. C., Rapin, I. and Moore, C. L. (1978). Neurologic complications of renal failure. In Edelman, C. M. (ed.) *Pediatric Kidney Disease*, pp. 408–421. (Boston: Little, Brown and Company)

258 Klinger, M. (1954). EEG observations in uremia. *Electroencephalogr. Clin. Neurophysiol.*, **6**, 519

259 Kiley, J. E. and Hines, O. (1965). EEG evaluation of uremia: wave frequency evaluation on 40 uremic patients. *Arch. Intern. Med.*, **116**, 67

260 Hampers, C. L., Doak, P. B., Callaghan, M. D., Tyler, H. R. and Merrill, J. P. (1966). The EEG and spinal fluid during hemodialysis. *Arch. Intern. Med.*, **118**, 340

261 Depner, T. A. and Gulyassy, P. F. (1979). Chronic renal failure. In Earley, L. E. and Gottschalk, C. W. (eds.) *Strauss and Welt's Disease of the Kidney*. 3rd Edn., pp. 211–261. (Boston: Little, Brown and Company)

262 Cuttelod, S. (1974). Effect of age and role of kidneys and liver on thyrotropin turnover in man. *Metabolism*, **23**, 101

263 Asbury, A. K., Victor, N. and Adams, R. D. (1962). Uremic polyneuropathy. *Trans. Am. Neurol. Assoc.*, **87**, 100

264 Asbury, A. K., Victor, M. and Adams, R. D. (1963). Uremic polyneuropathy. *Arch. Neurol.*, **8**, 413

265 Callaghan, N. (1966). Restless legs syndrome in uremic neuropathy. *Neurology*, **16**, 359

266 Nielsen, V. K. (1971). The peripheral nerve function in chronic renal failure. *Acta Med. Scand.*, **190**, 105

267 Thomas, O. K. (1976). Uraemic neuropathy. *Proc. Eur. Dial. Transplant. Assoc.*, **13**, 109

268 Freeman, R. B., Sheff, M. F., Maher, J. F. and Schreiner, G. E. (1962). The blood cerebrospinal fluid barrier in uremia. *Ann. Intern. Med.*, **56**, 233

269 Triger, D. R. and Jockes, A. M. (1969). Severe muscle cramps due to acute hypomagnesemia in haemodialysis. *Br. Med. J.*, **2**, 804

270 Arieff, A. I. and Massry, S. G. (1976). Dialysis disequilibrium syndrome. In Massry, S. G. and Sellers, A. L. (eds.) *Clinical Aspects of Uremia and Dialysis*, pp. 34–52. (Springfield, Ill.: C. C. Thomas)

271 Caruso, G., Spadetta, V. and Labianca, O. (1970). Subclinical uremic neuropathy. In Walton, J. N., Canel, N. and Scarlato, G. (eds.) *Muscle Diseases*, p. 173. (Amsterdam: Excerpta Medica)

272 Cavanagh, J. B. (1964). The significance of the 'dying back' process in experimental and human neurological disease. *Int. Rev. Exp. Pathol.*, **3**, 219

273 Forno, L. and Alston, W. (1967). Uremic polyneuropathy. *Acta Neurol. Scand.*, **43**, 640

274 Kornfeld, M. and Appenzeller, O. (1970). Pathology of sural nerve in uremic neuropathy. In *Proceedings V Congress of Neuropathology* (Paris)

275 Dinn, J. J. and Crame, D. L. (1970). Schwann cell disfunction in uraemia. *J. Neurol. Neurosurg. Psychiatry*, **33**, 605

276 Thomas, P. K., Hollinrake, K., Lascelles, R. G., O'Sullivan, D. J., Baillod, R. A., Moorhead, J. F. and Mackenzie, J. C. (1971). The polyneuropathy of chronic renal failure. *Brain*, **94**, 761

277 Dyck, P. I., Johnson, W. I., Lambert, E. H. and O'Brien, P. C. (1971). Segmental demyelination secondary to axonal degeneration in uremic neuropathy. *Mayo Clin. Proc.*, **46**, 400

278 Nielsen, V. K. (1974). The peripheral nerve function in chronic renal failure. X. Decremental nerve conduction in uremia? *Acta Med. Scand.*, **196**, 83

279 Nielsen, V. K. (1974). The peripheral nerve function in chronic renal failure. IX. Recovery after renal transplantation. Electrophysiological aspects (sensory and motor nerve conduction). *Acta Med. Scand.*, **195**, 171

280 Caruso, G., Santoro, L., Peretti, A., Serlenga, L., Usberti, M. and Andreucci, V. E. (1978). Uremic polyneuropathy: electrophysiological and histopathological aspects. *Dial. Transplant.*, **7**, 320

281 Thomas, P. K. (1971). The morphological basis for alteration in nerve conduction in peripheral neuropathy. *Proc. R. Soc. Med.*, **64**, 295

282 Andreucci, V. E., Usberti, M., Calderaro, V., Federico, S., Santoro, L. and Caruso, G. (1978). The need for dialysis. *Dial. Transplant.*, **7**, 313

283 Weidman, P. and Maxwell, M. H. (1976). Hypertension. In Massry, S. G. and Sellers, A. L. (eds.) *Clinical Aspects of Uremia and Dialysis*, pp. 100–145. (Springfield, Ill.: C. C. Thomas)

284 Davidson, R. C. and Scribner, B. H. (1979). Cardiovascular manifestations of renal failure. In Earley, L. E. and Gottschalk, C. W. (eds.) *Strauss and Welt's Diseases of the Kidney*. 3rd Edn., pp. 263–275. (Boston: Little, Brown and Company)

285 Ledingham, J. H. and Cohen, R. D. (1964). Changes in the extracellular fluid volume and cardiac output during the development of experimental renal hypertension. *Can. Med. Assoc. J.*, **90**, 292

286 Coleman, T. G., Bower, J. D., Langford, H. G. and Guyton, A. C. (1970). Regulation of arterial pressure in the anephric state. *Circulation*, **42**, 509

287 Guyton, A. C., Coleman, T. G., Cowley, A. W. Jr., Scheel, K. W., Manning, R. D. Jr. and Norman, R. A. Jr. (1972). Arterial pressure regulation. Overriding dominance of the kidneys in long-term regulation and hypertension. *Am. J. Med.*, **52**, 584

288 Selkurt, E. E. (1951). Effect of pulse pressure and mean arterial pressure modification on renal hemodynamics and electrolyte and water excretion. *Circulation*, **4**, 541

289 Koch, K. M., Aynedjian, H. S. and Bank, N. (1968). Effect of acute hypertension on sodium reabsorption by the proximal tubule. *J. Clin. Invest.*, 47, 1969

290 Bank, N. E., Koch, K. M., Aynedjian, H. S. and Aras, M. (1969). Effect of changes in renal perfusion pressure on the suppression of proximal tubular sodium reabsorption due to saline loading. *J. Clin. Invest.*, 48, 271

291 Aperia, A. C., Broberger, C. G. O. and Soderlund, S. (1971). Relationship between renal artery perfusion pressure and tubular sodium reabsorption. *Am. J. Physiol.*, 220, 1205

292 Navar, L. G. (1972). Distal nephron diluting segment responses to altered arterial pressure and solute loading. *Am. J. Physiol.*, 22, 945

293 Borst, J. G. and Borst-de Geus, A. (1963). Hypertension explained by Starling's theory of circulatory homeostasis. *Lancet*, 2, 677

294 Ulvila, J. M., Kennedy, J. A., Lamberg, J. D. and Scribner, B. H. (1972). Blood pressure in chronic renal failure: effect of sodium intake and furosemide. *J. Am. Med. Assoc.*, 220, 233

295 Tobian, L. Jr., Olson, R. and Chesley, G. (1969). Water content of arteriolar wall in renovascular hypertension. *Am. J. Physiol.*, 216, 22

296 Sivertsson, R. (1970). The hemodynamic importance of structural vascular changes in essential hypertension. *Acta Physiol. Scand.* (Suppl.), 343, 1

297 Folkow, B. (1971). The hemodynamic consequences of adaptive structural changes of the resistance vessels in hypertension. *Clin. Sci.*, 41, 1

298 Tobian, L. Jr. (1972). A viewpoint concerning the enigma of hypertension. *Am. J. Med.*, 52, 595

299 Seidel, C. L. and Bohr, D. F. (1971). Calcium and vascular smooth muscle contraction. *Circ. Res.*, 28 and 29 (Suppl. 11), 88

300 Brunner, H. R., Chang, P., Wallach, R., Sealey, J. E. and Laragh, J. H. (1972). Angiotensin II vascular receptors: their avidity in relationship to sodium balance, the autonomic nervous system and hypertension. *J. Clin. Invest.*, 51, 58

301 Symonds, E. M., Stanley, M. A. and Skinner, S. L. (1968). Production of renin by *in vitro* cultures of human chorion and uterine muscle. *Nature (London)*, 217, 1152

302 Ganten, D., Hayduk, K., Brecht, H. M., Boucher, R. and Genest, J. (1970). Evidence of renin release or production in splanchnic territory. *Nature (London)*, 226, 551

303 Vertes, V., Cangiano, J. L., Berman, L. B. and Gould, A. (1969). Hypertension in endstage renal disease. *N. Engl. J. Med.*, 280, 978

304 Stokes, G. S., Mani, M. K. and Stewart, J. H. (1970). Relevance of salt, water and renin to hypertension in chronic renal failure. *Br. Med. J.*, 3, 126

305 Wilkinson, R., Scott, D. F., Uldall, P. R., Kerr, D. N. S., Swinney, J. and Robson, V. (1970). Plasma renin and exchangeable sodium in the hypertension of chronic renal failure. The effect of bilateral nephrectomy. *Q. J. Med.*, 39, 377

306 Kotchen, T. A., Knight, E. L., Kashgarian, M. and Mulrow, P. J. (1970). A study of the renin–angiotensin system in patients with severe chronic renal insufficiency. *Nephron*, 7, 317

307 Brown, J. J., Dusterdieck, G., Fraser, R., Lever, A. F., Robertson, J. I. S., Tree, M. and Weir, R. J. (1971). Hypertension and chronic renal failure. *Br. Med. Bull.*, 27, 128

308 Weidmann, P., Maxwell, M. H., Lupu, A. N., Lewin, A. J. and Massry, S. G. (1971). Plasma renin activity and blood pressure in terminal renal failure. *N. Engl. J. Med.*, 285, 757

309 Medina, A., Bell, P. R. F., Briggs, J. D., Brown, J. J., Fine, A., Lever, A. F., Morton, J. J., Paton, A. M., Robertson, J. I. S., Tree, M., Waite, M. A., Weir, R. and Winchester, J. (1972). Changes in blood pressure, renin and angiotensin after bilateral nephrectomy in patients with chronic renal failure. *Br. Med. J.*, 4, 694

310 Lazarus, J. M., Hampers, C. L., Bennett, A. H., Vandam, L. D. and Merrill, J. P. (1972). Urgent bilateral nephrectomy for severe hypertension. *Ann. Intern. Med.*, 76, 733

311 Mahoney, J. F., Gibson, G. R., Sheil, A. G. R., Storey, B. G., Stokes, G. S. and Stewart, J. H. (1972). Bilateral nephrectomy for malignant hypertension. *Lancet*, **1**, 1036

312 Lee, J. B., Covino, B. G., Takman, B. H. and Smith, E. R. (1965). Renomedullary vasodepressor substance medullin: isolation, chemical characterization, and physiological properties. *Circ. Res.*, **17**, 57

313 Higgins, C. B., Vatner, S. F., Franklin, D., Patrick, T. and Braunwald, E. (1971). Effects of prostaglandin A, on the systemic and coronary circulations in the conscious dog. *Circ. Res.*, **28**, 638

314 Carr, A. A. (1970). Hemodynamic and renal effects of a prostaglandin, PGA_1 in subjects with essential hypertension. *Am. J. Med. Sci.*, **259**, 21

315 Westura, E. E., Kannegiesser, H., O'Toole, J. D. and Lee, J. B. (1970). Antihypertensive effects of prostaglandin A_1 in essential hypertension. *Circ. Res.*, **27** (Suppl.), 131

316 Lee, J. B., McGiff, J. C., Kannegiesser, H., Aykent, Y. Y., Mudd, G. and Frawley, T. F. (1971). Prostaglandin A_1: antihypertensive and renal effects. *Ann. Intern. Med.*, **74**, 703

317 Lee, S. J., Johnson, J. G., Smith, C. J. and Hatch, F. E. (1972). Renal effects of prostaglandin A_1 (PGA_1) on renal and adrenal function in man. *Circ. Res.*, **31** (Suppl.), 19

318 Fichman, M. P., Littenberg, G., Brooker, G. and Horton, R. (1972). The effect of prostaglandin A_1 (PGA_1) on renal and adrenal function in man. *Circ. Res.*, **31** (Suppl.), 19

319 Kaplan, N. M. (1978). *Clinical Hypertension*. 2nd End., p. 405. (Baltimore, MD: The Williams & Wilkins Co.)

320 Pabico, R. C. and Freeman, R. B. (1976). Pericarditis and myocardiopathy. In Massry, S. G. and Sellers, A. L. (eds.) *Clinical Aspects of Uremia and Dialysis*, pp. 69–99. (Springfield, Ill.: C. C. Thomas)

321 D'Cruz, I. A., Bhatt, G. R., Cohen, H. C. and Glick, G. (1978). Echocardiographic detection of cardiac involvement in patients with chronic renal failure. *Arch. Intern. Med.*, **138**, 720

322 Gibson, D. G. (1966). Hemodynamic factors in the development of acute pulmonary edema in renal failure. *Lancet*, **2**, 1217

323 Parisi, A. F., Tow, D. E., Felix, W. R. Jr. and Sasahara, A. A. (1977). Non-invasive cardiac diagnosis. (Third of three parts.) *N. Engl. J. Med.*, **296**, 427

324 Horowitz, M. S., Schultz, C. S., Stinson, E. B., Harrison, D. C. and Popp, R. L. (1974). Sensitivity and specificity of echocardiographic diagnosis of pericardial effusion. *Circulation*, **50**, 239

325 Edwards, K. D. G. and Whyte, H. M. (1959). Plasma creatinine level and creatinine as tests of renal function. *Aust. Ann. Med.*, **8**, 218

326 Jeliffe, R. W. (1971). Estimation of creatinine clearance when urine cannot be collected. *Lancet*, **1**, 975

327 Cockcroft, D. W. and Gault, M. H. (1976). Prediction of creatinine clearance from serum creatinine. *Nephron*, **16**, 31

328 Hamburger, J., Richet, G., Crosnier, J., Funck-Brentano, J. L., Antoine, B., Ducrot, H., Mery, J. P., De Montera, H. and Royer, P. (1966). *Nephrologie*. (Paris: Flammarion)

329 Goldsmith, D. I. (1978). Clinical and laboratory evaluation of renal function. In Edelmann, C. M. Jr. (ed.), *Pediatric Kidney Disease*, pp. 213–224. (Boston: Little, Brown and Company)

330 Rosenthall, L. (1966). Orthoiodohippurate I^{131} kidney scanning in renal failure. *Radiology*, **87**, 298

331 Freeman, L. M., Goldman, S. M., Shaw, R. K. and Blaufox, M. D. (1969). Kidney visualization with ^{131}I-orthoiodohippurate in patients with renal insufficiency. *J. Nucl. Med.*, **10**, 545

332 Schoutens, A., Dupuis, F. and Toussaint, C. (1972). ^{131}I-hippuran scanning in severe renal failure. *Nephron*, **9**, 275

333 Reba, R. C., Poulose, K. P. and Kirchner, P. T. (1974). Radiolabeled chelates for visualization of kidney function and structure with emphasis on their use in renal insufficiency. *Semin. Nucl. Med.*, **4**, 151

334 Sanders, R. C. and Jeck, D. L. (1976). B-scan ultrasound in the evaluation of renal failure. *Radiology*, **119**, 199

335 Baum, G. (1974). Applications of ultrasound. *J. Am. Med. Assoc.*, **229**, 1065

336 Koenigsberg, M., Freeman, L. M. and Blaufox, M. D. (1978). Radionuclide and ultrasound evaluation of renal morphology and function. In Edelmann, C. M. Jr. (ed.), *Pediatric Kidney Disease*, pp. 236–261. (Boston: Little, Brown and Company)

337 Ferrucci, J. T. Jr. (1979). Body ultrasonography. *N. Engl. J. Med.*, **300**, 538 and 590

338 Sanders, R. C. and Bearman, S. (1973). B-scan ultrasound in the diagnosis of hydronephrosis. *Radiology*, **108**, 375

339 Hasch, E. (1974). Ultrasound in the diagnosis of hydronephrosis in infants and children. *J. Clin. Ultrasound*, **2**, 21

340 Sanders, R. C. and Conrad, M. R. (1977). The ultrasonic characteristics of the renal pelvicalyceal echo complex. *J. Clin. Ultrasound*, **5**, 372

341 Pollack, H. M., Arger, P. H., Goldberg, B. B. and Mulholland, S. G. (1978). Ultrasonic detection of non-opaque renal calculi. *Radiology*, **127**, 233

342 Edell, S. and Zegel, H. (1978). Ultrasonic evaluation of renal calculi. *Am J. Roentgenol. Radium Ther. Nucl. Med.*, **130**, 261

343 Giordano, C. (1963). Use of exogenous and endogenous urea for protein synthesis in normal and uremic subjects. *J. Lab. Clin. Med.*, **62**, 231

344 Giovannetti, S. and Maggiore, Q. (1964). A low nitrogen diet with proteins of high biological value for severe chronic uraemia. *Lancet*, **1**, 1000

345 Schloerb, P. R. (1966). Essential L-amino acid administration in uremia. *Am. J. Med. Sci.*, **252**, 650

346 Richards, P., Metcalfe-Gibson, A., Ward, E. E., Wrong, O. and Houghton, B. J. (1967). Utilisation of ammonia nitrogen for protein synthesis in man, and the effect of protein restriction and uraemia. *Lancet*, **2**, 845

347 Varcoe, R., Halliday, D., Carson, E. R., Richards, P. and Tavill, A. S. (1975). Efficiency of utilization of urea nitrogen for albumin synthesis by chronically uraemic and normal man. *Clin. Sci. Mol. Med.*, **48**, 379

348 Walser, M. (1978). Keto-analogues of essential amino acids in the treatment of chronic renal failure. *Kidney Int.*, **13** (Suppl. 8), S-180

349 Walser, M. (1975). Ketoacids in the treatment of uremia. *Clin. Nephrol.*, **3**, 180

350 Cohen, B. D. (1978). Disturbances of nitrogen, carbohydrate and lipid metabolism. In Edelmann, C. M. (ed.) *Pediatric Kidney Disease*, pp. 432–442. (Boston: Little, Brown and Company)

351 Kopple, J. D. (1976). Dietary requirements. In Massry, S. G. and Sellers, A. L. (eds.) *Clinical Aspects of Uremia and Dialysis*, pp. 453–489. (Springfield, Ill.: C. C. Thomas)

352 Kopple, J. D. (1978). Nutritional management of chronic renal failure. *Postgrad. Med.*, **64**, 135

353 Anderson, C. F., Nelson, R. A., Margie, J. D., Johnson, W. J. and Hunt, J. C. (1973). Nutritional therapy for adults with renal disease. *J. Am. Med. Assoc.*, **223**, 68

354 Hyne, B. E. B., Fowell, E. and Lee, H. A. (1972). The effect of caloric intake on nitrogen balance in chronic renal failure. *Clin. Sci.*, **43**, 679

355 Gulyassy, P. F., Yamauchi, H. and Depner, T. A. (1979). Conservative management of chronic renal failure. In Earley, L. E. and Gottschalk, C. W. (eds.) *Strauss and Welt's Diseases of the Kidney*. 3rd Edn., pp. 395–420. (Boston: Little, Brown and Company)

356 Margie, J. D., Anderson, C. F., Nelson, R. A. and Hunt, J. C. (1974). *The Mayo Clinic Diet Cookbook*. (New York: Golden Press)

357 David, D. S., Rubin, A. L., Hochgelerent, E. and Stenzel, K. H. (1972). Dietary management in renal failure. *Lancet*, **1**, 34

358 Broyer, M. (1974). Renal failure and arterial hypertension. Chronic renal failure. In Royer, P., Habib, R., Mathieu, H. and Broyer, M. (eds.) *Pediatric Nephrology*. Part IV, pp. 371–377. (Philadelphia: Saunders)

359 Aronson, A., Furst, S., Kuylenstierna, P. and Nyberg, G. (1975). Essential amino acids in the treatment of advanced uremia: twenty-two months' experience in a five-year-old girl. *Pediatrics*, **56**, 538

360 Kopple, J. D., Sorensen, M. K., Coburn, J. W., Gordon, S. and Rubini, M. E. (1968). Controlled comparison of 20-g and 40-g protein diets in the treatment of chronic uremia. *Am. J. Clin. Nutr.*, **21**, 553

361 Kopple, J. D., Shinaberger, J. H., Coburn, J. W., Sorensen, M. K. and Rubini, M. E. (1969). Evaluating modified protein diets for uremia. *J. Am. Diet. Assoc.*, **54**, 481

362 Sorensen, M. K. and Kopple, J. D. (1968). Assessment of adherence to protein-restricted diets during conservative management of uremia. *Am. J. Clin. Nutr.*, **21**, 631

363 Kopple, J. D. and Coburn, J. W. (1974). Evaluation of chronic uremia. *J. Am. Med. Assoc.*, **227**, 41

364 Kopple, J. D. and Swendseid, M. E. (1977). Amino acid and keto acid diets for therapy in renal failure. *Nephron*, **18**, 1

365 Kopple, J. D. and Swendseid, M. E. (1974). Nitrogen balance and plasma amino acids levels in uremic patients fed an essential amino acid diet. *Am. J. Clin. Nutr.*, **27**, 806

366 Noree, L. O. and Bergstrom, J. (1975). Treatment of chronic uremic patients with protein-poor diet and oral supply of essential amino acids. II. Clinical results of long-term treatment. *Clin. Nephrol.*, **3**, 195

367 Walser, M., Coulter, A. W., Dighe, S. and Crantz, F. R. (1973). The effect of keto-analogues of essential amino acids in severe chronic uremia. *J. Clin. Invest.*, **52**, 678

368 Rose, W. C. (1957). The amino acid requirements of an adult man. *Nutr. Rev.*, **27**, 631

369 Kopple, J. D. (1978). Treatment with low protein and amino acid diets in chronic renal failure. In *Proceedings VII International Congress of Nephrology* (Montreal, June 18–23, 1978), pp. 497–507. (Basel: S. Karger)

370 Chantler, C. and Holliday, M. A. (1973). Growth in children with renal disease, with particular reference to the effects of calorie malnutrition: a review. *Clin. Nephrol.*, **1**, 230

371 Betts, P. R. and Magrath, G. (1974). Growth pattern and dietary intake of children with chronic renal insufficiency. *Br. Med. J.*, **2**, 189

372 Diaz, M., Kleinknecht, C. and Broyer, M. (1975). Growth in experimental renal failure. Incidence of calorie and amino acid intake. *Kidney Int.*, **8**, 349

373 Scharer, K. (1978). Growth in children with chronic renal failure. *Kidney Int.*, **13** (Suppl. 8), S-68

374 Abitrol, C. L. and Holliday, M. A. (1978). The effect of energy and nitrogen intake upon urea production in children with uremia and undernutrition. *Clin. Nephrol.*, **10**, 9

375 Kerr, D., Ashworth, A., Picou, D., Poulter, N., Seakin, A., Spady, D. and Wheeler, E. (1973). Accelerated recovery from infant malnutrition with high calorie feeding. In Gardner, L. L. and Amacher, P. (eds.) *Endocrine Aspects of Malnutrition*, pp. 467–479. (Santa Ynez: Kroc Foundation)

376 Abitbol, C. and Holliday, M. A. (1974). Nitrogen-sparing effect of essential amino acids in uremia. *Kidney Int.*, **6**, 15A

377 Giordano, C., De Santo, N. G., Di Toro, R., Pluvio, M. and Perrone, L. (1978). Amino acid and keto acid diet in uremic children and infants. *Kidney Int.*, **13** (Suppl. 8), S-83

378 Furst, P., Bergstrom, J. and Norée, L. O. (1975). Treatment of chronic uremic patients with protein poor diet and oral supply of essential amino acids. *Clin. Nephrol.*, **3**, 187

379 Holt, E. and Snyderman, S. (1961). The amino acid requirements of infants. *J. Am. Med. Assoc.*, **175**, 125

380 Bergstrom, J., Furst, P., Josephson, B. and Norée, L. (1970). Improvement of nitrogen balance in a uremic patient by the addition of histidine to essential amino acid solutions given intravenously. *Life Sci.*, **9**, 787

381 Furst, P. (1972). Studies in severe renal failure. II. Evidence for the essentiality of histidine. *Scand. J. Clin. Lab. Invest.*, **30**, 307

382 Walser, M., Mitch, W. E. and Collier, V. U. (1978). Effects of protein restriction plus keto analogues of essential amino acids of the course of chronic renal failure. In *Proceedings VII International Congress of Nephrology* (Montreal, June 18–23, 1978), pp. 483–487. (Basel: S. Karger)

383 Collier, V. U., Mitch, W. E. and Walser, M. (1978). The effect of spontaneous or induced lowering of plasma Ca × P product on progression of chronic renal failure. *Clin. Res.*, **26**, 564A

384 Erslev, A. J. (1974). Management of the anemia of chronic renal failure. *Clin. Nephrol.*, **2**, 174

385 Feldman, H. A. and Singer, I. (1975). Endocrinology and metabolism in uremia. *Medicine*, **54**, 351

386 Cattran, D. C., Steiner, G., Fenton, S. S. A. and Wilson, D. R. (1974). Hypertriglyceridemia in uremia and the use of triglyceride turnover to define pathogenesis. *Trans. Am. Soc. Artif. Intern. Organs*, **20**, 148

387 Murase, T., Cattran, D. C., Rubenstein, B. and Steiner, G. (1975). Inhibition of lipoprotein lipase by uremic plasma: a possible cause of hypertriglyceridemia. *Metabolism*, **24**, 1279

388 Sanfelippo, M. L., Swenson, R. S. and Reaven, G. M. (1977). Reduction of plasma triglycerides by diet in subjects with chronic renal failure. *Kidney Int.*, **11**, 54

389 Ginsberg, H., Olefsky, J., Kimmerling, G., Crapo, P. and Reaven, G. (1976). Induction of hypertriglyceridemia by a low fat diet. *J. Clin. Endocrinol. Metab.*, **42**, 729

390 Nestel, P. J., Carroll, K. F. and Havenstein, N. (1970). Plasma triglyceride response to carbohydrates, fats and calorie intake. *Metabolism*, **19**, 1

391 Grundy, S. (1975). Effects of polyunsaturated fats on lipid metabolism in patients with hypertriglyceridemia. *J. Clin. Invest.*, **55**, 269

392 Pierides, A. M., Alvarez-Ude, A. F. and Kerr, D. N. S. (1975). Clofibrate-induced muscle damage in patients with chronic renal failure. *Lancet*, **2**, 1279

393 Goldberg, A. P., Sherrad, D. J., Haas, L. B. and Brunzell, J. D. (1977). Control of clofibrate toxicity in uremic hypertriglyceridemia. *Clin. Pharmacol. Ther.*, **21**, 317

394 Goldberg, A., Brunzell, J. and Sherrard, D. (1975). Clofibrate effective treatment for uremic hypertriglyceridemia. *Kidney Int.*, **8**, 412

395 Di Giulio, S., Boulu, R., Drueke, T., Nicolai, A., Zingraff, J. and Crosnier, J. (1977). Clofibrate treatment of hyperlipidemia in chronic renal failure. *Clin. Nephrol.*, **8**, 504

396 Calderaro, V., Federico, S., Conte, G., Memoli, B. and Andreucci, V. E. (1977). Treatment of uremic hypertriglyceridemia with clofibrate. *Abstracts of XIV Congress of European Dialysis and Transplant Association*, May 31–June 3, Helsinki, p. 185

397 Committee of Principal Investigators (Oliver, M. F., Heady, J. A., Morris, J. N. and Cooper, H.) (1978). A co-operative trial in the primary prevention of ischaemic heart disease using clofibrate. *Br. Heart J.*, **40**, 1069

398 Oliver, M. F. (1978). Cholesterol, coronaries, clofibrate and death. *N. Engl. J. Med.*, **299**, 1360

399 Editorial (1978). Clofibrate and the primary prevention of ischaemic heart disease. *Br. Med. J.*, **2**, 1585

400 Einarsson, K., Hellstrom, K. and Leijd, B. (1977). Bile acid kinetics and steroid balance during nicotinic acid therapy in patients with hyperlipoproteinemia types II and IV. *J. Lab. Clin. Med.*, **90**, 613

401 Rocha, J., Davidson, R. C. and Scribner, B. H. (1972). The concept of basal sodium excretion in the management of hypertension in primary renal disease. In Onesti, G., Kim, K. E. and Moyer, J. H. (eds.) *Hypertension: Mechanisms and Management*, pp. 791–803. (New York: Grune & Stratton)

402 Nemati, M., Kyle, M. C. and Freis, E. D. (1977). Clinical study of ticrynafen: a new diuretic, antihypertensive and uricosuric agent. *J. Am. Med. Assoc.*, 237, 652

403 Huang, C. M., Chock, D., del Greco, F., Armstrong, M., Kroc, J. and Quintanilla, A. (1979). Antihypertensive and hemodynamic effects of ticrynafen compared with hydrochlorothiazide. *Nephron*, 23 (Suppl. 1), 51

404 Beg, M. A., Zuccarello, W., Donikian, M. A., Ragland, R. and Ziv, D. S. (1979). Renal function during ticrynafen therapy. *Nephron*, 23 (Suppl. 1), 64

405 Bauer, J. H. and Brooks, C. S. (1979). Comparative effects of ticrynafen and hydrochlorothiazide on blood pressure, renal function, serum uric acid and electrolytes, and body fluid spaces in hypertensive man. *Nephron*, 23 (Suppl. 1), 57

406 Veterans Administration Cooperative Study Group on Antihypertensive Agents (1979). Comparative effects of ticrynafen and hydrochlorothiazide in the treatment of hypertension. *N. Engl. J. Med.*, 301, 293

407 Stote, R. M., Dubb, J. W., Familiar, R., Erb, B., Weiherer, S. and Alexander, F. (1979). Ticrynafen: site of natriuretic activity. *Nephron*, 23 (Suppl. 1), 25

408 Friedman, A. and Steele, T. H. (1977). Supersaturation of urine with uric acid and monosodium urate: response to a uricosuric diuretic. *Clin. Res.*, 25, 621

409 Lelievre, G., Raviart, B. and Lepontre, E. (1978). Insuffisance rénale aiguë lors de l'administration d'un diurétique hypouricémiant, l'acide tiénilique. *Nouv. Presse Med.*, 7, 2654

410 Bennett, W. M. and Van Zee, B. E. (1979). Acute renal failure from ticrynafen. *N. Engl. J. Med.*, 301, 1179

411 Cohen, L. H., Norby, L. H., Champion, C. and Spargo, B. (1979). Acute renal failure from ticrynafen. *N. Engl. J. Med.*, 301, 1180

412 Selby, T. (1979). Acute renal failure from ticrynafen. *N. Engl. J. Med.*, 301, 1180

413 Ahlquist, R. P. (1948). A study of the adrenotropic receptors. *Am. J. Physiol.*, 153, 586

414 Koch-Weser, J. (1979). Drug therapy. Metoprolol. *N. Engl. J. Med.*, 301, 698

415 Ablad, B., Carlsson, E. and Ek, L. (1973). Pharmacological studies of two new cardioselective adrenergic beta-receptors antagonists. *Life Sci.*, 12, 107

416 Johnson, G., Regardh, C. G. and Solvell, L. (1975). Combined pharmacokinetic and pharmacodynamic studies in man of the adrenergic beta$_1$-receptor antagonist metoprolol. *Acta Pharmacol. Toxicol.*, 36 (Suppl. 5), 31

417 Brown, H. C., Carruthers, S. G., Johnston, G. D., Kelly, J. G., McAinsh, J., McDevitt, D. G. and Shanks, R. G. (1976). Clinical pharmacology of atenolol, a new beta-adrenoceptor blocking drug. *Clin. Pharmacol. Ther.*, 20, 524

418 McAinsh, J. (1977). Clinical pharmacokinetics of atenolol. *Postgrad. Med. J.*, 53 (Suppl. 3), 74

419 Bengtsson, C. (1976). Comparison between metoprolol and propranolol as antihypertensive agents: a double-blind cross-over study. *Acta Med. Scand.*, 199, 71

420 Singh, A. N., Paul, L. and Elie, R. (1978). Double blind comparison clinical trial of metoprolol versus propranolol in the long-term treatment of uncomplicated hypertensive patient. *Curr. Ther. Res.*, 24, 571

421 Zacharias, F. J., Mayes, P. J. and Cruickshank, J. M. (1977). Atenolol in hypertension: a double-blind comparison of the response to three different doses. *Postgrad. Med. J.*, 53 (Suppl. 3), 114

422 Prichard, B. N. C. (1978). Beta-adrenergic receptor blockade in hypertension, past, present and future. *Br. J. Clin. Pharmacol.*, 5, 379

423 Castleden, C. M., Danthan, J. R. E. and George, C. (1977). A comparison of once and twice daily atenolol in hypertension. *Postgrad. Med. J.*, **53**, 679

424 Keusch, G. W., Weidmann, P., Compere, V., Lee, D. B. N., Upham, A. T. and Massry, S. G. (1978). Minoxidil therapy in refractory hypertension. Analysis of 155 patients. *Nephron*, **21**, 1

425 Mitchell, H. C. and Pettinger, W. A. (1978). Long-term treatment of refractory hypertensive patients with minoxidil. *J. Am. Med. Assoc.*, **233**, 2131

426 Andreucci, V. E., Usberti, M., Federico, S., Pecoraro, C., Balletta, M. and Meccariello, S. (1981). Effectiveness of minoxidil in treating refractory hypertension in patients with various degrees of renal insufficiency. (In preparation)

427 Usberti, M., Federico, S., Dal Canton, A., Pecoraro, C., Meccariello, S., Stanziale, P. and Andreucci, V. E. (1980). Il minoxidil nel controllo rapido e protratto nell'ipertensione grave del bambino. (In preparation)

428 Graham, R. M. and Pettinger, W. A. (1979). Prazosin. *N. Engl. J. Med.*, **300**, 232

429 Chidsey, C. A. and Gottlieb, T. B. (1974). The pharmacologic basis of antihypertensive therapy: the role of vasodilator drugs. *Prog. Cardiovasc. Dis.*, **17**, 99

430 Graham, R. M., Thornell, I. R., Gain, J. M., Bagnoli, C., Oates, H. F. and Stokes, G. S. (1976). Prazosin: the first-dose phenomenon. *Br. Med. J.*, **2**, 1293

431 Curtis, J. A. and Bateman, F. J. A. (1975). Use of prazosin in management of hypertension in patients with chronic renal failure and in renal transplant recipients. *Br. Med. J.*, **4**, 432

432 Stokes, G. S. and Oates, H. F. (1978). Prazosin: new alpha-adrenergic blocking agent in treatment of hypertension. *Cardiovasc. Med.*, **3**, 41

433 Henning, M. (1978). Mechanism of action of methyldopa: an overview. In Zanchetti, A. (ed.) *Methyldopa in Hypertension*, pp. 175–179. (Rahway, New Jersey: Merck Sharp and Dohme International)

434 Hansson, L. and Humyor, S. N. (1973). Blood pressure overshoot due to acute clonidine (Catapres) withdrawal: studies on arterial and urinary catecholamines and suggestions for management of the crisis. *Clin. Sci. Mol. Med.*, **45** (Suppl. 1), 181

435 Jain, A. K., Ryan, J. R. and McMahon, F. G. (1973). The effect of single working doses of methyldopa on blood pressure. *Clin. Pharmacol. Ther.*, **14**, 137

436 McLeod, P. J. (1978). Single-dose methyldopa. In Zanchetti, A. (ed.) *Methyldopa in Hypertension*, pp. 253–257. (Rahway, New Jersey: Merck Sharp and Dohme International)

437 Bricker, N. S. and Fine, L. G. (1978). The trade-off hypothesis: current status. *Kidney Int.*, **13** (Suppl. 8), 5

438 Fiaschi, E., Maschio, G., D'Angelo, A., Bonucci, E., Tessitore, N. and Messa, P. (1978). Low protein diets and bone disease in chronic renal failure. *Kidney Int.*, **13** (Suppl. 8), 79

439 Baker, L. R. I., Akrill, P., Cattell, W. R., Stamp, T. C. B. and Watson, L. (1974). Iatrogenic osteomalacia and myopathy due to phosphate depletion. *Br. Med. J.*, **3**, 150

440 Dent, C. E. and Winter, C. S. (1974). Osteomalacia due to phosphate depletion from excessive aluminium hydroxide ingestion. *Br. Med. J.*, **1**, 551

441 Knochel, J. P. (1977). The pathophysiology and clinical characteristics of severe hypophosphatemia. *Arch. Intern. Med.*, **137**, 203

442 Clarkson, E. M., Luck, V. A., Hynson, W. V., Bailey, R. R., Eastwood, J. B., Woodhead, J. S., Clements, V. R., Oriordan, J. L. H. and de Wardener, H. E. (1972). The effect of aluminum hydroxide on calcium, phosphorus and aluminum balances, the serum parathyroid hormone concentration and the aluminum content of bone in patients with chronic renal failure. *Clin. Sci.*, **43**, 519

443 American Academy of Pediatrics: Report of the Committee on Nutrition, Infantile Scurvy and Nutritional Rickets in the United States. *Pediatrics*, **29**, 646

444 Dent, C. E. and Smith, R. (1969). Nutritional osteomalacia. *Q. J. Med.*, **38**, 195

445 Kleeman, C. R., Better, O. S., Massry, S. G. and Maxwell, M. H. (1967). Divalent ion metabolism and osteodystrophy in chronic renal failure. *Yale J. Biol. Med.*, **40**, 1

446 Liu, S. G. and Chu, H. I. (1943). Studies of calcium and phosphorus metabolism with special reference to the pathogenesis and effect of dihydrotachysterol (AT 10) and iron. *Medicine*, **22**, 103

447 Kaye, M. and Sagar, S. (1972). Effect of dihydrotachysterol on calcium absorption in uremia. *Metabolism*, **21**, 815

448 Brickman, A. S., Coburn, J. W., Massry, S. G. and Norman, A. W. (1974). 1,25-dihydroxyvitamin D_3 in normal man and patients with renal failure. *Ann. Intern. Med.*, **80**, 161

449 Henderson, R. G., Ledingham, J. G. G., Oliver, D., Small, D. G., Russell, R. G. G., Smith, R., Walton, R. J., Preston, C. and Warner, G. T. (1974). Effects of 1,25-dihydroxycholecalciferol on calcium absorption, muscle weakness and bone disease in chronic renal failure. *Lancet*, **1**, 379

450 Coburn, J. W., Brickman, A. S., Sherrard, D. J., Singer, F. R., Wong, E. G. C., Baylink, D. J. and Norman, A. W. (1977). Use of 1,25($OH)_2$-vitamin D_3 to separate types of renal osteodystrophy. *Proc. Eur. Dial. Transplant. Assoc.*, **14**, 442

451 Chalmers, T. M., Hunter, J. O., Davie, M. W., Szaz, K. F., Pelc, B. and Kodicek, E. (1973). 1-Alpha hydroxycholecalciferol as a substitute for the kidney hormone; 1,25-dihydroxycholecalciferol in chronic renal failure. *Lancet*, **2**, 696

452 Peacock, M., Gallagher, J. C. and Nordin, B. E. C. (1974). Action of 1-alpha-hydroxyvitamin D_3 on calcium absorption and bone resorption in man. *Lancet*, **1**, 385

453 Pechet, M. M. and Hesses, R. H. (1974). Metabolic and clinical effects of pure crystalline 1-alpha hydroxyvitamin D_3 and 1-alpha dihydroxyvitamin D_3. *Am. J. Med.*, **57**, 13

454 Fournier, A., Bordier, P., Gueris, J., Sebert, J. L., Marie, P., Ferriere, C., Bedrossian, J. and De Luca, H. F. (1979). Comparison of 1-alpha-hydroxycholecalciferol and 25-hydroxycholecalciferol in the treatment of renal osteodystrophy: greater effect of 25-hydroxycholecalciferol on bone mineralization. *Kidney Int.*, **15**, 196

455 Teitelbaum, S. L., Bone, J. M., Stein, P. M., Gilden, J. J., Bates, J., Boisseau, V. C. and Avioli, L. V. (1976). The skeletal response of patients with chronic renal insufficiency to 25-hydroxycholecalciferol. *J. Am. Med. Assoc.*, **235**, 164

456 Witmer, G., Margolis, A., Fontaine, O., Fritsch, J., Lenoir, G., Broyer, M. and Balsan, S. (1976). Effects of 25-hydroxycholecalciferol on bone lesions of children with terminal renal failure. *Kidney Int.*, **10**, 395

457 Avioli, L. V. (1973). Collagen metabolism, uremia and bone. *Kidney Int.*, **4**, 105

458 Miller, E. J. and Matukas, V. J. (1974). Biosynthesis of collagen. *Fed. Proc.*, **33**, 1198

459 Jowsey, J. and Riggs, B. L. (1968). Bone changes in a patient with hypervitaminosis. *Am. J. Clin. Endocrinol.*, **28**, 1833

460 Frame, B., Jackson, C. E., Reynolds, W. A. and Umphrey, J. E. (1974). Hypercalcemia and skeletal effects in chronic hypervitaminosis. A. *Ann. Intern. Med.*, **80**, 44

461 Havivi, E. and Guggenheim, K. (1975). Effect of hypervitaminosis A on composition of chick cartilage. *Int. J. Vitam. Nutr. Res.*, **45**, 307

462 Chertwo, B. S., Williams, G. A., Kiani, R., Stewart, K. L., Hargis, G. K. and Glayter, R. I. (1974). The interactions between vitamin A, vinblastine, and cytochalasin B in parathyroid hormone secretion. *Proc. Soc. Exp. Biol. Med.*, **147**, 16

463 Kleeman, C. R., Okun, R. and Heller, R. J. (1966). The renal regulation of sodium and potassium in patients with chronic renal failure and the effects of diuretics on the excretion of these ions. *Ann. N.Y. Acad. Sci.*, **139**, 520

464 Migone, L. and Borghetti, A. (1968). Aspetti fisiopatologici e clinici dell'insufficienza renale. In *69th Congress of Italian Society of Internal Medicine*, pp. 1–595. (Roma, Italy: L. Pozzi)

465 Garella, S., Dana, C. L. and Chazan, J. A. (1973). Severity of metabolic acidosis as a determinant of bicarbonate requirements. *N. Engl. J. Med.*, **289**, 121

466 Arieff, A. I. (1972). Principles of parenteral therapy. A. Principles of parenteral therapy and parenteral nutrition. In Maxwell, M. H. and Kleeman, C. R. (eds.) *Clinical Disorders of Fluid and Electrolyte Metabolism.* 2nd Edn., pp. 567–589. (New York: McGraw-Hill)

467 Posner, J. B. and Plum, F. (1967). Spinal-fluid pH and neurologic symptoms in systemic acidosis. *N. Engl. J. Med.*, **277**, 605

468 Finch, C. A. and Lenfant, C. (1972). Oxygen transport in man. *N. Engl. J. Med.*, **286**, 407

469 Duke, M. and Abelmann, W. H. (1969). The hemodynamic response to chronic anemia. *Circulation*, **39**, 503

470 Neff, M. S., Kim, K. E., Persoff, M., Onesti, G. and Swartz, C. (1971). Hemodynamics of uremic anemia. *Circulation*, **43**, 876

471 Mitchell, T. R. and Pegrum, G. D. (1971). The oxygen affinity of haemoglobin in chronic renal failure. *Br. J. Haematol.*, **21**, 463

472 Chillar, R. K. and Desforges, J. F. (1974). Red cell organic phosphates in patients with chronic renal failure on maintenance hemodialysis. *Br. J. Haematol.*, **26**, 549

473 Aljama, P., Ward, M. K., Pierides, A. M., Eastham, E. J., Ellis, H. A., Feest, T. G., Conceicao, S. and Kerr, D. N. S. (1978). Serum ferritin concentration: a reliable guide to iron overload in uremic and hemodialyzed patients. *Clin. Nephrol.*, **10**, 101

474 Fisher, J. W., Roh, B. L., Malgor, L. A., Samuels, A. I., Thompson, J., Noveck, R. and Espada, J. (1971). Chemical agents which stimulate erythropoietin production. In Fisher, J. W. (ed.) *Kidney Hormones*, pp. 343–371. (London: Academic Press)

475 Duckham, J. M. and Lee, H. A. (1976). The treatment of refractory anemia of chronic renal failure with cobalt chloride. *Q. J. Med.*, **178**, 277

476 Alexanian, R. (1969). Erythropoietin and erythropoiesis in anemic men following androgens. *Blood*, **33**, 564

477 Mirand, E. A. and Murphy, G. P. (1971). Erythropoietin activity in anephric humans given prolonged androgen treatment. *J. Surg. Oncol.*, **3**, 59

478 Shaldon, S., Patyna, W. D., Kaltwasser, P., Werner, E., Koch, K. M. and Schoeppe, W. E. (1971). The use of testosterone in bilateral nephrectomized dialysis patients. *Trans. Am. Soc. Artif. Intern. Organs*, **17**, 104

479 Richardson, J. R. Jr. and Weinstein, M. B. (1971). Erythropoietic response of dialyzed patients to testosterone administration. *Ann. Intern. Med.*, **73**, 403

480 Choi, E. S. K., Chung, T. J., Morrison, R. S., Myers, C. and Greenberg, M. S. (1974). Hypertriglyceridemia in hemodialysis patients during oral dromostanolone therapy for anemia. *Am. J. Clin. Nutr.*, **27**, 901

481 Opelz, G., Mickey, M. R. and Terasaki, P. I. (1972). Identification of unresponsive kidney transplant recipients. *Lancet*, **1**, 868

482 Opelz, G. and Terasaki, P. J. (1974). Poor kidney survival in recipients with frozen blood transfusion or no transfusions. *Lancet*, **2**, 696

483 Opelz, G. and Terasaki, P. I. (1976). Prolongation effect of blood transfusions on kidney graft survival. *Transplantation*, **22**, 380

484 Strom, T. B. and Merrill, J. P. (1977). Hepatitis B, transfusions and renal transplantation. *N. Engl. J. Med.*, **296**, 225

485 Sirchia, G. (1978). Blood transfusion and kidney transplantation. *Dial. Transplant.*, **7**, 390

486 Alexandre, G. P. J. and Van Cangh, P. J. (1978). Influence of blood transfusion on kidney transplantation. *Dial. Transplant.*, **7**, 392

487 Brynger, H., Frisk, B., Ahlmen, J., Attman, P. O., Blohme, I., Sandberg, L. and Gelin, L. E. (1977). Graft survival and blood transfusion. *Proc. Eur. Dial. Transplant. Assoc.*, **14**, 290

488 Brynger, H., Frisk, B., Ahlmen, J., Blohme, I., Sandberg, L. and Gelin, L. E. (1978). Blood transfusions and graft survival in living related donor transplantation. *Dial. Transplant.*, 7, 396

489 Giordano, C., Esposito, R., Randazzo, G. and Pluvio, M. (1972). Oxystarch as a gastrointestinal sorbent in uremia. In Kluthe, R. (ed.) *Uremia*, p. 132. (Stuttgart: Georg Thieme Verlag)

490 Giordano, C., Esposito, R. and Pluvio, M. (1973). The effects of oxidized starch on blood and faecal nitrogen in uremia. *Proc. Eur. Dial. Transplant. Assoc.*, 10, 136

491 Giordano, C., Esposito, R., Di Leo, V. A. and Pluvio, M. (1979). Oxycellulose as oral sorbent in uremia. *Clin. Nephrol.*, 11, 142

492 Yatzidis, H. (1978). Preliminary studies with locust bean gum, a new sorbent with great potential. *Kidney Int.*, 13 (Suppl. 8), 152

493 Yatzidis, H., Koutsicos, D. and Digenis, P. (1979). Newer oral sorbents in uremia. *Clin. Nephrol.*, 11, 105

494 Setälä, K. (1978). Bacterial enzymes in uremia management. *Kidney Int.*, 13 (Suppl. 8), S-194

495 Setälä, K. (1979). Treating uremia with soil bacterial enzymes: further developments. *Clin. Nephrol.*, 11, 156

496 Blythe, W. B. (1979). The management of intercurrent medical and surgical problems in the patient with chronic renal failure. In Earley, L. E. and Gottschalk, C. W. (eds.) *Strauss and Welt's Diseases of the Kidney*. 3rd Edn., pp. 517–537. (Boston: Little, Brown and Company)

497 Anderson, R. J., Gambertoglio, J. G. and Schrier, R. W. (1976). *Clinical Use of Drugs in Renal Failure*. (Springfield, Ill.: C. C. Thomas)

498 Cutler, R. E. and Christopher, T. G. (1976). Drug therapy during renal insufficiency and dialytic treatment. In Massry, S. G. and Sellers, A. L. (eds.) *Clinical Aspects of Uremia and Dialysis*, pp. 427–452. (Springfield, Ill.: C. C. Thomas)

499 Weinstein, L. (1970). Antibiotics. I. The penicillins. In Goodman, L. S. and Gilman, A. (eds.) *The Pharmacological Basis of Therapeutics*. 4th Edn., pp. 1204–1241. (London: The Macmillan Company)

500 Kampmann, J., Hansen, J. M., Siersbock-Nielsen, K. and Laursen, H. (1972). Effect of some drug on penicillin half-life in blood. *Clin. Pharmacol. Ther.*, 13, 516

501 Schrier, R. W., Bulger, R. J. and Van Arsdel, P. P. (1966). Nephropathy associated with penicillin and homologues. *Ann. Intern. Med.*, 64, 116

502 Baldwin, D. S., Levine, B. B., McCluskey, R. T. and Gallo, G. R. (1968). Renal failure and interstitial nephritis due to penicillin and methicillin. *N. Engl. J. Med.*, 279, 1245

503 Love, D. W. and Salter, F. J. (1971). Penicillin and carbenicillin induced neuro-encephalopathy. *Drug. Intell. Clin. Pharm.*, 5, 361

504 Curtis, J. R. and Williams, G. B. (1975). *Clinical Management of Chronic Renal Failure*. (Oxford: Blackwell Scientific Publications)

505 Bryan, C. S. and Stone, W. J. (1975). Comparably massive penicillin G therapy in renal failure. *Ann. Intern. Med.*, 82, 189

506 Bulger, R. J., Lindholm, D. D., Murray, J. S. and Kirby, W. M. (1964). Effect of uremia on methicillin and oxacillin blood levels. *J. Am. Med. Assoc.*, 187, 319

507 Kunin, C. M. and Finkelberg, Z. (1970). Oral cephalexin and ampicillin: antimicrobial activity, recovery in urine and persistence in blood of uremic patients. *Ann. Intern. Med.*, 72, 349

508 Jusko, W. J., Lewis, G. P. and Schmitt, G. W. (1973). Ampicillin and hetacillin pharmacokinetics in normal and anephric subjects. *Clin. Pharmacol. Ther.*, 14, 90

509 Tannenberg, A. M., Wicher, K. J. and Rose, N. R. (1971). Ampicillin nephropathy. *J. Am. Med. Assoc.*, 218, 449

510 Whelton, A., Carter, G. G., Garth, M. A., Darwish, M. A. and Walker, W. G. (1971). Carbenicillin-induced acidosis and seizures. *J. Am. Med. Assoc.*, **218**, 1942

511 Cox, C. E. (1973). Pharmacology of carbenicillin-inadyl sodium in renal insufficiency. *J. Infect. Dis.*, **127** (Suppl.), 157

512 Bran, J. L., Karl, D. M. and Kaye, D. (1971). Human pharmacology and clinical evaluation of an oral carbenicillin preparation. *Clin. Pharmacol. Ther.*, **12**, 525

513 Hinman, A. R. and Wolinsky, E. (1967). Nephrotoxicity associated with the use of cephaloridine. *J. Am. Med. Assoc.*, **200**, 724

514 Kaplan, K., Reisberg, B. and Weinstein, L. (1968). Cephaloridine. *Arch. Intern. Med.*, **121**, 17

515 Perkins, R. L., Apicella, M. A., Lee, I., Cuppage, F. E. and Saslaw, S. (1968). Cephaloridine and cephalotin: comparative studies of potential nephrotoxicity. *J. Lab. Clin. Med.*, **71**, 75

516 Linton, A. L., Bailey, R. R. and Turnbull, D. I. (1972). Relative nephrotoxicity of cephalosporin antibiotics in an animal model. *Can. Med. Assoc. J.*, **107**, 414

517 Silverblatt, F., Turck, M. and Bulger, R. (1970). Nephrotoxicity due to cephaloridine: a light and electronmicroscopic study in rabbits. *J. Infect. Dis.*, **122**, 33

518 Silverblatt, F., Harrison, W. O. and Turck, M. (1973). Nephrotoxicity of cephalosporin antibiotics in experimental animals. *J. Infect. Dis.*, **128** (Suppl.), 367

519 Dodds, M. G. and Foord, R. D. (1970). Enhancement by potent diuretics of renal tubular necrosis induced by cephaloridine. *Br. J. Pharmacol.*, **40**, 227

520 Lawson, D. H., Macadam, R. F., Singh, H., Gavras, H. and Linton, A. L. (1970). The nephrotoxicity of cephaloridine. *Postgrad. Med. J.*, **46** (Suppl.), 36

521 Norrby, R., Stengvist, K. and Elgefors, B. (1976). Interaction between cephaloridine and furosemide in man. *Scand. J. Infect. Dis.*, **8**, 209

522 Kleinknecht, P., Ganeval, D. and Droz, D. (1973). Acute renal failure after high doses of gentamicin and cephalothin. *Lancet*, **1**, 1129

523 Fillastre, J. P., Laumonier, R., Humbert, G., Dubois, D., Metayer, J., Delpech, A., Leroy, J. and Robert, M. (1973). Acute renal failure associated with combined gentamicin and cephalothin therapy. *Br. Med. J.*, **2**, 396

524 Seldin, D. W., Carter, N. W. and Rector, F. C. Jr. (1971). Consequences of renal failure and their management. In Strauss, M. B. and Welt, L. G. (eds.) *Disease of the Kidney*. 2nd Edn., pp. 211–272. (Boston: Little, Brown and Company)

525 Levison, M. E., Levison, S. P., Ries, K. and Kaye, D. (1973). Pharmacology of cefazolin in patients with normal and abnormal renal function. *J. Infect. Dis.*, **128** (Suppl.), 354

526 Onishi, H. R., Zimmerman, S. B. and Stapley, E. O. (1974). Observations on the mode of action of cefoxitin. *Ann. N.Y. Acad. Sci.*, **235**, 406

527 Geddes, A. M., Schnurr, L. P., Ball, A. P., McGhie, D., Brookes, G. R., Wise, R. and Andrews, J. (1977). Cefoxitin: a hospital study. *Br. Med. J.*, **1**, 1126

528 Une, T. and Mitsuhashi, S. (1977). Antimicrobial evaluation of cefoxitin, a new semi-synthetic cephamycin. *Arzneimitt. Forsch.*, **27**, 89

529 Bach, V. T., Roy, J. and Thadepalli, H. (1977). Susceptibility of anaerobic bacteria to cefoxitin and related compounds. *Antimicrob. Agents Chemother.*, **11**, 912

530 Thadepalli, H., Webb, D., Roy, I. and Bach, V. (1978). Evaluation of cefoxitin sodium therapy in anaerobic infections. *J. Antimicrob. Chem.*, **4** (Suppl. B), 203

531 Wilson, P., Leung, T. and Williams, J. D. (1978). Antibacterial activity, pharmacokinetics and efficacy of cefoxitin in patients with abdominal sepsis and other infections. *J. Antimicrob. Chem.*, **4** (Suppl. B), 127

532 Trollfors, B., Norrby, R. and Kristianson, K. (1978). Effects on renal function of treatment with cefoxitin sodium alone or in combination with furosemide. *J. Antimicrob. Chem.*, **4** (Suppl. B), 85

533 Baylis, C., Rennke, M. R. and Brenner, B. M. (1977). Mechanisms of the defect in glomerular ultrafiltration associated with gentamicin administration. *Kidney Int.*, 12, 344

534 Warner, W. A. and Sanders, E. (1971). Neuromuscular blockade associated with gentamicin therapy. *J. Am. Med. Assoc.*, 215, 1153

535 Schultze, R. G., Winters, R. E. and Kauffman, H. (1971). Possible nephrotoxicity in gentamicin. *J. Infect. Dis.*, 124 (Suppl.), 145

536 Wilfert, J. N., Burke, J. P., Bloomer, H. A. and Smith, C. B. (1971). Renal insufficiency associated with gentamicin therapy. *J. Infect. Dis.*, 124 (Suppl.), 148

537 Cutler, R. E. and Orme, B. M. (1969). Correlation of serum creatinine concentration and kanamycin half-life. *J. Am. Med. Assoc.*, 209, 539

538 Whelton, A., von Wittenau, M. S., Twomey, T. M., Walker, W. G. and Bianchine, J. R. (1974). Doxycycline pharmacokinetics in the absence of renal function. *Kidney Int.*, 5, 365

539 Phillips, M. E., Eastwood, J. B., Curtis, J. R., Gower, P. E. and de Wardener, H. E. (1974). Tetracycline poisoning in renal failure. *Br. Med. J.*, 2, 149

540 Singer, I. and Rotenberg, D. (1973). Demeclocycline-induced nephrogenic diabetes insipidus. *Ann. Intern. Med.*, 79, 679

541 Frimpter, G. W., Timpanelli, A. E., Eisenmenger, W. J., Stein, H. S. and Ehrlich, L. I. (1963). Reversible Fanconi syndrome caused by degraded tetracycline. *J. Am. Med. Assoc.*, 184, 11

542 Kanfer, A., Daniel, F., Vigeral, Ph. and Mery, J. P. (1979). Surdité transitoire chez des insuffisants rénaux traités par l'érithromycine. *Nouv. Presse Med.*, 8, 2283

543 Mery, J. P. and Kanfer, A. (1979). Ototoxicity of erythromycin in patients with renal insufficiency. *N. Engl. J. Med.*, 301, 944

544 Revert, L. (1977). Fosfomycin in patients subjected to periodic hemodialysis. *Chemotherapy*, 23 (Suppl. 1), 204

545 Gobernado, M. and Garcia, J. (1977). Renal insufficiency and fosfomycin. *Chemotherapy*, 23 (Suppl. 1), 200

546 Kalowski, S., Nanra, R. S., Mathew, T. H. and Kincaid-Smith, P. (1973). Deterioration in renal function in association with co-trimoxazole therapy. *Lancet*, 1, 394

547 Mohring, K. and Madsen, P. O. (1971). Treatment of urinary tract infections with oxolinic acid in patients with normal and impaired renal function. *Delaware Med. J.*, 43, 376

548 Grüneberg, R. N. (1974). Oxolinic acid in urinary infections. *Lancet*, 2, 1088

549 Meers, P. D. (1974). Oxolinic acid in urinary infections. *Lancet*, 2, 721

550 Virtanen, S., Kasanen, A., Forsstrom, J., Karmakoski, J. and Kaarsalo, E. (1978). Oxolinic acid in the treatment of the urinary tract infection. *Curr. Ther. Res.*, 23, 376

551 Guyer, B. M. (1974). Drug profile: Prodoxol (oxolinic acid). *J. Int. Med. Res.*, 2, 458

552 Shimizu, M., Nakamura, S., Takase, Y. and Kurobe, N. (1975). Pipemidic acid: absorption, distribution and excretion. *Antimicrob. Agents Chemother.*, 7, 441

553 Humbert, G., Fillastre, J. P. and Leroy, A. (1976). Etude de l'élimination urinaire d'un nouvel antibactérien de synthèse, l'acide pipémidique, chez le sujet normal et l'insuffisant rénal. *Sem. Hop. Paris Thérapeutique*, 52, 32

554 Calabresi, P. and Parks, R. E. (1970). Alkylating agents, antimetabolites, hormones and other antiproliferative agents. In Goodman, L. S. and Gilman, A. (eds). *The Pharmacological Basis of Therapeutics*, pp. 1348–1395. (London: The Macmillan Company)

3

Peritoneal dialysis

D. G. Oreopoulos

Studies on the permeability of the peritoneal membrane and the factors which influence it[1] started as early as 1877, and a significant amount of information had accumulated before 1923 when Ganter[2] performed the first peritoneal dialysis (PD) on uraemic rabbits and later on a uraemic patient. Since this pioneer work, many investigators have studied PD and the technique has prolonged the lives of many renal failure patients. Those who wish a review of the early literature on PD are referred to Boen[3].

Although peritoneal dialysis was discovered long before haemodialysis, the significant morbidity and mortality associated with PD persuaded physicians to choose haemodialysis when it became available, despite its complexity and the need for specialized personnel. Subsequently, however, PD was rediscovered and became the object of renewed interest in the late 1950s and early 1960s. In 1964, Boen wrote a book[3] which firmly established the various applications of peritoneal dialysis in clinical medicine. In 1965, Weston and Roberts[4] introduced the 'acute' or stylet catheter, which made acute PD easy and safe. It is still in use. Perhaps the single most important development in the establishment of chronic PD was the introduction of the permanent peritoneal catheter, designed by Palmer[5] in 1964 and modified to its present form by Tenckhoff[6] in 1968. In 1971, Lasker[7] introduced his automatic peritoneal cycler which permitted the automation of PD, and, for the first time, made home PD feasible. In 1972, Tenckhoff et al.[8] introduced their reverse osmosis (RO) PD system, which not only increased the safety of the method but also lowered its cost to a level competitive with chronic haemodialysis. With permanent access to the peritoneal cavity secured and the automated devices available, chronic PD became an important adjunct in the treatment of end-stage renal disease, and experience at the Toronto Western Hospital[9,10] demonstrated the feasibility of long-term chronic intermittent PD. However, this enthusiasm apparently was not shared by most nephrologists; for example, in 1977 in the United States only a small percentage (2%) of chronic dialysis patients were maintained on chronic PD[11].

The next important step in the progress of chronic PD was the introduction in 1976 by Popovich and his colleagues[12] of the concept of continuous ambulatory peritoneal dialysis (CAPD). On the basis of peritoneal kinetics data, they predicted that five changes of 2-litre peritoneal dialysate a day, 7 days a week, would provide an excellent control of both small (urea, creatinine, etc.) and middle (inulin B_{12}, etc.) molecules. Clinical trials of this method confirmed these theoretical predictions and showed that this technique provided excellent biochemical control and several other advantages[13]. The obvious advantages of CAPD were overshadowed by three defects: cumbersome equipment and time-consuming technique, a high incidence of peritonitis (one episode every 10 patient weeks), and increased protein losses (13–20 g/day). The introduction of a new technique at the Toronto Western Hospital[14] in 1978 removed the first two disadvantages. Since then there has been a world-wide increase in interest in PD, and specifically in CAPD, and the number of patients treated on CAPD is increasing steadily. However, only the passage of time will show whether CAPD will become the treatment of choice for most patients requiring chronic dialysis.

PERITONEAL DIALYSIS TECHNIQUES

Acute (or stylet) peritoneal catheter

This catheter is now established as the device of choice for acute OD. It can be introduced into the peritoneal cavity at the bedside if it is done under strict sterile conditions. The patient is asked to empty his bladder and have a bowel movement. If constipated he should be given an enema. After preparation and draping of the abdomen, a point in the middle third of the space between the umbilicus and symphysis pubis is infiltrated with a local anaesthetic down to the peritoneum. Dialysate solution, 2–3 l, is introduced via a 14- or 15-gauge needle to distend the peritoneal cavity. This step is not always necessary, and instead the patient may be asked to 'blow up' his abdomen just before the catheter is introduced. The catheter is inserted through the skin and underlying fascia by applying firm pressure with a twisting motion. When the tip enters the peritoneal cavity, there is a sudden decrease in resistance and dialysis fluid appears in the catheter. The trocar is removed completely and the catheter is advanced as far as possible into the right (preferably) or left iliac fossa, or into the minor pelvis. The catheter is connected to the administration tubing through a connection tube and the dialysis fluid is drained from the abdomen to determine whether dialysis is feasible. If drainage is unsatisfactory, the catheter must be repositioned or replaced.

The first few exchanges may be blood-stained but they usually clear later. If it persists, occasionally bleeding will stop when pressure is applied around the catheter. If there is leakage of dialysis fluid around the catheter, a purse string suture in the skin around the catheter may prevent further leakage. If the dialysate does not drain easily, the patient may assist by changing position. If none of these measures helps, the catheter should be replaced through the same perforation or a new hole in one flank, preferably the left.

At the end of the procedure, the catheter is replaced by a Dean's prosthesis later if the patient will require more dialysis.

Complications of the acute peritoneal catheter

The principal complications of the acute peritoneal catheter are visceral perforations, namely bowel, bladder or aortic. After bowel perforation, the patient will experience severe pain and perhaps watery diarrhoea. At drainage time, the dialysate may contain faecal material. After bladder perforation, the patient may feel urgency, and, in aortic perforation, blood appears in the catheter and the patient may go into shock.

In most cases, removal of the catheter is sufficient to control the complication. Occasionally, when faecal peritonitis ensues, the patient should be dialysed through another abdominal hole. Surgical intervention is rarely necessary.

Dean's prosthesis

This device consists of a blunt-ended stem and a disc-shaped head; it maintains a permanent fistulous tract through the abdominal wall into the peritoneal cavity, which permits easy catheter replacement (Figure 1).

The prosthesis can stay in place until another dialysis is required.

Permanent peritoneal catheter

This catheter has been one of the main innovations in chronic PD and has contributed more than any other device to the establishment of chronic PD. Originally designed by Palmer, it was modified by Tenckhoff. The catheter, as it is supplied at present, is made of silastic Teflon at least 25 cm long. Two Dacron felt cuffs divide the structure into three parts: intra-abdominal, subcutaneous – between the two cuffs (approximately 9 cm), and the external part. The cuffs, through tissue ingrowth, stabilize the catheter and prevent leakage of dialysate and bacterial invasion along the subcutaneous tunnel.

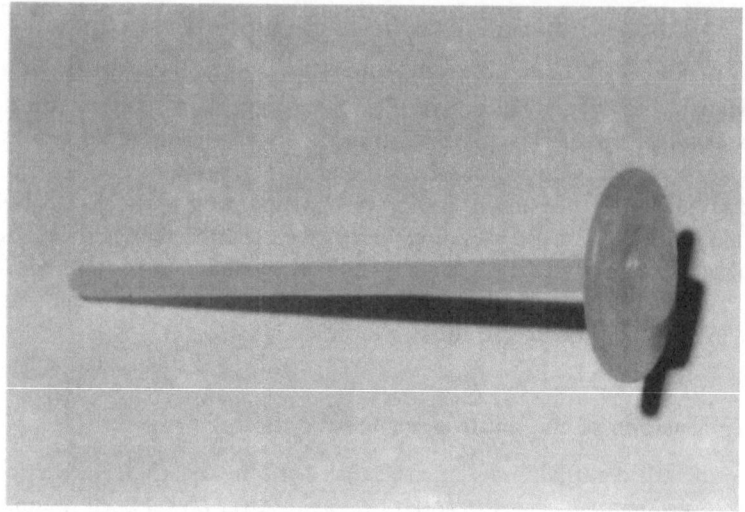

Figure 1 The Dean's prosthesis

The catheter can be implanted at the patient's bedside under local anaesthesia or in the operating room under general or local anaesthesia.

On the night before the insertion, the patient is given an enema, and, immediately before implantation, asked to empty his bladder. In addition, before implantation, we give 1 g of cephalothin and 1.5 mg/kg body weight of tobramycin intravenously.

Catheter implantation at the bedside is as follows. After preparation and draping, the abdomen is filled with dialysate to at least moderate distension, using either a No. 15 needle or the acute (stylet) catheter. After anaesthesia at the midline, a 2–3 cm skin incision is made 3–4 cm below the umbilicus, and the subcutaneous fat is dissected away to expose the fascia. The linea alba and peritoneum are then perforated with the special trocar, which is composed of a thin and a thick segment. The perforation is performed perpendicularly to the abdomen wall while the patient tightens his abdominal muscles. Often a small vertical stab into the fascia will facilitate trocar insertion.

After the thin segment of the trocar is introduced, the stylet is removed and the silicone rubber catheter with its obturator is introduced into the trocar. Once the catheter tip has entered the peritoneal cavity, the trocar is flattened cephaloid as far as possible, and then the catheter is gently advanced to the deeper pelvis, until the patient reports irritation of his bladder or rectum. If the catheter encounters resistance (probably due to entanglement with omentum), it is pulled back and reinserted at an even flatter angle.

Once the catheter is in place, the solid upper segment of the trocar is removed and its bivalve tip is split slightly; the two halves are then removed.

The catheter is checked, and, if it is patent, a subcutaneous tunnel is created. Once the exact skin exit site has been determined, the catheter is directed through the subcutaneous tunnel. The stab wound should be approximately 5 mm, since a narrow fit may lead to skin necrosis and a loose fit may lead to infection. The subcutaneous cuff should be 1 cm away from the skin. Dialysis should be instituted as soon as possible after catheter placement.

When the catheter is to be implanted surgically, a slightly larger incision is made to include the fascia and the peritoneum, and the catheter is implanted in the minor pelvis under vision. Following that, the peritoneum and the muscles are sewn around the first cuff and the catheter comes out through the subcutaneous tunnel as in the medical implantation. Again, dialysis starts immediately after implantation so that any problems will be detected early and solved immediately.

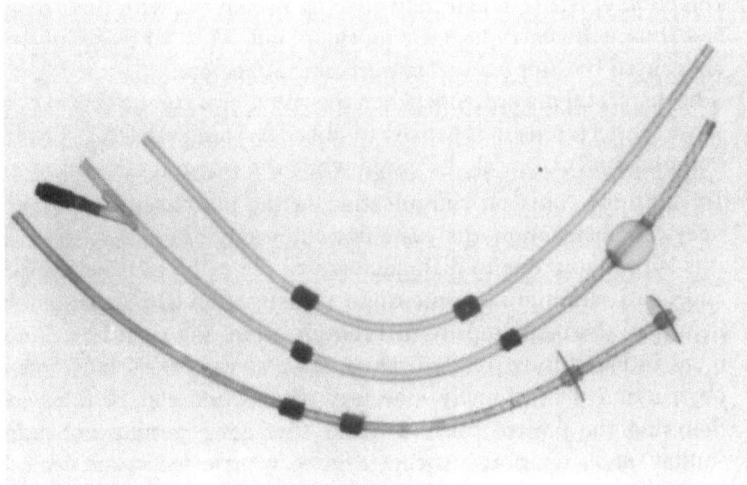

Figure 2 The three types of permanent peritoneal catheters: top – the Tenckhoff catheter; middle – the Goldberg catheter; bottom – the Toronto Western Hospital catheter

To avoid some of the complications associated with the permanent Tenckhoff catheter (described below), two new catheters have been introduced (Figure 2). The first, the Goldbert catheter, has a balloon in the middle of its intra-abdominal part which can be inflated from outside the body with 20 ml of saline to keep the omentum away from the catheter. This catheter is no longer in production. The second device, the Toronto Western Hospital catheter, has two discs made of silastic Teflon sheets (1 mm thick and 28 mm diameter) on its intra-abdominal part. In addition, the distance between the two cuffs is only 2.5 cm and the catheter comes straight out through a skin exit 1–2 cm away from the midline incision. Both of these catheters must be implanted in the operating room.

Table 1 shows some of the complications related to the permanent peritoneal catheter:

(1) Bloody effluent usually appears immediately after implantation and occasionally during the first exchange of chronic dialysis. It is benign and rarely leads to clotting.

(2) Abdominal pain is common during the first few weeks after catheter implantation, after prolonged use of concentrated dialysate solution and in certain patients using the RO machines (described below).

(3) Some patients may experience pain near the tip of the catheter during inflow when it is displaced from the pelvis to one of the hypochondria.

(4) Occasionally, a patient with subcutaneous leak may develop swelling of the abdominal wall, the penis or the scrotum. Usually, the leak seals off spontaneously if dialysis can be postponed for 7–10 days.

(5) Infection of the skin exit may develop in persons with poor hygiene and those who carry bacteria on their skin. Most of these infections are caused by *Staphylococcus aureus* or *S. epidermidis*.

(6) The distal cuff may extrude when the cuff is close to the skin exit, and, if the tunnel is long, it is usually followed by tunnel abscess. The latter complication can rarely be cured while the catheter is in place.

(7) In the most common complication of the permanent catheter, the one-way obstruction, dialysate flows in easily but cannot drain out; this is probably due to dislodgement of the catheter from the pelvis and/or its wrapping by omentum. Constipation and slight paralytic ileus may also contribute to this complication. Vigorous bowel movement induced by strong laxatives, such as castor oil, may free this obstruction. Occasionally, one-way obstruction can be relieved by dialysing the patient for 1–2 weeks through a permanent catheter (inflow) and a temporary catheter (outflow) inserted in one flank. Use of the Toronto Western Hospital catheter has a significantly lower frequency of this complication.

(8) Finally, permanent catheter obstruction may follow one-way obstruction or an episode of peritoneal infection, or it may develop *de novo*, especially in those who have a tendency to form fibrin clots. Addition of heparin to the dialysate and to the catheter between dialyses may prevent this complication. We usually give heparin at a concentration of 500 units per litre immediately after catheter implantation and continue it for 2 months. At the end of this period, we decrease heparin and eventually stop it if the patient is not forming macroscopic fibrin clots. At least 75% of patients can be dialysed without heparin. Fibrin clot formation is very common among the diabetic patients. In those patients who tend to form fibrin clots, we usually continue dialysing with heparin at an average concentration of 500 units per litre. In all patients, between dialyses, we instil 3 ml of

heparin solution (1000 units per ml) in the catheter and seal it with a rubber cap. If this is done under sterile conditions in the unit, it is usually sufficient to prevent clot formation in the catheter.

Recently, it has been reported that the use of 'Beta-Caps' (Quinton Company, Seattle) between dialyses reduces the incidence of peritonitis. In this system, the end of the catheter is filled up with an iodine solution (Betadine-Proviodine) and sealed with a cap that keeps the iodine solution in place. Despite this claim, I see no indication for their use.

Table 1 Complications related to the peritoneal catheter

Bloody effluent
Abdominal pain
Dialysate leakage
Infection of the skin exit
Extrusion of the distal (subcutaneous) cuff
Tunnel abscess
One-way obstruction
Permanent catheter obstruction

Automatic peritoneal dialysis machines

Cyclers

In Europe, where dialysate is available in 10-litre containers, a variety of simple cyclers are in use. In North America, the Lasker cycler, which is manufactured by American Medical Products Corporation, is used almost exclusively (Figure 3). This gravity-operated cycler retains all the simplicity of manual PD. It has a central pole with eight hooks from which an equal number of dialysate containers can be suspended, a heater box, a cycler, and a final drainage container which is used if a floor drain is not available. On its front, the cycler has two timers: one determines the duration of the 'fill cycle' (the time the fluid takes to run into the peritoneal cavity and stay in it), the other determines the duration of the 'drain cycle' (the time during which the fluid drains out of the peritoneal cavity). On one side of the cycler there is a special metal bar with four holders which accept four tubes. Two motor-driven T-shaped plungers move outwards or inwards and compress or release these tubes in pairs. The timers determine how long each plunger will compress a pair of these tubes. On the other side of the cycler, a counterbalanced scale monitors the volume of fluid draining from the peritoneal cavity.

The advantages of the Lasker cycler are that it is simple, noiseless, mobile, small, has a low initial capital cost, and its operation can be easily learned for home dialysis. However, its running costs are high because it uses commercial dialysate. In addition, because it is an open system, it is associated with a high rate of peritonitis (one episode per 300 dialyses).

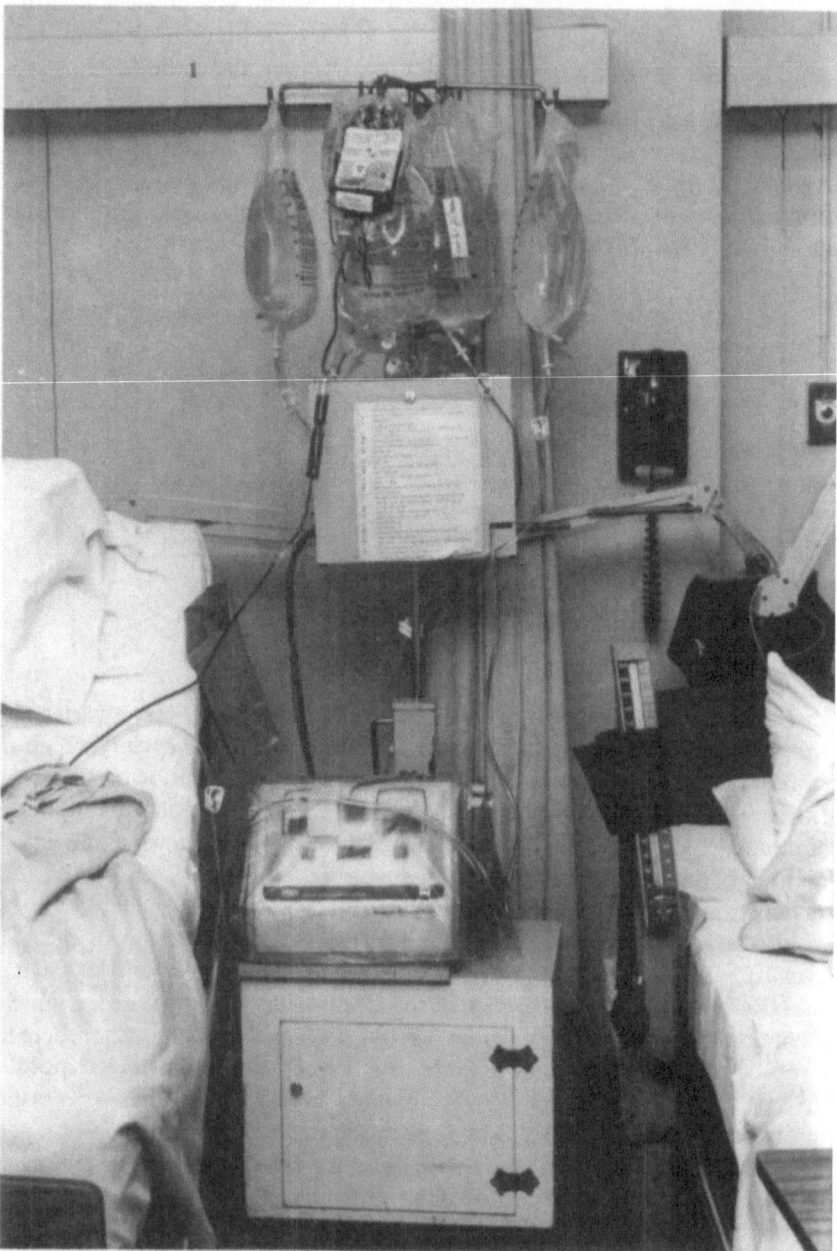

Figure 3   The Lasker-Automatic peritoneal catheter (American Medical Products Corporation)

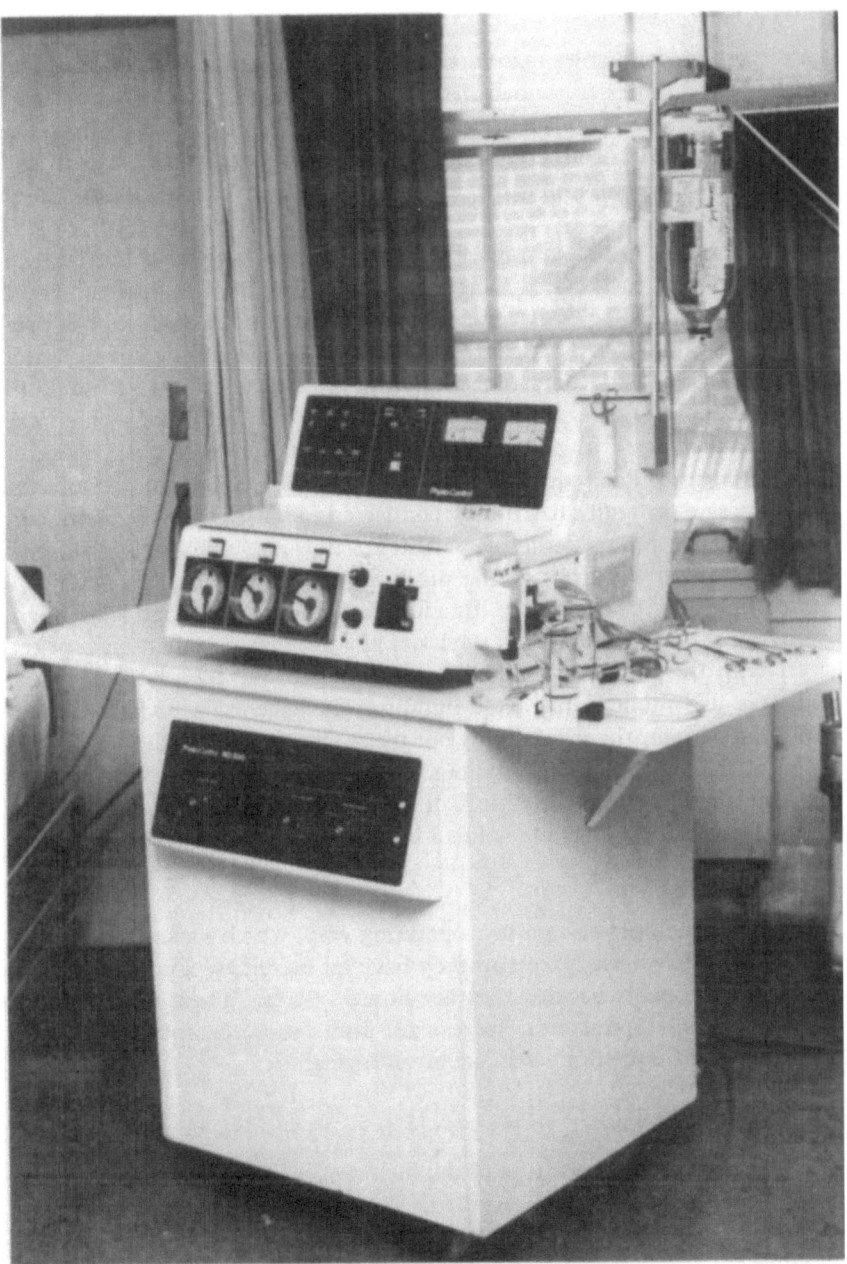

Figure 4   The 'Physio-Control' reverse osmosis peritoneal dialysis system

Reverse osmosis machines

Although two companies manufacture this type of machine, that in widest use in North America is manufactured by Physio-Control Company of Seattle (Figure 4). This device produces sterile, deionized water from tap water by passing it through a RO membrane. The integrity of the membrane is monitored by comparing the conductivity of the water before and after passage through it.

After it leaves the membrane, the sterile deionized water is passed over long ultraviolet light tubes which provide 'back-up' sterilization. From there, it is warmed to body temperature and stored in a reservoir. A proportioning pump mixes 19 parts of the warm, sterile and deionized water with one part of a concentrated solution of electrolytes and dextrose. This concentrated solution is available in two dextrose concentrations which will provide a dialysate with a final dextrose concentration of 1.5 g/100 ml or of 2.5 mg/100 ml. If it is required, additional dextrose can be pumped into the final dialysate through extra tubing connected to a 50% dextrose container. The dialysate is pumped into the patient at a flow rate of 200 or 400 ml/min. Three timers at the front of the machine control the infusion time, the 'dwell' time and the drain time. In addition, two monitors control dialysate temperature and conductivity; the latter ensures appropriate mixing of the water with the concentrate. The pressure inside the tube leading to the patient is also monitored to avoid pumping dialysate against a kinked tube. From the patient, the fluid drains out by gravity to a sump tank and from there to a floor drain. Other functions monitored are the power supply to the machine and UV lamp, the supply of water and changes in its quality.

Once a week, the machine is filled with a formaldehyde solution for 2.5 hours to sterilize it. After sterilization, the system is rinsed and can be used safely for a week.

The RO machines have a low operating cost, which makes them competitive with haemodialysis, and they have an extremely low incidence of peritonitis, probably because they are closed systems. Their disadvantages are high initial capital cost, large size, immobility, complex and noisy operation and frequent mechanical breakdowns.

Peritoneal dialysate

Table 2 shows the composition of the Baxter–Dianeal dialysate used at our hospital; it is available commercially in 2- or 3-litre plastic bags. Since most patients are slightly acidotic at this concentration, Tenckhoff recommended a higher concentration of lactate (38 mmol/l). Hypermagnesaemia is common in most of our patients, and some may reach serum levels of up to 2.5 mmol/l. The provision of a dialysate with a lower magnesium concentration may permit a more effective removal and hence prevent hypermagnesaemia.

During PD, most renal failure patients receive a potassium-free dialysate because the peritoneal membrane clears potassium slowly[15], and these patients have a tendency to hyperkalaemia. However, if a patient is receiving digitalis or digoxin, especially during the initial dialyses, potassium should be added to the dialysate to avoid sudden changes in serum potassium and prevent myocardial irritability and a potentially fatal arrhythmia. The dextrose concentration of the dialysate is either 1.5 or 4.25 g/100 ml. Higher dextrose concentrations confer no advantage and may even be dangerous because of the risk of hyperglycaemia, hyperosmolar coma and abdominal pain. A dextrose concentration of 1.5% is still hypertonic in comparison with plasma (320 mmol/l), and, even with this relatively low hypertonicity, certain patients may lose significant amounts of fluid. If these patients do not receive enough fluid by mouth or parenterally to replace that which is removed, we use a dialysate with a dextrose concentration of 0.5 g/100 ml. With the latter, the patient is actually gaining weight because this dialysate is hypotonic compared with the blood.

Table 2 Composition of Baxter–Dianeal solution employed by Toronto Western Hospital

	Concentration (mmol/l)
Na	132
Cl	101.5
Lactate	35
Ca	1.5
Mg	0.75

Peritoneal clearances

The peritoneal membrane has a surface area[16] of approximately 1 m², and it appears that only a small part of this area actively participates in dialysis. As a result, the peritoneum can clear urea from the blood stream at a rate of 20–30 ml/min and creatinine at a rate of 15–20 ml/min; these rates are only one-quarter to one-sixth of those obtained by haemodialysis[16]. Because of the peritoneal membrane's larger pore size, clearance of middle molecules – those with a molecular weight of 300–1500 daltons – like inulin, is significantly higher in PD (approximately 6 ml/min) than in haemodialysis (1 ml/min). Since we do not know which uraemic substances are responsible for the manifestations of uraemia, this more effective clearance of middle molecules may explain why patients on PD do as well as those on haemodialysis, despite higher levels in the former of small molecular weight substances, such as creatinine (see 'middle molecule theory')[17].

Hypertonic dialysate (4.25%) produces a higher clearance than an isotonic fluid (1.5%), a fact which can be only partially explained by the larger volume of fluid removed by 4.25% than by 1.5% dextrose dialysate. The increased extraction by the more concentrated solution has been attributed to a 'solvent-drag' effect exerted by the hypertonic dialysate, associated with ultrafiltration and an increase in peritoneal permeability[18].

The length of time during which the fluid stays in the peritoneal cavity (the 'dwell' or 'equilibration' time) also influences the concentration (or amount) of solutes removed; most of the solvent is removed during the first 10 min and thereafter there is only a small increase in concentration[19].

Initially, some workers were concerned that continuous irritation of the peritoneal membrane by the dialysate might lead to a decline in the peritoneal clearance[20]. However, serial measurements of peritoneal clearances for periods of up to 6 years in patients who had no or infrequent episodes of peritonitis showed no such decline[21]. Despite low peritoneal clearances, patients on chronic PD have biochemical values similar to those on chronic haemodialysis.

Factors that may increase or decrease peritoneal clearance are shown in Table 3.

Table 3 Factors affecting peritoneal clearances

Factors increasing:
  High dialysate temperature
  High flow rate of the dialysate
  Increase in the dialysate dextrose concentration
  Vasodilators added to the dialysate
  Albumin added to the dialysate
  Alternating hypertonic with hypotonic dialysate solution

Factors decreasing:
  Use of dialysate at room temperature
  Administration of vasoconstrictive agents
  Renal failure secondary to systemic or vascular disease (lupus, hypertension)
  Ileus
  Acute renal failure secondary to heat stress or exercise
  In men, a 'small abdominal cavity and tight muscular abdominal walls'

A dialysate temperature of 37 °C produces[22] a 35% greater clearance than a dialysate temperature of 20 °C. The higher the concentration gradient between blood and dialysate, the higher the peritoneal clearance. A higher concentration gradient can be achieved by using larger volumes of dialysate or by inducing more rapid exchange. However, dialysate volume above 2 l is impractical and flow rates above 4 l/h are painful and produce little further increase[19].

Hypertonic dialysate increases[18] peritoneal clearance because it removes greater volumes of fluid and also because it exerts a 'solvent drag'. The addition of vasodilators to the dialysate has only a small effect on the peritoneal clearance apart from nitroprusside[23] which, at a concentration of 5 mg/l, increases the average extraction by approximately 20%. Nitroprusside has a greater effect on large molecules, such as albumin, than on the small ones. Finally, the addition of albumin to the dialysate will increase the clearance of protein-bound substances, such as calcium, bilirubin, salicylates and barbiturates.

Factors which may decrease peritoneal clearance include use of a dialysate at room temperature (20°C) and the systemic administration of vasoconstrictive agents. For example, antidiuretic hormone, a vasoconstrictive agent, leads to a fall in the peritoneal membrane area (consistent with a decreasing splanchnic blood flow) and an increase in mean pore radius[24]. Patients with collagen vascular disease, systemic arterial hypertension and paralytic ileus show a similar selective reduction in the clearance of high molecular weight solutes, suggesting that they have suffered a selective reduction in the permeability of peritoneal capillaries or mesothelium[25].

Peritoneal dialysis requirements

Most patients require 40 h of dialysis per week, usually as two periods of 20 h or four periods of 10 h. DeSanto and his colleagues[26] have reported excellent results with daily 'short' dialyses with 10 l of dialysate each night.

Patients who have an endogenous creatinine clearance of 3–5 ml/min may be maintained in good health with only 30 h of PD each week.

To compensate for serum proteins lost in the dialysate, we recommend a diet supplement of 60–80 g of protein/day.

A significant percentage of patients (20–30%) form fibrin clots in the dialysate which threaten the survival of the permanent catheter. Heparin added to the dialysate will prevent these clots.

Table 4 Drug removal by peritoneal dialysis

	Drugs removed by peritoneal dialysis	*Drugs not removed by peritoneal dialysis*
(a) Antimicrobial agents	5-fluorocytosine, isoniazid, amikacin, gentamicin, tobramycin, kanamycin, cephalothin, cephalexin, colistin, sulfisoxazole	cefamandole, chloramphenicol, clindamycin, erythromycin, lincomycin, ampicillin, carbenicillin, penicillin-G, methicillin, nafcillin, quinine, tetracycline, doxycycline, vancomycin
(b) Analgesics	aspirin	acetaminophen, methadone, propoxyphene
(c) Sedatives	phenobarbital, ethchlorvynol, lithium carbonate, meprobamate, glutethimide	pentobarbital, secobarbital, chlorpromazine, amitriptyline, imipramine, nortriptyline
(d) Cardiovascular agents	quinidine, diazoxide, methyldopa, nitroprusside	hydralazine, reserpine, digoxin, digitoxin
(e) Miscellaneous	diphenylhydantoin	chlorpropamide

Peritoneal dialysis and drugs

Table 4 lists those drugs which are and are not removed by PD[27]. Knowledge of this list is important so that if a patient on PD is receiving any of the drugs that are removed by PD, its dose can be adjusted upward while he is on dialysis.

If a patient is suffering from overdose of any of the drugs that move freely through the peritoneal membrane, PD may be considered for treatment, although haemodialysis and haemoperfusion give better results. Addition of various substances to the dialysate, such as albumin, lipid, THAM and the use of hypertonic solutions, may enhance removal of poisons.

Acute peritoneal dialysis

Peritoneal dialysis is adequate for the treatment of most patients with acute renal failure and this constitutes the major indication for acute PD. Table 5 shows some other indications for acute peritoneal dialysis:

(a) Severe intractable congestive heart failure: in these patients large amounts of fluid can be removed over 24–48 h.

(b) Internal haemorrhage: heparinization of haemodialysis may be hazardous so PD is safer.

(c) Peritonitis after bowel perforation, either before or after operation: patients may benefit from continuous lavage with fluid containing antibiotics.

(d) Pancreatitis: large amounts of amylase can be removed by PD.

(e) Hypercalcaemia or hyperuricaemia: in these cases, temporary control of hypercalcaemia is important, especially if treatment of the under-lying disease has been started and one expects this to control the hypercalcaemia. Since most dialysis solutions contain calcium, one can make a solution by mixing

$NaHCO_3$ (7%)	75 ml
2/3 + 1/3 (Dextrose–Saline)	1000 ml
NaCl (0.9 g/100 ml)	1000 ml
Dextrose 50%	50 ml

This mixture will contain

HCO_3	35 mmol/l
Na	135 mmol/l
Cl	100 mmol/l
Dextrose	12.5 g/l

(f) Severe hypothermia: here one can raise the temperature with warm dialysate during PD.

(g) Few investigators believe that PD has any place in the treatment of hepatorenal syndrome.

(h) Other conditions, such as Reye's syndrome, hyaline membrane disease of the newborn, oxalosis, cystinosis and leucinosis, but little is known concerning its precise role in these conditions.

Table 5 Indications for acute peritoneal dialysis

Acute renal failure
Severe intractable congestive heart failure
Patients with internal haemorrhage (brain trauma or surgery, pericarditis) requiring dialysis
Patients with unstable cardiovascular system requiring dialysis
Faecal peritonitis
Hypercalcaemia
Acute uric acid nephropathy
Hypothermia
Other: Reye's syndrome, hyaline membrane disease of the newborn, oxalosis, cystinosis, leucinosis, lactic acidosis

Contraindications to acute PD include hypercatabolism with acute renal failure, recent abdominal surgery and shock. In the first case, peritoneal removal of urea and potassium cannot usually keep pace with production. However, the only way to find out whether PD will be adequate is to start PD and follow the BUN and serum K levels daily. If these levels increase despite dialysis, this method should be stopped and the patient transferred to haemodialysis. Similarly, after recent abdominal surgery, dialysate leakage through the drains or the incision may threaten fluid balance, make skin care difficult and set the stage for infection. Finally, in incipient shock, the peritoneal clearance of small molecules, which depends on blood flow rates, is low and will decrease even further if vasoconstrictive agents are used.

Chronic peritoneal dialysis

The contribution of chronic PD to treatment of end-stage renal disease varies from country to country. In the United States, in 1977, only 2% of the total dialysis population were maintained on PD, but, in the same year in Canada, 16% of the patients were on PD. In the city of Toronto, this figure was 55%.

Home dialysis, which is one of the most important indications for PD, can be learned by almost any patient (Table 6). In contrast to the long training period needed to prepare a patient for home haemodialysis, PD can be learned in 10–15 dialysis days. Although the cost of home peritoneal dialysis is higher than that of home haemodialysis, it is competitive with the cost of hospital haemodialysis.

Whereas home haemodialysis requires a selected population, home PD can be performed by patients living alone and with limited living space, and by those living with relatives who may be unwilling or unable to help. Home PD imposes little strain on the relatives.

Table 6   Indications for chronic peritoneal dialysis

For home dialysis
Diabetics with renal failure
Patients over 60 years of age
Patients with unstable cardiovascular system
Patients without vascular access
Patients who prefer PD
Patients awaiting kidney transplant or fistula maturation

It is an important advantage of PD that the patient can sleep while dialysing overnight; this feature partially offsets the disadvantages of the long dialysis time required with this method.

Peritoneal dialysis is indicated in diabetics with renal failure. Because of generalized atherosclerosis, it is often difficult in these patients to achieve vascular access for haemodialysis, and, in addition, PD avoids heparinization which, in some diabetic patients on haemodialysis, may precipitate blindness. Although no controlled study has been done, experience to date suggests that progression to blindness during chronic PD is rare, whereas the literature contains several reports of patients who have become blind on haemodialysis. However, once established, neuropathy and vascular calcifications tend to progress on PD. For these reasons, it is our policy to start PD earlier in diabetics than in non-diabetics (i.e. when serum creatinine is 5–6 mg/100 ml).

Older patients, especially if cardiovascular function is unstable, seem to tolerate PD better than haemodialysis. The peritoneal route also offers many advantages to children and should be considered in their treatment. In addition, despite the advances being made in the technology of vascular access, patients will be encountered who do not have suitable vessels for haemodialysis, and, in these patients, PD is indicated absolutely. Finally, patients who require dialysis for a short period only, for example while awaiting kidney transplantation, can be maintained equally well with either haemodialysis or peritoneal dialysis.

All the indications noted in the foregoing paragraphs refer to chronic intermittent PD, but this picture will probably change with the introduction of continuous ambulatory peritoneal dialysis – CAPD (described later). This technique of dialysis is more efficient than intermittent PD, and, in time, will be preferred for almost all patients on chronic PD at home. In addition, because of its many advantages, CAPD may replace chronic haemodialysis in a significant number of patients[28].

COMPLICATIONS OF PERITONEAL DIALYSIS

The complications of PD can be divided into acute (during the dialysis) and chronic. The acute complications include those related to the catheter (described earlier) and those related to dialysis. The chronic include: abdominal or shoulder pain, dehydration, hypokalaemia, disequilibration syndrome, overheating of dialysate and peritonitis.

Abdominal pain

This may be the dominant symptom in patients on the RO machine, and is usually due to infusion of dialysate under pressure. Some workers have proposed the use of a pressure dampener to eliminate this complaint[29]. Such pain usually disappears spontaneously after 6–8 weeks on dialysis. Prolonged use of dialysate with a high concentration of dextrose may also induce an abdominal pain which may mimic peritonitis – a complication which must be excluded each time a patient complains of abdominal pain.

Shoulder pain

This is probably due to diaphragmatic irritation. It is rarely serious, responds to oral analgesics, and disappears after the end of dialysis.

Dehydration

This may be induced by the use of large volumes of 4.25% dextrose dialysate particularly early in the course of treatment, before the therapist has established the pattern of the patient's fluid removal. This complication can be handled easily by oral or intravenous administration of fluids. The common consequences of excessive fluid removal are hypotension and muscle cramps, and certain patients may develop transient hypertension.

Hypokalaemia. This may develop in patients dialysed for long periods with potassium-free dialysate and may be particularly hazardous in those on digitalis or digoxin. If dialysis is planned for more than 24 h, potassium should be added to the dialysate in concentrations of 2–4 mmol/l.

Disequilibration syndrome. This is a very rare complication of PD and results from oedema of the brain when the solute concentrations in the cerebrospinal fluid cannot keep pace with the rapid changes in blood solutes such as urea.

Overheating of dialysate. This has become a serious risk since the introduction of automatic machines. As soon as the patient complains that the dialysate is hot, it should be drained out as quickly as possible. The abdominal pain associated with this complication may persist for a few days. One of our patients, after exposure to 2 l of overheated dialysate, had increased bowel sounds for a time and developed paralytic ileus which lasted for 5 days. After the paralytic ileus resolved and normal bowel motility returned, the patient developed severe metabolic acidosis and respiratory failure from which she recovered completely.

Peritonitis

This is the most important acute complication associated with PD. At the Toronto Western Hospital[9], its incidence among patients dialysed in hospital is low – 0.2% of all dialyses performed, but, among home dialysis patients served by this hospital, the incidence is higher – 0.3%. Clinical peritonitis is characterized by abdominal pain, cloudy effluent and rebound tenderness. In addition, some patients may have fever, vomiting or ileus, but these symptoms are not always present.

In addition to bacterial peritonitis, we have encountered a number of patients with aseptic peritonitis. These episodes can be divided into three groups: those due to the presence of endotoxin in the dialysate; those due to dialysate of a low pH; and those that show no growth of organisms because they are receiving concurrent antibiotics. On one occasion, at this hospital, the presence of endotoxin in the dialysate gave rise to an epidemic (48 episodes among 28 patients) of abdominal pain, cloudy fluid with many leukocytes, and mild fever, but no rigors[30]. Dialysate of abnormally low pH can also mimic peritonitis.

No agreement has been reached concerning the significance of positive cultures of ascitic fluid in the patient who has no symptoms. Some workers suggest that it indicates occult infection and that it heralds permanent obstruction of the catheter[31]. However, when we reviewed 78 patients, 11 of whom had episodes of permanent catheter obstruction, we found that only four episodes had been preceded by asymptomatic positive bacterial culture.

Management of peritonitis

The optimal treatment of peritonitis in PD patients is still uncertain, and methods in current use include prolonged lavage with intraperitoneal (IP) antibiotics or continuation of PD with IP antibiotics. It may be unnecessary to continue IP administration of antibiotics once effluent cultures have become negative, and some units recommend conversion to oral antibiotic therapy at this time. In March 1980 we changed our policy in the treatment of peritonitis from prolonged lavage with antibiotics to brief lavage without antibiotics followed by PD with added antibiotics. The details of this protocol are as follows: once the diagnosis of peritonitis is established, the PD tubing is changed and the adapter and distal end of the catheter are immersed in Proviodine for 15 minutes. Thereafter, three exchanges (preferably using 1.5% Dianeal) are instilled and drained as fast as possible, without the addition of antibiotics. Exchanges are then performed every 6 hours. The first exchange contains 1.7 mg/kg body weight of tobramycin, 1000 mg of cephalothin and 1000 units of heparin per 2 litres; each subsequent exchange contains 16 mg of tobramycin, 500 mg of cephalothin and 1000 units of heparin per 2 litres. Tobramycin and cephalothin should not be mixed in the same syringe but can be safely mixed in the same dialysate bag. The resolution of peritonitis should be monitored clinically, by daily effluent cultures and by serial effluent white cell counts. We have found the latter to be a very valuable diagnostic tool – 'normal' effluents contain up to 50 cells/mm^3 and in the presence of peritonitis counts range from 100 to several thousand/mm^3. With effective treatment they fall to normal levels within a few days. We do not give phosphate binders or other constipating drugs during the treatment of peritonitis and we usually stop treatment 7 days after the first negative culture. This protocol may need to be modified for (a) fungal, (b) tuberculous, (c) 'surgical' or multiple organism peritonitis or (d) tunnel abscess or severe exit site infection.

In a study comparing the first 12 patients treated as above with 12 patients treated by prolonged lavage we found that there was a trend towards more rapid bacteriological and clinical resolution in the group treated by brief lavage followed by PD with added antibiotics. We concluded that treatment of peritonitis by PD with IP antibiotics is at least as effective and certainly less costly in terms of hospital stay, nursing time and dialysis solutions, as treatment by prolonged lavage with IP antibiotics. The apparent clinical benefit may be explained by the fact that the low pH and high osmolality of dialysate (Dianeal) inhibits the phagocytic and bactericidal defences of the peritoneum. During lavage, the peritoneum and its polymorphonuclear cells are repeatedly exposed to fresh dialysate which has a low pH and a high osmolality whereas, with PD, the prolonged dwell time allows both pH and osmolality to reach an equilibrium with blood. This equilibrium allows the peritoneal defence mechanisms to work in conjunction with the added antibiotics. We still employ a brief period of lavage without antibiotics, which seems to produce some clinical improvement, possibly by removing inflammatory products such as histamine and serotonin which may be responsible for the abdominal pain seen in peritonitis.

We have now treated 30 patients by this technique. The outcome has been satisfactory with continuation of PD in all, although two patients have required catheter reimplantation due to concurrent severe exit site infection. We have not found it necessary to use parenteral antibiotics in the treatment of peritonitis as the combination of cephalothin and tobramycin given intra-peritoneally is effective in the treatment of the majority of episodes of peritonitis. If loading and maintenance doses of tobramycin are given as suggested above, then adequate serum levels can be rapidly reached and maintained. Even when tobramycin therapy is discontinued, adequate bactericidal levels are maintained for several days. The need for prolonged IP antibiotics once effluent cultures are negative is uncertain, and we have previously shown that oral cephalosporins, given 30 minutes prior to CAPD exchanges, give adequate blood and effluent levels. It may then be feasible to give oral antibiotics once the effluent cultures have become negative and this would further reduce inpatient stay.

Patients who develop paralytic ileus (absent bowel sounds) must fast, and we usually give an intravenous infusion of albumin to replace the protein losses which are increased by the peritonitis. If the patient can eat, he is given extra amounts of protein.

In the presence of clinical peritonitis, we continue to dialyse until three to four consecutive daily cultures have been negative. On rare occasions, the dialysate culture remains positive, or, after transient improvement, becomes positive again. These cases represent one of the following possibilities: chronic contamination of the catheter, intraperitoneal abscess formation, and bowel perforation. The last should be suspected if cultures of dialysate yield anaerobic organisms. In our experience, bowel perforation is often secondary to faecal impaction following heavy ingestion of antacids, especially those combining aluminium hydroxide and calcium carbonate.

The incidence of peritonitis can be decreased if PD is carried out in a separate unit by trained personnel, and especially by using the closed RO system.

Chronic complications of peritoneal dialysis

Renal osteodystrophy

Hyperphosphataemia is a frequent finding because PD gives poor control of phosphorus levels[32]. As a result, the osteitis form of renal osteodystrophy is also common, and, probably for the same reason, these patients have a high incidence of vascular calcification and soft-tissue (including articular) calcification. The latter can produce a variety of rheumatological complaints which present chiefly as gout or pseudogout. Commonly, the hyperparathyroidism is progressive and difficult to treat with vitamin D or its analogues because of the presence of hyperphosphataemia. Often these patients require parathyroidectomy.

Recently, we reported that the osteomalacic form of renal osteodystrophy was rare among PD patients[33], but we have since encountered several patients who developed osteomalacia and pseudofractures. This syndrome is most common among patients following total parathyroidectomy or those receiving anticonvulsants and barbiturates.

Uraemic neuropathy

Contrary to an earlier view that patients on chronic PD do not develop neuropathy, we have seen four patients who developed severe neuropathy while on chronic PD and several others who showed minimal progression of this symptom[34]. Two of our patients developed dementia similar to that described after chronic haemodialysis and both died.

Anaemia

This finding is common among patients on chronic peritoneal dialysis and some will require transfusions. Occasionally, they receive benefit from treatment with androgenic steroid.

Constipation and bowel perforation secondary to faecal impaction

Chronic constipation is a serious problem in these patients because they receive large amounts of antacids in an attempt to control hyperphosphataemia, and a serious complication of this chronic constipation is bowel perforation due to faecal impaction. The physician should avoid combined administration of aluminium hydroxide and calcium carbonate, especially in patients with polycystic kidneys, because four of our six patients who perforated had polycystic kidneys[35].

Pericarditis

Pericarditis is almost as common in PD patients as it is among those on chronic haemodialysis, but tamponade is uncommon[36].

Renal stones

Four patients on chronic PD who had chronic glomerulonephritis formed small recurrent calcium oxalate stones. Although the concentration of calcium in their urine was low, it was supersaturated with calcium oxalate.

Hypertriglyceridaemia

This state, which may predispose to accelerated cardiovascular disease, has been reported[37] in patients on chronic PD. However, others[38] have not been able to confirm this.

Sexual function

The effect of chronic PD on sexual function has not been studied extensively, mainly because most of these patients are elderly. The presence of the catheter may occasionally inhibit the partner, but, on most occasions, sexual intercourse is feasible and painless. Many of the younger female patients menstruate, but the use of contraceptives is probably unnecessary because pregnancy has never been reported.

PERITONEAL DIALYSIS AND HEPATITIS

If the patient's blood is positive for Australia antigen, the dialysate effluent will also be positive[39] and hence the nurses handling it will be exposed to hepatitis. For this reason, the fluid should be drained directly into a floor drain, and the cycler, which operates with disposable tubing, should be preferred to the RO machines. Whenever possible, these patients should be trained for home dialysis.

PERITONEAL DIALYSIS IN DIABETICS

In the treatment of diabetics in end-stage renal failure, PD may have an advantage over haemodialysis because diabetic retinopathy, which seems to progress in patients on haemodialysis, does not progress during chronic PD. However, once established, other complications, such as neuropathy and vascular calcifications, usually progress.

During PD, blood sugar can be controlled by intraperitoneal insulin administration in addition to the patient's regular insulin requirements. Usually, we start with 4–6 units of crystalline insulin per litre of 1.5% dextrose and 8–10 units per litre of 4.25% dextrose. Then, after each blood sugar measurement, every 6 h during the first few days, the dose of insulin is individualized for each patient. The insulin should be omitted from the last four or five exchanges to avoid postdialysis hypoglycaemia.

The prognosis of diabetics on PD is significantly worse than that of non-diabetics, chiefly because of a high incidence of cardiovascular death and progression of diabetic complications – we had only a 44% 1-year survival among 31 diabetic patients. It is now our policy to start these patients on PD much earlier than we start non-diabetics, that is when serum creatinine is 5–6 mg/100 ml, and thus we hope to anticipate the diabetic complications. In addition, maintaining a tight blood sugar control (fasting and post-prandial blood sugar levels below 200 mg/100 ml) may be important in preventing the progression of these complications.

PERITONEAL DIALYSIS AND TRANSPLANTATION

During the years 1976 and 1977, we performed kidney transplants in 70 patients who were maintained on chronic PD. In 36 of these, PD was continued for some time after transplantation, usually in the early stages. In these patients, the concurrent use of immunosuppressive treatment did not increase the incidence of peritonitis. Seventeen patients with transplanted kidneys had to be returned to PD after nephrectomy. Comparison of the results of transplantation between patients maintained on haemodialysis and those maintained on PD showed no significant differences[40]. Those who suffer from ureteral reflux or have polycystic kidneys require nephrectomy before transplantation. They are usually maintained on haemodialysis for 2–3 weeks after the operation. However, because the residual kidney function makes a significant contribution to the patient's well-being, the nephrectomy should be performed immediately before the transplantation.

PERITONEAL DIALYSIS AND HAEMODIALYSIS

A successful haemodialysis programme makes an important contribution to the success of peritoneal dialysis. Haemodialysis may be required temporarily – for example, when the catheter must be removed, as in the presence of persistent or fungal peritonitis or in case of abdominal operations. Haemodialysis may be required permanently – for example, when the peritoneal clearance has decreased significantly and PD can no longer maintain life. In certain centres, nephrologists prefer to create an AV fistula in all patients on chronic PD so that, whenever haemodialysis is required, vascular access is available at once. We have found this to be unnecessary because we can perform acute haemodialysis for as long as 3–4 months through the subclavian route using the catheter developed by Uldall and his colleagues[41].

HOME PERITONEAL DIALYSIS

Since the introduction of CAPD, most patients who are candidates for home PD should be maintained on it. Exceptions are those who have specific contraindications for this technique, such as patients with lumbar disc protrusion, hypertriglyceridaemia, recurrent peritonitis and loss of ultrafiltration capacity.

CONTINUOUS AMBULATORY PERITONEAL DIALYSIS

Popovich *et al.*[12] introduced CAPD in 1976. Its advantages include efficiency in removing small and middle molecules; efficient removal of sodium, potassium and water; excellent control of hypertension and anaemia; low cost; and a significant psychological improvement resulting from independence from the machine and a limited number of dietary or fluid restrictions.

However, until recently, these advantages were overshadowed by three major disadvantages, namely, the high incidence of peritonitis, the cumbersome and time-consuming nature of the technique, and the high rate of protein losses (10 or 20 mg/day). The last flaw can probably be overcome by an increased protein intake. The first two difficulties have been solved with the introduction of a new technique (the Toronto Western Hospital technique for CAPD) which has made CAPD simpler and safer[14].

Technique for CAPD

For this technique the dialysate must be in plastic bags (Baxter–Dianeal). The permanent peritoneal catheter is connected to the bags through simple plastic tubing with appropriate spikes at each end. After the dialysate has run into the peritoneal cavity, the empty bag, still connected to the tubing, is folded and carried under the patient's clothes in a cloth waist-pocket. After 6 h, the patient drains the dialysate into the same plastic bag, removes the spike from the used bag and connects it to the fresh one. Most patients tolerate dialysate at room temperature. If the patient has to use hypertonic dialysate, the volume of ultrafiltration will exceed the capacity of the 2-litre bags, hence we underfill 3-litre bags with 2 litres of dialysate. If these are not available, the patient has to use extra sterile drainage bags.

Table 7   Complications among 66 patients on CAPD

Cardiovascular	
Hypotension	31
Dizziness	11
Oedema	17
Atrial fibrillation	2
Pericarditis	1
Impaired blood supply – legs (gangrene in two)	4
Gastrointestinal	
Nausea and vomiting	11
Poor appetite (transient)	5
Deterioration in haemorrhoids	4
Rectal prolapse	2
Constipation	5
Musculoskeletal	
Arthritis	16
Back pain	14
Cramps	11
Cutaneous	
Skin-exit site infections	15
Pruritus	10
Dermatitis	6
Dialysate leak	3
Miscellaneous	
Tiredness	10
Insomnia	4

Most of the patients exchange four bags a day, 7 days a week. If, on this scheme, the serum creatinine remains below 13 mg/100 ml, the patients are advised to exchange three bags a day (every 8 hours). If, on the other hand, with this scheme, the serum creatinine rises above 17 mg/100 ml, the patient is advised to have five exchanges a day.

On the four exchanges a day, the intervals between exchanges are 2×6 hours, 4 hours and 8 hours, the last interval being timed to allow uninterrupted sleep.

Table 7 shows the complications that may be encountered in patients on CAPD. Most of them can be handled and the patients do not have to interrupt CAPD. To date, our experience suggests that lumbar-disc protrusion is the main contraindication to CAPD.

At this hospital, the infection rate has been one episode every 8.9 patient months in an unselected population. Since a few patients had two or three episodes of peritonitis, and since these infections were probably due to incorrect technique, we believe that results in patients selected for CAPD will be much better. The severity of peritonitis varies from a mild form, with cloudy fluid and mild abdominal tenderness, to severe inflammation, with abdominal tenderness, fever, vomiting, pain and ileus. This variability may be related to the host defences or to the length of time which passes between the appearance of symptoms and the beginning of treatment. As soon as they develop unusual abdominal pain accompanied by cloudy fluid, our patients are directed to take a sample for a gram stain and to start immediately on a combination of cephalosporins and tobramycin which will control both Gram-negative and Gram-positive organisms.

If a patient with peritonitis is very sick, he is admitted to hospital and treated as described earlier. If the symptoms are mild, he can continue on CAPD with the addition of appropriate antibiotics to the dialysate for a total of 10 days.

We believe that once the incidence of peritonitis is brought down to one episode every 16–18 months, the many advantages of CAPD will establish this method as the treatment of choice for the majority of patients requiring chronic dialysis.

References

1 Wegner, G. (1877). Chirurgische Bemerkungen über die Peritonealhöhle, mit besonderer Berücksichtigung der ovariotomie. *Arch. Klin. Chir.*, **20**, 51
2 Ganter, G. (1923). Ueber die Beseitigung giftiger stroffe aus dem Blute durch Dialyse. *Münch. Med. Wochschr.*, **70-11**, 1478
3 Boen, S. T. (1964) *Peritoneal Dialysis in Clinical Medicine*. (Springfield, Ill.: Charles C. Thomas)
4 Weston, R. E. and Roberts, M. (1965). Clinical use of stylet-catheter for peritoneal dialysis. *Arch. Intern. Med.*, **115**, 659
5 Palmer, R. A., Quinton, W. E. and Gray, J. E. (1964). Prolonged peritoneal dialysis for chronic renal failure. *Lancet*, **1**, 700
6 Tenckhoff, H. and Schechter, H. (1968). A bacteriologically safe peritoneal access device. *Trans. Am. Soc. Artif. Intern. Organs*, **14**, 181
7 Lasker N. (1971). Chronic peritoneal dialysis. *Pennsylvania Med.*, **74**, 67
8 Tenckhoff, H., Meston, D. and Shilipetar, G. (1972). A simplified automatic peritoneal dialysis system. *Trans. Am. Soc. Artif. Intern. Organs*, **18**, 436
9 Karanicolas, S., Oreopoulos, D. G., Pylypchuk, G., Fenton, S. S. A., Cattran, D. C., Rapoport, A. and deVeber, G. A. (1977). Home peritoneal dialysis: three years' experience in Toronto. *Can. Med. Assoc. J.*, **116**, 266

10 Oreopoulos, D. G. (1977). The coming of age of home peritoneal dialysis (Editorial). *Can. Med. Assoc. J.*, **116**, 232

11 Friedman, E. A., Delano, B. G. and Butt, K. M. H. (1978). Pragmatic realities in uremia therapy. *N. Engl. J. Med.*, **298**, 368

12 Popovich, R. P., Moncrief, J. W., Dechard, J. B., Bomar, J. B. and Pyle, W. K. (1976). The d efinition of a novel portable/wearable equilibrium peritoneal dialysis technique. *Abstr. Am. Soc. Artif. Intern. Organs*, **5**, 64

13 Popovich, R. P., Moncrief, J. W., Nolph, K. D., Gjods, A. J., Twatdowsky, A. J. and Pyle, W. K. (1978). Continuous ambulatory peritoneal dialysis. *Ann. Intern. Med.*, **88**, 449

14 Oreopoulos, D. G., Robson, M., Izatt, S., Clayton, S. and deVerber, G. A. (1978). A simple and safe technique for continuous ambulatory peritoneal dialysis. *Trans. Am. Soc. Artif. Intern. Organs*, **24**, 484

15 Brown, S. T., Ahearn, D. J. and Nolph, K. D. (1973). Potassium removal with peritoneal dialysis. *Kidney Int.*, **4**, 67

16 Henderson, L. W. (1973). The problem of peritoneal membrane area and permeability. *Kidney Int.*, **3**, 409

17 Babb, A. L., Farrell, P. C. and Uveli, D. A. (1972). Hemodialyzer evaluation by examination of solute molecular septra. *Trans. Am. Soc. Artif. Intern. Organs*, **18**, 98

18 Henderson, L. W. (1966). Peritoneal ultrafiltration dialysis enhanced urea transfer using hypertonic peritoneal dialysis fluid. *J. Clin. Invest.*, **45**, 950

19 Robson, M., Oreopoulos, D. G., Izatt, S., Ogilvie, R., Rapoport, A. and deVeber, G. A. (1978). The influence of exchange volume and dialysate flow-rate on solute clearances in peritoneal dialysis. *Kidney Int.*, **14**, 486

20 Finkelstein, F. O., Klinger, A. S., Bastle, C. and Yap, P. (1977). Sequential clearance and dialysance measurements in chronic peritoneal dialysis patients. *Nephrology*, **18**, 342

21 Tenckhoff, H. (1974). Peritoneal dialysis today: a new look. *Nephron*, **12**, 420

22 Miller, R. B. and Tassistro, C. R. (1969). Peritoneal dialysis. *N. Engl. J. Med.*, **281**, 945

23 Nolph, K. D. M., Ghods, A. J., Brown, P., Vanstone, J., Miller, F. N., Weigmann, D. L. and Harris, P. D. (1977). Factors affecting peritoneal dialysis efficiency. *Dial. Transplant.*, **6**, 52

24 Henderson, L. W. and Kintzel, J. E. (1971). Influence of antidiuretic hormone on peritoneal membrane area and permeability. *J. Clin. Invest.*, **50**, 2437

25 Nolph, K. D. M., Stoltz, M. L. and Maher, J. F. (1971). Altered peritoneal permeability in patient with systemic fasculitis. *Ann. Intern. Med.*, **75**, 753

26 DeSanto, N. G., Cirillo, D., Senatore, R., Cicchetti, T., Manzo, M., Capasso, G. and Giordano, C. (1978). Comparing schedules of daily peritoneal dialysis. *J. Dial.*, **2**, 311

27 Bennett, W. M., Singer, I., Golper, T., Feig, P. and Goggins, C. J. (1977). Guidelines for drug therapy in renal failure. *Ann. Intern. Med.*, **86**, 754

28 Oreopoulos, D. G., Robson, M., Faller, B., Ogilvie, R., Rapoport, A. and deVeber, G. A. (1980). Continuous ambulatory peritoneal dialysis: a new era in the treatment of chronic renal failure. *Clin. Nephrol.* (In press)

29 Ivanovich, P. and Jones, K. M. (1976). Pulse dampener for elimination of automatic peritoneal dialysis abdominal pain. *Dial. Transplant.*, **5**, 54

30 Karanicolas, S., Oreopoulos, D. G., Izatt, S., Shimizu, A., Manning, R. F., Sepp, H., deVeber, G. A. and Darby, T. (1977). Epidemic of aseptic peritonitis caused by endotoxin during chronic peritoneal dialysis. *N. Engl. J. Med.*, **296**, 1336

31 Devine, H., Oreopoulos, D. G., Izatt, S., Raymond, M. and deVeber, G. A. (1975). The permanent Tenckhoff catheter for chronic peritoneal dialysis. *Can. Med. Assoc. J.*, **113**, 219

32 Oreopoulos, D. G., Izatt, S. and Ogilvie, R. (1977). Phosphate kinetics in patients undergoing peritoneal dialysis (abstract). In *Third International Workshop on Phosphate and Other Minerals*, July, Madrid, Spain

33 Oreopoulos, D. G., Rabinovich, S. and Meema, H. E. (1973). Contrasting bone changes in patients on chronic hemodialysis and chronic peritoneal dialysis. In Frame, B., Prafitt, a. m. and Duncan, H. (eds.) *Linical Aspects of Metabolic Bone Disease*, p. 628. (Detroit: Excerpta Medica)

34 Oreopoulos, D. G., Blair, G. R., Meema, H. E. and deVeber, G. A. (1975). Evolution of uremic neuropathy and renal osteodystrophy in patients undergoing chronic peritoneal dialysis. *Abstr. Am. Soc. Artif. Intern. Organs*, **4**, 47

35 Karanicolas, S., Oreopoulos, D. G., Dombros, N., Pierratos, A., Mathews, R. E. and Vas, S. (1979). Intestinal obstruction and bowel perforation in patients undergoing chronic peritoneal dialysis. *Abstr. Am. Soc. Artif. Intern. Organs*, **8**, 46

36 Silverberg, S., Oreopoulos, D. G., Wise, D. J., Uden, D. E., Meindok, H., Jones, M., Rapoport, A. and deVeber, G. A. (1977). Pericarditis in patients undergoing long-term hemodialysis and peritoneal dialysis. *Am. J. Med.*, **63**, 874

37 Cattran, D. C., Fenton, S. S. A., Wilson, D. R. and Steiner, G. (1976). Defective triglyceride removal in lipemia associated with peritoneal and hemodialysis. *Am. J. Med.*, **85**, 29

38 Oreopoulos, D. G., Karanicolas, S., Izatt, S. and deVeber, G. A. (1967). Dialysis and triglycerides. *Ann. Intern. Med.*, **85**, 679

39 Oreopoulos, D. G. (1972). Hepatitis and treatment of chronic renal failure by peritoneal dialysis. *Lancet*, **2**, 1256

40 Cardella, C. J., Oreopoulos, D. G., Uldall, P. R., Harding, M. and deVeber, G. A. (1979). Renal transplantation in patients on maintenance intermittent peritoneal dialysis. *Abstr. Am. Soc. Artif. Intern. Organs*, **8**, 70

41 Uldall, P. R., Dyck, R. F., Woods, F., Merchant, N., Martin, G. S., Cardella, C. J., Sutton, D. and de Veber, G. A. (1979). A subclavian cannula for temporary vascular access for haemoodialysis or plasmapheresis. *Dial. Transplant.*, **8**, 963

4

Vascular access

G. Williams

There is an increasing requirement for both short- and long-term access to the circulation. Knowledge of this subject should not be confined to those surgeons specializing in the diseases where it might be required. Considerable onus is placed on referring doctors, anaesthetists and nurses to ensure that potentially useful peripheral vessels are not damaged or thrombosed and, that after a vascular access procedure has been performed, it is not lost by inadvertent hypotension, occlusion by a blood pressure cuff, or by its use for administration of intravenous fluids. Conservation of possible blood access sites by thoughtful long-term planning is necessary from the very beginning of the illness to ensure that the patient need never be deprived of treatment because of lack of suitable vessels. Despite the accumulation of considerable experience, with a great variety of blood access methods now

Table 1 Vascular access systems

External cannulae and shunts	*Internal arteriovenous fistulae*
Cannulae	Arm
Shaldon catheter	Radial cephalic
Teflon catheter	End-to-end
	Side-to-side
Shunts	Antecubital
Quinton Scribner	Saphenous vein autograph
Ramirez winged shunt	
Buselmeier shunt	Leg
Thomas shunt	Sapheno-popliteal
Allen Brown shunt	Sapheno-femoral
	Arm or leg allo- or xenografts
	Human umbilical vein
	Sparks Mandril
	Bovine arterial graft
	Dacron velour
	Expanded polytetrafluoroethylene (PTFE)

available, the initial approach to the patient requiring vascular access remains controversial. Short-term access may be required for exchange transfusion, haemodialysis in the treatment of acute renal failure, and for haemoperfusion in the treatment of various types of poisoning[1,2]. Plasma exchange is being increasingly used for both short- and long-term management of a variety of immunologically mediated disorders[3-5]. Patients with chronic renal failure, maintained on home dialysis, are surviving for many years, and, for this, require effective long-term access to their circulation. The range of techniques available (Table 1) includes direct vessel cannulation[6-9], external shunts[10-12], subcutaneous arteriovenous fistulae using the patient's own vessels[13-15], and implantable vascular conduits[16-20]. If immediate access is required, either direct vessel cannulation or an external arteriovenous shunt should be used. In uncomplicated cases, where treatment can be planned in advance, the aim is to create a subcutaneous arteriovenous fistula which will have fully matured by the time dialysis is required. There are particular problems in patients where the majority of vascular sites have been used or where no suitable vessels are available for an external shunt or subcutaneous fistula.

Anaesthesia

Before embarking on any form of vascular access surgery, the procedure is fully explained to the patient. For those patients in whom long-term haemodialysis is the proposed form of treatment, it is our practice before surgery to introduce the patient to others who are well established on dialysis and have a successfully functioning arteriovenous shunt or fistula.

Either local infiltration, regional or general anaesthesia can be used. Patients who are particularly restless or anxious may be given a sedative preoperatively. Particular care should be taken with those patients who are seriously ill and require ventilation. It should never be assumed that they are also unconscious and anaesthetized.

Local anaesthetics are ineffective in some patients with chronic renal failure[21] and general anaesthesia is required even for simple procedures. It has been shown in patients with chronic renal failure where anaesthesia had been induced by a supraclavicular brachial plexus block that the overall duration of the anaesthetic was 38% less than in normal patients[22]. No specific biochemical lesion has been found to account for this.

For the creation of a simple arteriovenous fistula or the insertion of an arteriovenous shunt, 1% lignocaine by direct infiltration can be used with a maximum dose of 20 ml to ensure no untoward effect on myocardial contractility and cardiac output. Lignocaine with adrenaline is never used as this results in vasoconstriction and increases the difficulties of surgery. The disadvantages of local infiltrational anaesthesia are that the duration of action may be short and there is no vasodilating effect. However, these disadvantages are minor when compared with the problems associated with regional blockade. Brachial plexus blockade using the supraclavicular route can cause a pneumothorax, Horner's syndrome and phrenic nerve paralysis. The use of the safer axillary route has the disadvantage that, if the musculo-cutaneous nerve arises high in the neck, the anaesthesia may be ineffective over the radial aspect of the wrist, the area most likely to be operated upon in the creation of a subcutaneous arteriovenous fistula. This type of anaesthesia takes longer to perform, and, even in expert hands, an overall incidence of failure of 5–7% occurs[23].

General anaesthesia

General anaesthesia is required for patients in whom a local anaesthetic agent is ineffective or who are particularly anxious. It is also necessary in those patients undergoing more complicated types of vascular access surgery, particularly where extensive exposure may be required and where it may be necessary to explore more than one set of vessels. The management of patients with a functioning fistula and shunt who need to undergo a general anaesthetic is described later in the chapter.

VASCULAR ACCESS IN THE ADULT

Techniques for immediate vascular access

Direct vessel cannulation

Cannulation of a large peripheral vessel was the only method available for vascular access prior to the development of the external arteriovenous shunt[10] in 1960. Until recently, direct vessel cannulation has had limited use. It has been used mainly for short-term dialysis or plasma exchange or to give time while an arteriovenous fistula matures. However, with the development of Teflon cannulae and single-needle dialysis, adequate vascular access can be obtained for periods of months without significant complications[9] and modifications of this technique will probably supersede the use of the external shunt in the majority of patients. Cannulation of the subclavian vein is to be preferred as there is a lower incidence of infection and the patient retains mobility. Cannulation of both the subclavian and femoral vessels will be described as it may, particularly in children, be impossible to use the subclavian route.

Subclavian vein cannulation

The vein can either be cannulated by the supra- or infraclavicular route. When using a long-term indwelling Teflon catheter, the infraclavicular route is to be preferred so that the catheter can be threaded through a long subcutaneous tunnel to reduce the incidence of infection.

Method of insertion. The cannula is inserted using a local anaesthetic and a meticulous aseptic technique. The patient lies completely flat with the head turned to the opposite side. The skin above and below the clavicle is prepared with an antiseptic solution and the area draped. Local anaesthetic is infiltrated 5 cm in all directions from the insertion site at the junction of the clavicle and the first rib. A full thickness skin incision is made and a subcutaneous tunnel created in the direction of the anterior axillary fold. A 16-gauge angio-cath is inserted into the subclavian vein through the incision and a guidewire passed through it into the superior vena cava. The angio-cath is then removed. The proximal end of the guidewire is passed through the subcutaneous tunnel and the Teflon catheter threaded over it into the subclavian vein so that it eventually lies in the superior vena cava. After removal of the guidewire, the skin incision is closed and the cannula is fixed to the skin with adhesive tape. When the cannula is not being used for dialysis or plasma exchange, heparin saline is injected through it twice daily. To reduce the incidence of infection, the cannula is changed at weekly intervals by passing a fresh guidewire through it so that it can be withdrawn over the guidewire and a new cannula inserted. Since the introduction of this technique[9], no patient with terminal renal failure in this series has required the insertion of a Silastic Teflon shunt or temporary peritoneal dialysis because of lack of a vascular access site. Though infection of the cannula was frequent, it was eradicated in all cases, allowing dialysis to continue uneventfully. The authors report no cases of air embolus or venous thrombosis.

Femoral vein catheterization

Because of a higher incidence of infection and venous thrombosis, the femoral vein should only be used when subclavian vein cannulation is not possible. It has been used with some success in children who have required short-term vascular access[8], and, in the original description[6], two cannulae were inserted using the Seldinger technique[24], one cannula acting as the 'arterial' line and the other the venous line. The use of a single caval catheter to withdraw blood and any suitable peripheral vein for its return has also been described[25]. However, with the development of single-needle dialysis, it is now only necessary to insert one catheter into the femoral vein.

Technique for the introduction of femoral vein catheter. The patient is placed in the prone position with the thigh externally rotated. The skin is cleaned thoroughly and local anaesthetic infiltrated over the femoral vessels. A 16-gauge needle is inserted into the femoral vein and a guidewire passed through it. The needle is then removed and a Teflon catheter passed over the guidewire which is removed. The catheter is passed up to lie in the inferior vena cava, and, if necessary, a second catheter inserted using the same technique to lie in a lower part of the vena cava. The cannula is filled with heparin saline until it is required. After dialysis, the catheter is removed and pressure exerted over the femoral vessels for at least 10 minutes to ensure adequate haemostasis.

Femoral artery cannulation

Using exactly the same technique as for cannulation of the femoral vein, a catheter can be inserted into the femoral artery. In view of the potential hazards to the arterial wall and possible emboli or thrombosis, use of the femoral artery is to be avoided where possible.

External shunts

External arteriovenous shunts are of two main types:

(a) Those derived from that described by Quinton et al.[10], consisting of a Teflon vessel tip and a Silastic conduit, and

(b) Those comprising Thomas's shunt[12], which consists of a Dacron collar attached to a straight Silastic cannula, and the Allen Brown shunt, which consists of a knitted Dacron collar and a silicone rubber tube. A Dacron elbow sleeve covers the silicone tube beyond the Dacron to provide a bacterial barrier.

The properties of the ideal external shunt were described[10] in 1960 (Table 2). The Quinton–Scribner shunt currently in use is shown in Figures 1 and 2. A straight-winged Ramirez shunt[26] (Figure 3) is particularly useful in

Table 2 Properties of an ideal external shunt[9]

1. The inner surface should minimize clotting
2. Minimal tissue reaction
3. Adequate fixation to subcutaneous tissue
4. Good seal at exit site
5. Cannula material elastic and moves with limb
6. Able to withstand external trauma
7. Should not occlude blood vessels at the cannula site
8. Easily replaceable tip
9. Easy to attach to the dialyser circuit
10. Should not project any appreciable distance above the skin

children. The Buselmeier shunt (Figure 4) has limited applications and is described later. Arteriovenous shunts are relatively easy to insert and can be used immediately. However, their effectiveness in the longer term, when compared to direct subclavian vein cannulation, requires further study. The life expectancy of a shunt is usually limited to that of the venous end and is on average 7–10 months[27]. A shunt is more prone to thrombosis and infection than a subcutaneous arteriovenous fistula which is the method of choice for long-term vascular access. The use of the arteriovenous shunt may be superseded in future by direct subclavian vein cannulation using a Teflon catheter[9].

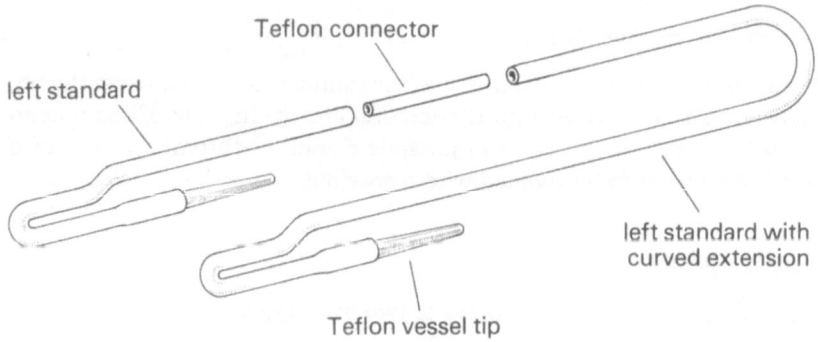

Figure 1 The Quinton–Scribner shunt, showing the Teflon tip, Silastic tubing and Teflon connecting piece

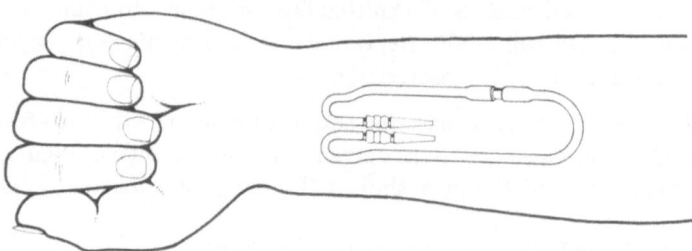

Figure 2 An ST-series shunt with moulded silicone rubber cannulae with integral silicone rubber vessel tips

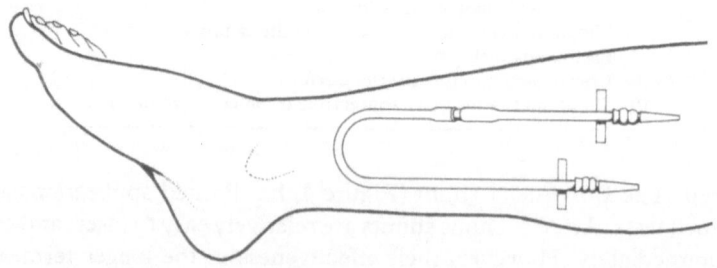

Figure 3 The winged Ramirez silicone rubber shunt

Insertion of shunts. In the adult, there is a choice of two main sites for insertion of an arteriovenous shunt: the radial artery and cephalic vein at the wrist, and the posterior tibial artery and the long saphenous vein at the ankle, thus making four peripheral sites available for each patient. Where possible, sites in the leg should be used first, enabling the vessels at the wrist to be converted into an arteriovenous fistula if the patient requires long-term treatment. There is no difference in survival of shunts placed in the leg compared with those in the arm[28]. Should vessels in the leg be unsuitable, the possibility of creating a shunt and a fistula at the wrist, at the same or a subsequent operation, should be considered[29] (see later).

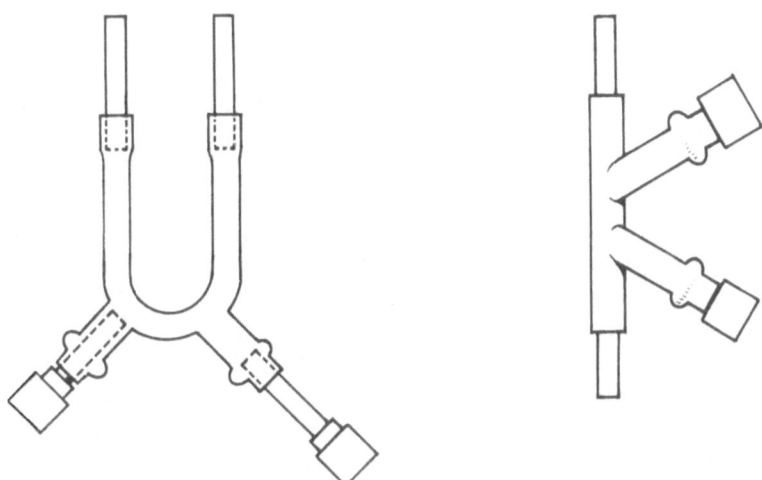

Figure 4 The straight and curved Buselmeier shunt with two access ports, each of which is fitted with a removable occluding plug

The technique for insertion of an arteriovenous shunt. The greatest possible attention should be paid to detail, particularly in selection of the site for the shunt, handling of tissues and correct alignment of the cannulae to avoid any kinking or distortion of vessels. The procedure should be carried out under strictly aseptic conditions, though if the patient is too ill to move there is no reason why it should not be carried out in the ward[10]. In the majority of cases, local anaesthesia is satisfactory. Certain general principles apply to the insertion of all shunts. If possible, only one incision should be used to ensure that the area between the two shunts is not devitalized, and, where possible, the non-dominant limb should be used to allow the patient maximum mobility. If the shunt is inserted in the leg, the incision should be high enough to enable the patient to comfortably wear a shoe. When selecting the shunt tips, the largest which will fit comfortably into the vessel should be selected and the tubing should never be clamped with crushing forceps.

The insertion of an arteriovenous shunt at the ankle. A single incision is made midway between the long saphenous vein and the posterior tibial artery and carried down to the periosteum of the medial malleolus. The subcutaneous tissue is undermined on either side and the artery is exposed first. The fibrous sheath surrounding the posterior tibial vessels is incised and the artery cleared, taking care not to tear the venae commitantes which surround it. It is only necessary to clear 2–3 cm of the artery as any extensive mobiliz-ation will lead to a loss of support for the artery and a tendency to kink when the shunt tip is inserted. Two non-absorbable ligatures are passed round the artery. Traction on these provides haemostasis. The most suitable shunt tip is selected and secured in the Silastic tubing. This is then filled with heparin saline. A small transverse arteriotomy is made in the more proximal part of the artery and the shunt tip inserted so that it lies in that part of the artery which is still surrounded by its supporting tissue. The shunt is secured as shown in Figure 5. A subcutaneous pouch is made to allow the curved or winged part of the shunt to lie comfortably. A small incision is made in the skin and the shunt tubing drawn through it to the exterior. Once the shunt has been inserted into the artery, it is necessary to clamp the tube with a small bulldog clamp. Heparinized saline should be injected intermittently down the tubing while the vein is mobilized and the procedure repeated. The shunt is joined together using a Teflon connecting piece (Figure 1). The joint is further protected by wrapping Elastoplast around it. A light crepe bandage is applied, with part of the shunt tubing projecting so that this can be checked to ensure that clotting does not occur. Two bulldog clips are attached to the bandage and these are carried with the patient at all times in order to occlude the shunt should it accidentally become disconnected.

Insertion of a shunt at the wrist. Before inserting a shunt at the wrist, it is

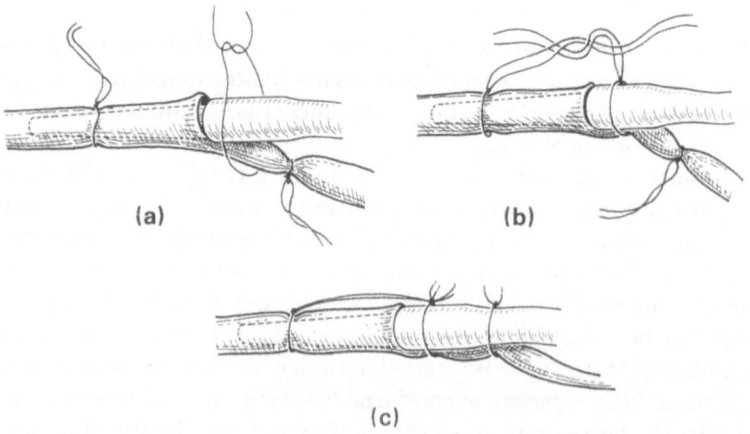

(a)   (b)

(c)

Figure 5   The method of inserting and securing an arteriovenous shunt

necessary to ensure that there is an adequate collateral circulation through the hand as the radial artery is tied during the procedure. To do this, the ulnar and radial arteries are occluded by pressure and the patient is then asked to open and close his fist until pallor occurs in the hand. Pressure is then released separately from each artery and by clinical observation a good assessment of collateral flow can be obtained. It is usually possible to feel blood pulsating in the radial artery after pressure has been released from the ulnar artery.

A single incision is again used at a high enough level to ensure that the subcutaneous tubing does not interfere with movements of the wrist. Care should be taken not to divide the dorsal branches of the radial nerves which usually lie immediately beneath the incision. The artery is mobilized first, and, again, it is only necessary to dissect free 2–3 cm to ensure that it has adequate support. The technique of insertion of the shunt is the same as that depicted in Figure 5. After the shunt has been inserted, it is important to ensure the shunt tip is correctly aligned and that the shunt tubing lies snugly beneath the skin in the subcutaneous pocket as early shunt failure is invariably due to bad alignment of the vessel and shunt tip.

In uncomplicated cases, experience has shown that the straight shunt is simpler to insert, causes less local trauma and allows a higher flow rate[30,31]. The other major advantage is the ease with which the straight shunt can be unblocked using a Fogarty embolectomy catheter.

Difficulties in shunt insertion. Difficulties in inserting a shunt may arise if the patient has no palpable vessels, if the vessels have been previously used for inserting shunts or intravenous cannulae, or if the patient's vessels are calcified or atheromatous. When these situations arise and direct vessel cannulation cannot be used, there is no alternative but to explore each potential vessel site in turn, starting with those in the leg, and, if necessary, extending the incisions proximally until suitable sized vessels are found. When the peripheral vessels are not suitable, the use of an alternative external shunt must be considered, using the larger proximal vessels (see later).

Postoperative care of arteriovenous shunts. In any patient, there are only a limited number of suitable sites for vascular access so that preservation and careful handling of a shunt is vital. The importance of the shunt should be impressed on the patient who should be fully aware of the possible complications and how they should be dealt with. Patients with any form of vascular access are particularly vulnerable when undergoing a general anaesthetic. The surgeon and anaesthetist should both be informed of the presence of a shunt or fistula so that they are not used for intravenous injections or infusions. Care must also be taken to protect the limb from pressure while the patient is unconscious and to ensure that it is not used for taking the blood pressure.

Prevention of bleeding due to disconnection.

(i) The site of division of the shunt should at all times be closed by several turns of Elastoplast or Steristrip. This should be checked, especially on return from theatre and after any procedure involving the shunt.

(ii) All patients with shunts should be provided with a pair of crocodile or bulldog clamps which should at all times be clipped to the bandage on the opposite side of the leg to the shunt. In this position the clips are prevented from accidentally occluding the shunt. In the event of the two ends becoming disconnected, the first action of the patient or nurse is to clamp both sides of the shunt with the clips.

(iii) The extra lengths of shunt tubing projecting above the bandage should be taped lightly to the skin of the leg to minimize the chance of the tubing catching on protruding objects.

(iv) In rare cases, the tip of the shunt may become dislodged from the artery or vein resulting in bleeding which may be controlled by the application of very firm pressure just above the exit hole of the shunt until surgical replacement of the tip is arranged.

Prevention of clotting.

(i) The patient's position in bed should be such that he/she does not lie with the weight of the limb compressing the shunt.

(ii) If the shunt is situated in the arm, the blood pressure should never be taken in that arm.

(iii) Bandages over the shunt tubing should not be tight or bulky and should be closed with Micropore or Elastoplast, as safety pins can easily transfix the shunt tubing.

Checking shunts and recognition of clotting. The shunt is carrying blood at arterial pressure and can therefore be regarded as an external pulse. The correct way to check it is firstly to *look*. If the column of blood is blue or interrupted by clear gaps of serum, it is clotted. Secondly, it should be checked by *touch*. If the index finger and thumb are pressed gently on either side of the shunt tubing without totally occluding it, the pulse can be felt like any other. In no circumstances should the shunt be pinched back on itself or twisted over. These measures are not only unnecessary but may cause clotting or cracking of the Silastic tubing. If the skin over the venous end is palpated, a definite thrill can be felt. Thirdly, it should be checked by *listening*. If the shunt is patent, a bruit will be heard proximal to the shunt tip.

Prevention of infection. Opinions vary as to the routine daily care of the shunt. We have not found it necessary to dress the shunt areas daily except when a shunt has been inserted in the thigh. In patients with a shunt in the wrist or ankle, it is only dressed when the patient attends for dialysis. The area where the tubing projects through the skin is cleaned with a mild antiseptic solution. After dialysis, a clean, dry dressing is placed over the shunt exit sites and a light crepe bandage applied. If there is any evidence of infection a combination of ampicillin and flucloxacillin is used until bacteriological sensitivities are available. Abscess development is treated by incision and drainage with appropriate antibiotics. It is not always necessary to remove the shunt.

Management of a thrombosed shunt. Clotting of the shunt may be the result of many factors, but poor surgical technique resulting in badly aligned shunt tips is probably the most important. Precipitating factors include periods of hypotension, shunt infection and successful renal transplantation[32]. The actual episode of clotting may be preceded by days or weeks of reduced blood flow and high venous pressure. When this situation arises angiograms should be performed through both ends of the shunt[33,34]. The most frequent finding is angulation of the vessel tip with a small amount of clot or thrombus in the vessel. This method of investigation also gives valuable information about the state of the vessels proximal to the shunt. If angulation of the shunt tip is demonstrated, the shunt should be revised as soon as possible, resiting the tip proximally. If there is poor shunt flow or repeated clotting episodes with no radiological evidence of a mechanical problem, long-term anticoagulation should be considered[35]. Once the shunt has clotted, flow should be restored as soon as possible using one of the following methods. If the clot is recent, it may be possible to simply aspirate it from the shunt and restore flow. Failing this, a fine polythene cannula can be inserted into the lumen of the shunt and the clot aspirated. When the shunt tubing has been completely cleared, 2 ml of heparin saline can be injected gently down the fine polythene cannula. This will usually dislodge the small amount of remaining thrombus. However, this should not be done until most of the clot has been removed. If this is not successful, then, using the same fine cannula inserted as far as possible into the shunt, one ampoule (5000 units) of urokinase is injected into the tubing so that it lies as near to the vessel tip as possible. Both ends of the shunt are then connected by an intravenous giving set to a litre of normal saline so that there is constant pressure keeping the urokinase at the site of the thrombosis. After 30 minutes in contact with the urokinase, it is usually possible to aspirate the clot. We have found this technique to be successful in 89% of the clotted shunts treated. It is important that the shunt is observed at frequent intervals while this procedure is being used to ensure that the patient does not receive a sudden large infusion of intravenous fluids through the venous limb of the shunt. After the shunt has been successfully unblocked, further investigation using angiography should be undertaken, so that, if necessary, the shunt can be revised and resited in a more proximal vessel. If a straight shunt has been used, and this is the main advantage of this type of shunt, a No. 3 Fogarty embolectomy catheter can be passed down the shunt into the vessel itself and the clot gently withdrawn after inflating the balloon. If a shunt has to be unblocked frequently, antibiotics will be needed to prevent septic emboli.

Forceful unblocking of a shunt by dislodging the thrombus into the general circulation can result in septic pulmonary emboli[36] or cerebral arterial occlusion[32].

Infections following shunts. Subacute bacterial endocarditis and mycotic aneurysm formation are rare complications but of great importance. Subacute bacterial endocarditis should be suspected in any patient with pyrexia and malaise in whom vascular access surgery has been performed. Mycotic aneurysms usually occur at the site of the shunt but may occur distally as a result of septic emboli. Septicaemia remains a major cause of death in patients on regular dialysis and faulty aseptic technique during the use of the shunt is probably the commonest cause. This is more frequent when the shunts are used for venous or arterial blood sampling by those who are not aware of the problems which may arise. It has been shown that, in patients undergoing plasma exchange for Goodpasture's syndrome, the development of an infection at the site of the shunt is associated with enhanced allergic tissue damage[37].

Removal of arteriovenous shunts. If the shunt has clotted and there is no evidence of infection, consideration should first be given to conversion of the vessels into an arteriovenous fistula. This can only be done at the wrist (see later). If this is not desired, the shunt can usually be removed by gentle traction. If this causes pain, the wound can be opened using a local anaesthetic, the vessels explored and the retaining ligatures divided. When the shunt tips have been removed, the vessels are ligated.

If the shunt is still functioning and no longer required, for example after successful renal transplantation, the shunt tubing should be clamped for 48 hours to ensure adequate thrombosis in the vessels. The shunt can then be dealt with as above. If the shunt is infected, a formal exploration of the shunt and ligation of the vessels should be performed using appropriate antibiotic cover.

Alternative types of shunts and indications for their use

In the small group of patients for whom immediate vascular access is required, there may be no suitable vessels for the insertion of a Scribner-type shunt or for direct vessel cannulation. In this situation, the use of one of the other three types of external shunt should be considered:

   (a) The Thomas shunt,
   (b) The Allen Brown shunt,
   (c) The Buselmeier shunt.

The Thomas shunt, introduced in 1969[12], consists of a Dacron skirt attached to a straight Silastic cannula. The arterial cannula has a slightly larger Dacron skirt than the venous limb. Two sizes are available for adults or children. The advantages of this shunt are that it does not interrupt blood flow in the artery to which it is attached and clotting is less frequent. When clotting does occur, it is relatively easy to deal with using a Fogarty embolectomy catheter. It does, however, have one major disadvantage in that the long-term survival of these shunts is not great, since over 50% are lost as a direct result of infection. It is necessary to attach the Thomas shunt on to the femoral vessels and any vascular access surgery performed in the thigh has a very high rate of infection. The incidence can be reduced by meticulous care of the shunt exit sites together with the use of antibiotic creams and waterproof dressings. When infection does occur, it is difficult to eradicate and secondary haemorrhage may arise. Infection and haemorrhage necessitate removal of the shunt and repair of the artery using either a vein patch or a Teflon patch, but this can be extremely difficult in the presence of infection.

Technique of insertion of the Thomas shunt. General anaesthesia is preferable, although the shunt can be inserted using local infiltration of anaesthetic if necessary. An incision is made over the femoral vessels below the inguinal ligament and the common femoral artery and vein isolated. The femoral artery is occluded and an arteriotomy made, preferably in an area free of atheroma, the size of the arteriotomy depending on the size of the Dacron skirt on the Thomas shunt. Using a 5 or 6/0 vascular suture, the skirt is sutured in place, and the distal clamp on the femoral artery is then released to enable retrograde flow to occur down the shunt and to clot the Dacron skirt. Once haemostasis has been secured, the proximal clamp is released. The femoral vein can then be clamped and the second shunt sutured into place in a similar manner. The shunts are then brought to the surface through separate stab incisions and the two ends joined with a suitable connector. It is vitally important that the whole operative area is kept clean and that antibiotic creams are used around the shunt exit sites.

The Allen Brown shunt (Figure 6). This shunt is similar to the Thomas shunt, consisting of silicone rubber tubing attached to a short length of knitted Dacron. A Dacron velour sleeve covering the silicone tube beyond the Dacron graft provides a bacterial barrier, and, as tissue ingrowth will occur into this sleeve, it gives the shunt greater stability. Because of its smaller size, it can be used both in the groin or arm, and also in children.

Technique for insertion. This is similar to that used for the Thomas shunt, though it may be sutured end-to-end on the vessel if required (Figure 6).

Femoral saphenous shunt. This shunt has the advantage of not having to use foreign material for the anastomosis on to the femoral artery. Three centimetres of the upper saphenous vein are removed and sutured end-to-side on

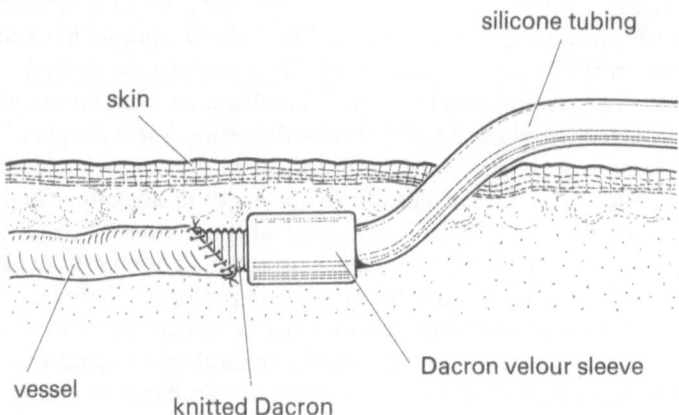

Figure 6   The Allen Brown shunt sutured end-to-end to the vessel

to the common femoral artery. A large Teflon tip with straight Silastic tubing or a Buselmeier shunt (Figure 7) is then inserted into this portion of the saphenous vein and tied in place. This acts as the arterial end while the venous end is inserted into the stump of the saphenous vein. Should the shunt become infected, it is, in theory, easier to deal with than an infected Thomas shunt. It also creates a smaller arteriovenous fistula, and so cardio-vascular side-effects, which are associated with the larger Thomas shunt, are reduced.

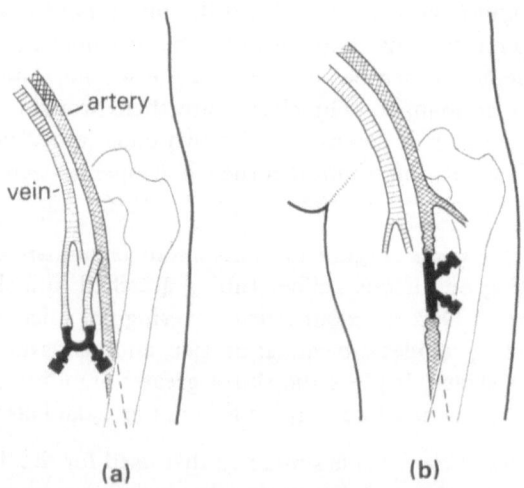

Figure 7   (a) A U-shaped Buselmeier shunt inserted into the terminal portion of the saphenous vein. The other end of the shunt has been inserted into an 8 cm portion of the saphenous vein which has been removed and sutured end-to-side to the femoral artery. (b) The Buselmeier shunt used as an interposition in the femoral artery

Femoro–femoro shunts. If there are no suitable veins available, a Buselmeier shunt can be used. The Buselmeier shunt and its uses are shown in Figures 4 and 7. The superficial femoral artery is exposed below the profunda femoris and the two vessel tips inserted, one in a proximal direction and one in a distal direction (Figure 7). The tips are joined by straight Silastic tubing and secured by ligatures.

Simultaneous creation of arteriovenous shunt and arteriovenous fistula

In the patient in whom long-term dialysis will be required and there is a paucity of potential sites the creation of a simultaneous arteriovenous shunt and fistula at the wrist should be attempted. Where there is a good collateral circulation from the ulnar into the radial artery, the radial artery and the adjacent superficial vein can be divided and sutured end-to-end, creating an arteriovenous fistula. A Quinton–Scribner shunt can be inserted into the distal ends of the vessels. I have used this technique with success in two patients.

Arteriovenous fistulae

Arteriovenous shunts, although still probably the most effective way of providing immediate short-term access to the circulation, have numerous disadvantages. The mean life of a shunt is approximately 10 months so that repeated clotting episodes become a considerable problem as more and more access sites are used when the shunts are resited. This may lead to the situation of a patient dying because no vascular access sites are available. The use of a subcutaneous arteriovenous fistula was first described in 1966[13]. Since then, successful dialysis has been carried out in patients with such a fistula for many years. A decision to create an arteriovenous fistula should be made as early as possible so that the fistula will have adequate time to mature before it is required for dialysis and so that suitable venous tributaries are not used up by repeated venepunctures. The longer a fistula can be left before it is used for dialysis purposes, the better. A period of 6 weeks should be allowed whenever possible.

Though fistulae in the leg have been described[38], there are certain disadvantages. The veins are usually deep and therefore difficult to cannulate, severe varicosities of the long saphenous system may develop, and there is a much higher incidence of infection. The most convenient site to construct an arteriovenous fistula is over the lateral border of the radius between the radial artery and the adjacent cephalic vein. The anastomosis between the artery and vein can either be performed side-to-side, end-to-side or end-to-end, particularly if distal vessels are to be used for creation of an arteriovenous shunt. Fistulae using the ulnar artery have been described but have a much higher incidence of thrombosis, and therefore use of the radial artery and cephalic vein is to be preferred[39].

Surgical technique. In most patients, this can be performed using local anaesthesia. A longitudinal incision is made midway between the radial artery and the adjacent superficial vein. Great care should be taken to handle the vessels as little as possible as they will constrict and make the anastomosis more difficult. The main trunk of the vein should be mobilized as little as possible, since excessive mobilization allows the vein to rotate while the anastomosis is performed and decrease its lumen. As few side branches of the main vein as possible should be divided, as these vessels will aid the development of alternative venous pathways. The artery should be carefully freed from its accompanying vena commitantes. Two linen sutures approximately 2 cm apart are drawn under the artery and vein and the vessels approximated. An incision 1–1.5 cm in length is made in the artery and vein and the anastomosis performed using a 6 or 7/0 vascular suture. If it is difficult to mobilize the vein, the possibility of creating an end-to-side anastomosis with the proximal end of the divided vein should be considered. The distal end of the vein is tied off. After ensuring that haemostasis is complete, the newly created fistula should be palpated to ensure that a thrill is present and that the proximal and distal limbs of the vein are filled, as failure to detect a thrill at this stage of the operation is frequently associated with non-functioning of the fistula. It is worth taking the anastomosis down and repeating it at this stage if no thrill is present. The skin is closed with interrupted sutures without drainage and a light crepe bandage applied.

The patient and nursing staff should understand that the blood pressure should never be taken on that arm and that the fistula should not be used for routine venepuncture. In the early postoperative period, the patient should keep the arm elevated when it is not in use, and normal light activities should be encouraged in the immediate postoperative period. The nursing staff should listen over the site of the fistula for the presence of a bruit at half-hourly intervals for the first 4 hours after creation of the fistula and then four-hourly until the fistula is well established. The sudden disappearance of the bruit or thrill is suggestive of venous thrombosis and the patient should be returned to theatre and the fistula explored. By adopting this policy of immediate exploration, if the fistula loses its thrill in the early postoperative period, it has been possible to reconstitute the majority of the fistulae re-explored.

Alternative fistulae

If the vessels at the wrist are not suitable, one should have no hesitation in using the vessels in the antecubital fossa.

Surgical technique. Again, this can be performed under local anaesthesia. Using a transverse incision, the brachial artery and adjacent veins are exposed. Because of the variable venous anatomy in the antecubital fossa, many alternative types of fistulae are possible. Surgical technique differs in three ways from the fistula at the wrist.

(1) Before completing the venous anastomosis, the valves in the veins of the forearm should be destroyed by the passage of a Fogarty catheter.
(2) The arteriotomy in the brachial artery should not be more than 1 cm or too large a fistula will develop, leading to high output cardiac failure.
(3) Where possible, the venous flow is encouraged to be in a distal rather than a proximal direction.

Where there are adequate veins in the forearm, the proximal vein in a side-to-side anastomosis should be tied off, or, alternatively, an end-to-side anastomosis can be performed using the distal end of the vein. If the veins of the forearm are not well developed, the proximal venous limb should be left alone as this will create a suitable channel in the upper arm. Cannulation in this area, however, is more difficult, particularly in a fat patient. We have used brachial fistulae in 45 patients, and, in 43 of these, the fistula was suitable for haemodialysis, the longest period of continuous use being 2 years and 3 months. A proximal forearm arteriovenous fistula, involving an end-to-side anastomosis between a perforating branch of the cephalic or median antecubital vein and the proximal radial artery, has been described[40]. The authors claim that they are less subject to direct injury during venepuncture because the arteriovenous connection is buried deep within the antecubital space. They describe 40 patients, 34 of whom had a patent functioning fistula at the time of report or until the time of transplantation or death, and the periods of function reported were from 1 to 38 months.

Conversion of a Scribner shunt to an arteriovenous fistula

This technique[29], described in 14 patients, is of considerable value in that potential vascular access sites are saved and used for the creation of an arteriovenous fistula. Though this cannot be done in every case, by adhering strictly to certain important points of technique a high degree of success should be obtained. The fistula between the radial artery and cephalic vein is constructed 2–3 cm proximal to the shunt tips. The intima and walls of vessels must look and feel normal in these areas. If thrombosis of the shunt is the indication for its conversion to a fistula, the thrombus is removed using a small Fogarty catheter and the vessels irrigated with heparin saline. The arteriotomy and venotomy used for inserting the Fogarty catheter can be used for the side-to-side anastomosis for the fistula. Once the fistula has been created, the vessels are ligated distally as near to the site of the anastomosis as possible. The shunt cannulae are removed through their original skin exits, thereby avoiding contamination of the wound and the patient is started on prophylactic antibiotics. In all 14 patients in the series reported, dialysis was resumed using the newly created fistula within 24–72 h of conversion from a shunt. I have used this technique in three patients with similar results.

End-to-end arteriovenous fistula without sutures

In this type of fistula, the end-to-end anastomosis is carried out by inserting the artery 4–5 mm into the vein and then cementing the vessels with an acrylic adhesive[41]. In this series, 56 arteriovenous end-to-end fistulae were created in 55 uraemic patients – 54 between the radial artery and cephalic vein and two between the ulnar artery and vein. Apart from one case of detachment of the anastomosis on the sixth day, all fistulae functioned, and, in nine, it was possible to use the fistula within 6 days of the surgical operation.

Other types of arteriovenous fistulae

In the majority of patients, it will be possible to create a satisfactory arteriovenous fistula using their own vessels in the forearm. In the remainder, alternative forms of vascular access will have to be considered (Table 1).

Sparks Mandril

This was first introduced in 1972 as a method of femoro–popliteal artery bypass. It was subsequently used as a method for vascular access, but has the disadvantage of having to be implanted at least 6 weeks before it can be used.

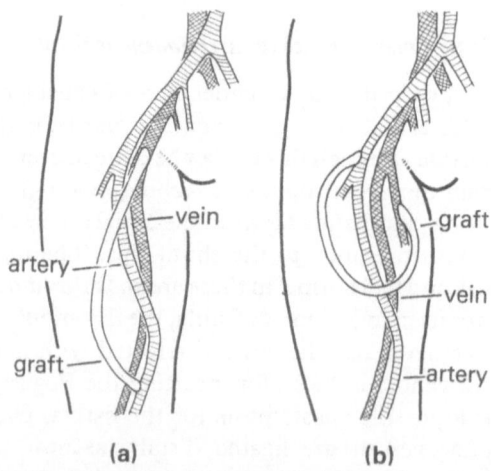

(a)   (b)

Figure 8   (a) Interposition graft between the distal femoral artery and the femoral vein. (b) The graft has been looped between the terminal portion of the saphenous vein and the femoral artery

The Mandril consists of a silicone rubber rod with a covering of a specially prepared siliconized knitted Dacron tube. The Mandril is inserted sub-cutaneously in the forearm or leg, either straight or in a loop (Figures 8 and 9) exactly where the a.v. fistula is required. Six weeks later, the silicone Mandril is removed, leaving a tissue tube containing knitted Dacron within its wall with a uniform diameter of 6 mm and a smooth lining. The arterial end is anastomosed end-to-side to the adjacent artery and the venous end is anastomosed end-to-side to the adjacent vein. In order to prevent serious

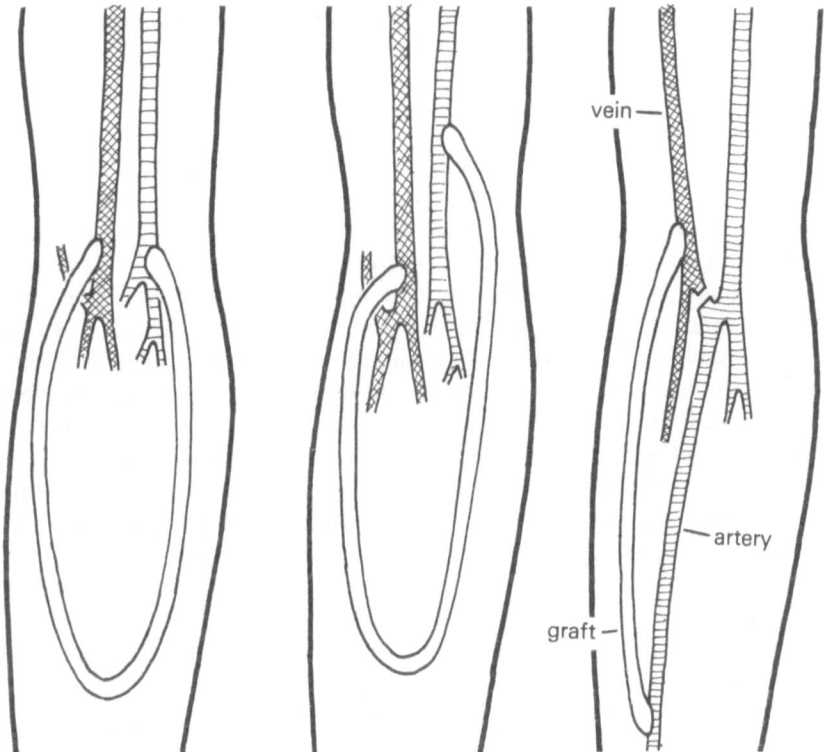

Figure 9 The alternative methods by which a graft or saphenous vein can be used to create a vascular access in the forearm

damage to the knitted Dacron substrate of the implanted graft by the sharp cutting edge of conventional dialysis needles, special cannulae with a pointed obturator must be used. The obturator passes between the inter-stices of the two knitted layers of Dacron. Because of the need for two operations to insert the graft and the delay of 6 weeks before it can be used, these grafts have not found great favour and there are few long-term reports of their use. In addition, a 75% failure at 12 months has been reported[36] due to thrombosis of the graft.

Autogenous vein grafts

In theory, part or all of the long saphenous veins, cephalic veins and external jugular veins can be used to provide a vascular bridge to create an arterio-venous fistula. The only time that I now use an autogenous venous fistula is when the upper thigh is the only suitable site available for vascular access. Accepting that any form of vascular access to the upper thigh is prone to infection, the incidence of infection is less when the patient's own saphenous vein, rather than an implanted device of foreign material, is used. In the arm, where infection is not so great a problem, I prefer to use an implanted PTFE graft (see later), as these have a higher patency rate than autogenous vein grafts. Using the saphenous vein, the fistula in the thigh can be made either in a loop or as a straight fistula (Figure 8).

Operative procedure. The operation is best performed under general anaes-thesia. The site of the procedure is chosen with regard to previous surgery in the leg, preference being given to a limb in which the distal portion of the saphenous vein has already been used for an a.v. shunt. The leg is positioned with the hip and knee flexed and the limb externally rotated and a transverse incision made over the sapheno–femoral junction and the vein isolated. All tributaries are tied but the sapheno–femoral junction is not ligated. The vein is mobilized distally and divided just below the knee. It is usually necessary to make three or four step-ladder incisions in the skin over the vein to allow for mobilization. The saphenous vein is then withdrawn to the groin in-cision. A bulldog clip is placed over the sapheno–femoral junction and a soft cannula inserted into the distal vein. The vein is irrigated with heparin saline and any leaks in it are sutured. The vein is then rerouted subcutaneously and anastomosed end-to-side to the popliteal artery. A small drain is left in the popliteal incision and the wound closed. The graft can be used within a week, but it is preferable to allow adequate healing and fixation of the vein for 3 or 4 weeks before it is used for dialysis. If the fistula is to be looped, a similar procedure is adopted, but the anastomosis is made to the proximal femoral artery rather than the popliteal artery (Figure 8).

Bovine heterografts

It is well known that untreated arterial xenografts function poorly when used as arterial substitutes and often lead to disastrous results[42]. There are, however, isolated reports in the older literature of long-term successes with such preparations[43,44].

A modified bovine heterograft has been available for use for vascular access since 1972[45]. Its availability, ease of handling, biocompatibility and durability has led to its extensive use as a vascular conduit for access for haemodialysis[6,46–48], although a number of problems are still encountered. These include frequent clotting at the venous anastomosis site and technical difficulty with implantation due to its large diameter (7.5–9 mm), together with the risk of infection and the relatively high cost. Before using the graft, the patient should be given antibiotics. The bovine graft can be used in any of the situations described in Figures 8 and 9. A cumulative 2-year function of 76% has been reported for the graft[49]. Thirty-nine per cent of the patients in this series experienced occlusion of the graft after the initial 6-week period. By far the most common cause of late thrombosis in patients with a bovine graft is venous outflow obstruction, secondary to pseudointimal proliferation at the venous anastomosis. Many of these obstructed bovine grafts can be salvaged by a thromboendarterectomy with a patch graft using PTFE rather than sacrificing one of the patient's own veins for a vein patch. As well as thrombosis, the risk of bleeding, ischaemic complications, infection and false aneurysm formation must be considered. Bleeding at the site of needle puncture frequently occurs if the graft is used within the first 10 days of its insertion. In most cases it will respond to pressure over the graft, but occasionally the bleeding may dissect along the graft tunnel causing a tunnel haematoma and graft occlusion. Ischaemic complications due to fistula 'steal' may occur because of the large size of the bovine graft, and, in this case, banding of the fistula may lead to successful relief of symptoms. In others, the fistula may have to be ligated or removed. When infection has been associated with the bovine graft, this has been most frequently seen, in our experience, when the graft has been inserted in the leg. Occasionally the infection will respond to systemic antibiotic therapy, but, in the majority of cases, it is necessary to remove the graft as anastomotic disruption may occur if the infected graft is left in place. The serious complication of false aneurysm formation occurs in approximately 10% of patients[16], and almost half such grafts have to be removed and replaced by a new one, although it is occasionally possible to resect the aneurysmal area and replace this with a PTFE graft. A small porportion of aneurysms can be resected and the hole in the wall of the graft can be closed. We have found straight grafts in the forearm to be less satisfactory than loop grafts, almost certainly because of the poor vessel flow which is insufficient to keep the bovine graft patent. Others[50] have reported an 81% patency rate when loop grafts were excluded and believe that straight grafts have a higher patency and that loop grafts are contraindicated.

Dacron arteriovenous fistulae

Both Dacron velour and seamless woven Dacron have been used for arteriovenous fistulae[20,51]. Of the two, seamless woven Dacron is harder to puncture and has a higher rate of occlusion and thrombus formation. An accumulative patency rate of 71% from between 12 and 30 months has been reported using the Dacron velour arteriovenous fistula.

Umbilical vein arteriovenous fistula

Preserved human umbilical vein has been used for the creation of arteriovenous fistulae for approximately 4 years[19]. Cost has limited its widespread
use and it does not appear to have any significant advantages over cheaper
synthetic grafts. In a series of 27 grafts, 20 were complication-free with a
follow-up period of 1–7 months. Complications were encountered in seven
of the 27 grafts, but six of these were resolved satisfactorily; 26 of the 27
grafts were therefore usable during this period of follow-up[52].

Polytetrafluoroethylene (PTFE) arteriovenous fistulae

Expanded polytetrafluoroethylene was introduced as a vascular prosthesis
in 1972 in the form of a venacaval graft[53] and later as an arterial conduit[54]. Its
possible use as an arteriovenous conduit for haemodialysis was first reported
in 1973[55]. The major defect of the expanded PTFE graft is its weakness in
tensile strength in a circumferential direction which makes the graft technically more difficult to suture and leads to a higher incidence of aneurysm
formation. It has since been modified by W. L. Gore and Associates, in an
attempt to overcome this defect, by spirally reinforcing the original graft
with PTFE tape. The graft manufactured by Impra does not have this
reinforcing second layer and the description given in this section relates to
the Gortex PTFE graft which has a wall thickness of 0.6 mm and a nominal
fibril length of 30 μm. A variety of internal diameters are available and one

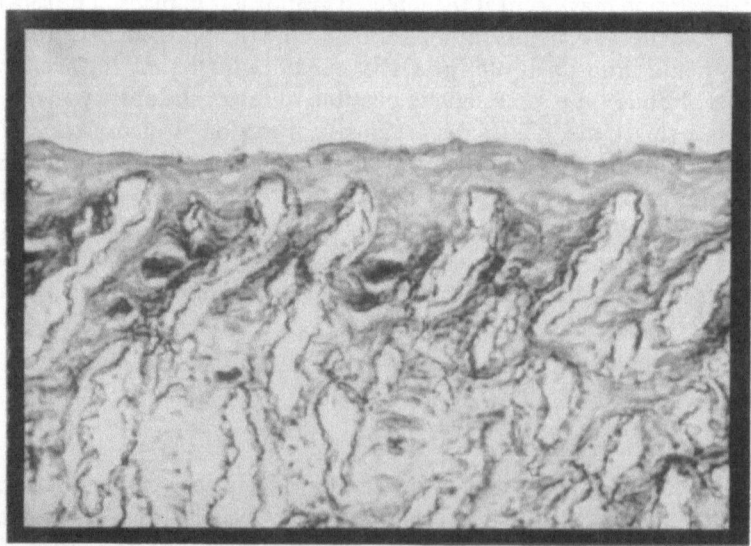

Figure 10 At 11 months this a.v. fistula demonstrates a well-healed collagenous flow lining
without obvious endothelialization. Trichrome, 400 ×

considerable advantage is the development of a tapered graft for ease of suture on to smaller peripheral vessels. This may also obviate the occurrence of a steal syndrome. Since the PTFE graft is non-crimped, it lies best in the straight position. Loop grafts can, however, be easily formed provided there are no acute angulations or kinks. The grafts develop minimal tissue ingrowth and a neo-intima composed of very thin amorphous proteinaceous material with little fibrin or cellular involvement (Figure 10). They are considerably less thrombogenic than woven Dacron[56, 57]. The potential uses of the graft are shown in Figures 8 and 9. Because there is increased potential for infection, we have not used a Gortex graft in the leg.

Operative technique. If possible, we try to use the distal radial artery and a convenient vein in the antecubital fossa (Figure 9). Our second choice is to use the brachial artery and loop the graft back to either a vena-commitantes or suitable superficial vein in the antecubital fossa (Figure 9). It is often necessary to perform an extensive dissection of the antecubital fossa to find a vein of suitable calibre. When the vessels have been isolated, the subcutaneous tunnel for the graft is made using a straight Hegar dilator one size smaller than the diameter of the graft, as, in this way, the graft gets immediate support from the surrounding subcutaneous tissues and, since the graft is porous, the postoperative oedema is considerably lessened. It is essential, when the graft is placed in the loop position, to ensure that it is not kinked or angulated in any way. Patients must receive prophylactive antibiotics prior to surgery, but we have not used prophylactic anticoagulation. Anastomosis has been accomplished with 6/0 vascular sutures.

Care of shunts and fistulae in patients undergoing general anaesthetic

There are potential hazards facing any patient with a shunt or fistula undergoing a general anaesthetic. The shunt may be compressed while the patient is anaesthetized, it may clot if the patient is subjected to periods of hypotension, or the anaesthetist may inadvertently use the fistula for the insertion of an intravenous cannula or use the limb for measurement of blood pressure. To prevent these problems, we ensure that the patients are themselves aware of the potential dangers which may arise, and insist that, when any patient undergoes a general anaesthetic, the anaesthetist and theatre staff are informed of the presence of the arteriovenous shunt or fistula and that the limb is labelled.

VASCULAR ACCESS PROCEDURES IN CHILDREN

A child who has been accepted for treatment of chronic renal failure by long-term haemodialysis potentially has a longer life on dialysis than an adult, and the planning of vascular access therefore takes on even greater importance. In general, for long-term dialysis, an arteriovenous fistula should be constructed whenever possible. Though repeated needling of a small child may create initial problems, an external shunt tends to clot more frequently in children because of the smaller vessel size, thus resulting in more frequent hospitalization and psychological trauma to the child and his parents. The life and activities of a child with a shunt are restricted because of the attendant risks of infection and trauma, and a subcutaneous arteriovenous fistula allows the child considerably greater freedom to indulge in normal activities.

Sapheno–femoral catheterization

This technique can be used in small children and infants where short-term dialysis or plasma exchange is required, but should not be used when long-term treatment is contemplated as valuable access sites will inevitably be destroyed. Using single needle dialysis techniques, it is only necessary to expose one saphenous vein under general anaesthesia and a long Teflon catheter can be inserted to lie in the inferior vena cava. In larger children, a Teflon catheter can be inserted directly into the femoral vein using the Seldinger technique.

External arteriovenous shunts

The main indications for an external shunt are in those children who require short-term haemodialysis for acute renal failure, and in some cases requiring plasma exchange. The site chosen for the arteriovenous shunt depends on the size of the child. In children over 30 kg, a radial artery to cephalic vein shunt should be possible. For those below this weight, a shunt between the brachial artery and cephalic vein should be feasible. In smaller children, an Allen Brown shunt in the arm or Thomas shunt in the leg may be required. As soon as the child reaches a suitable size, a subcutaneous arteriovenous fistula should be created. If a shunt has been inserted at the wrist, consideration should be given to converting this to an arteriovenous fistula.

Operative technique

Radial artery, cephalic vein shunt. The basic technique is similar to that described in adults; paediatric shunts and shunt tips are available. In older children, the shunt can be inserted at the wrist, but, in younger children, the incision should be placed higher in the forearm over the middle and distal third. It is preferable to use the straight Ramirez shunts as they take up considerably less space in the subcutaneous tissues and are much easier to declot. In small children, particularly if they are restless, it is preferable to enclose the arm, in the postoperative period, in a light plaster case to prevent the shunt being dislodged.

Brachial artery cephalic vein shunt. If a wrist shunt has failed or the vessels are too small, then an upper arm shunt can be performed when short-term dialysis is needed, although a thigh shunt will probably function for longer periods if it does not become infected.

Surgical technique. An incision is made on the medial aspect of the upper arm midway along the brachial artery. It is important to insert the shunt tips high enough to ensure that the shunt will not be traumatized by flexion of the elbow but low enough to avoid damage to the collateral vessels. As in an arteriovenous shunt at the wrist, a straight Ramirez winged shunt is most appropriate. A second incision is made under the lateral aspect of the upper arm, the cephalic vein exposed and the shunt tip inserted. Though this technique was not recommended by Buselmeier *et al*[58], successful dialysis from experience covering 40 shunts has been recorded[59], the longest functioning for 44 weeks.

Thigh shunts

These are preferable in young infants and babies. The choice of procedures is between a Thomas shunt small vessel appliqué, a sapheno–femoral shunt, and, in children where the saphenous vein is not available, a Buselmeier interposition shunt. There is a serious hazard of infection with all these techniques.

Operative technique

The technique for inserting a Thomas shunt is the same as for an adult. If a femoro–saphenous shunt is to be constructed, either the superficial or profundo–femoral arteries can be used. Ischaemia of the leg is theoretically more likely when the superficial femoral artery is used, but technically this is the easier operation. The superficial femoral artery is isolated below its bifurcation and the shunt tip inserted as in an adult. If the profundo–femoral artery is to be used, the shunt should be inserted so that the shunt tip does not lie within the lumen of the common femoral artery. Similarly, when inserting the venous end, this should lie within the saphenous vein and not protrude into the common femoral vein. It is preferable to use a Buselmeier shunt (Figure 7) with straight Silastic tubing rather than the curved type as there is little room in young infants to make an adequate subcutaneous bed. Postoperatively, the shunt exit wounds should be covered with antibiotic cream and the shunt, when not in use, should be covered with a waterproof dressing. (Bending at the hip must be prevented by the use of an appropriate splint.)

Femoral artery interposition shunt

The technique for inserting this shunt is the same as in adults and has been described earlier in the chapter.

Arteriovenous fistulae

If the child is of suitable size, it may be possible to construct a conventional Cimino–Brescia fistula at the wrist, and, whenever possible, this should be attempted. The subcutaneous arteriovenous fistula may require weeks or months following surgery before it is sufficiently developed for use for dialysis. This delay can be diminished by a programme of regular hand exercises, performed with a tourniquet lightly applied to the upper arm and begun 2 weeks after surgery. In the small child, the venous enlargement following a fistula may not be adequate for efficient dialysis. However, the vessel enlargement which does occur will usually allow for the later placement of a larger prosthetic shunt[60]. In children too small for creation of a conventional fistula and in whom vessel sites are being rapidly utilized to maintain an arteriovenous shunt, the feasibility of creating either a saphenous vein looped graft in the arm or a Gortex PTFE graft in the arm should be considered. The techniques required are exactly the same as those in adults. The operation is, however, technically far more difficult and should be performed only by those with considerable experience in this field.

Though there are no reports of the use of Gortex grafts in children, from comparison of the results of Gortex grafts and saphenous vein limb fistulae in adults, it would probably be better to attempt the creation of a Gortex fistula rather than a saphenous vein loop fistula.

SUMMARY

The substitution of a mature Cimino–Brescia radiocephalic arteriovenous fistula, with temporarizing subclavian or femoral vein catheterization and single-needle dialysis, for the Scribner arteriovenous shunt as the primary access route for haemodialysis or plasma exchange will lead to the sparing of superficial venous channels and permit trouble-free vascular access for 3 years or more[61]. A 100% 2-year mid-forearm and an almost 90% distal radiocephalic fistula survival has been reported[39]. This compares with a mean survival of 9 months for the venous cannula of an arteriovenous shunt and 11.2 months for the arterial cannula[27].

Thrombosis remains the major cause of late failure of an arteriovenous fistula, both during dialysis and after transplantation. Survival rates for arteriovenous fistulae are lower in women than in men, particularly after transplantation. When the patency of a fistula is threatened, the creation of other access routes becomes mandatory and is simplified when other superficial venous channels are available at the other wrist or at the antecubital fossa[40]. When the venous channels are inadequate, the alternatives are a saphenous vein graft, umbilical vein graft, Dacron velour graft, Sparks Mandril modified bovine graft or a PTFE graft. All of these conduits have achieved varying degrees of success, but they cannot be considered ideal and should not be used as a primary access procedure when the patient's own vessels are suitable for the creation of an arteriovenous fistula.

(1) The autologous saphenous vein graft, either in the arm or rerouting in the leg, involves an extensive dissection and a disappointing 50% 1-year failure rate has been reported[62]. This corresponds to the experience of other units[15,45].

(2) The cost of the umbilical vein graft compared with other grafts precludes its use at present.

(3) The Sparks Mandril requires a period of 6 weeks implantation before it can be used, making it unsuitable in the majority of patients.

(4) Bovine grafts have a patency rate of between 71% and 90% at 1 year[16,46,63], but a higher incidence of non-thrombotic complications has been reported than in any of the other grafts. These complications include distal ischaemia due to 'steal' bleeding, wound complications, infection and pseudointimal hyperplasia, resulting in venous obstruction and false aneurysm formation.

In studies comparing the modified bovine graft and expanded PTFE graft, the use of PTFE has been associated with a higher patency rate and lower complication rate[49,64,65]. While there have been no studies to compare the reinforced Gortex PTFE graft with the non-inforced Impra graft, for theoretical reasons alone, the Gortex graft is to be preferred as the vascular conduit for haemodialysis.

References

1 Vale, J. A., Rees, A. J., Widdop, B. and Goulding, R. (1975). Use of charcoal haemoperfusion in the management of severely poisoned patients. *Br. Med. J.*, 1, 5

2 Rees, A. J. and Widdop, B. (1977). Haemoperfusion in the treatment of acute drug overdose. *Riv. Tossicol. Sp. Clin.*, 2, 17

3 Peters, D. K., Rees, A. J. and Lockwood, C. M. (1977). Plasma exchange in glomerular and related auto allergic disease. *Proc. EDTA*, 14, 409

4 Lockwood, C. M., Rees, A. J., Russell, B. and Peters, D. K. (1977). Experience of the use of plasma exchange in the management of potentially fulminating nephritis and SLE. *Exp. Haematol.*, 5 (Suppl.), 117

5 Lockwood, C. M., Rees, A. J., Pearson, T. A., Evans, D. J., Peters, D. K. and Wilson, S. B. (1976). Immunosuppression and plasma exchange in the treatment of Goodpasture's syndrome. *Lancet*, 1, 711

6 Shaldon, S., Chiandussi, L. and Higgs, B. (1961). Haemodialysis by percutaneous catheterisation of the femoral artery and vein with regional heparinisation. *Lancet*, 2, 857

7 Erben, J., Kvasnicka, J., Bastecky, J. and Vortel, V. (1969). Experience with routine use of subclavian cannulation in haemodialysis. *Proc. Eur. Trans. Dial. Assoc.*, 6, 59

8 Anderson, J., Lee, H. A. and Stroud, C. E. (1965). Haemodialysis in infants and small children. *Br. Med. J.*, 1, 1405

9 Uldall, P. R., Dyck, R. F., Woods, F., Merchant, N., Martin, G. S., Cardella, C. J., Sutton, D. and de Veber, G. A. (1979). A subclavian cannula for temporary vascular access for hemodialysis or plasmapheresis. *Dial. Transplant.*, 8, 963

10 Quinton, W. E., Dillard, H. and Scribner, D. H. (1960). Cannulation of blood vessels for prolonged haemodialysis. *Trans. Am. Soc. Artif. Intern. Organs*, 6, 104

11 Buselmeier, T. J., Simmons, R. L., Najarian, J. S., Duncan, D. A., von Hartitzsch, B. and Kjellstrand, C. M. (1973). The clinical application of a new prosthetic arteriovenous shunt. *Nephron*, 12, 22

12 Thomas, G. I. (1970). Large vessel applique arteriovenous shunt for haemodialysis. *Am. J. Surg.*, 120, 244

13 Brescia, M. J., Cimino, J. E., Appel, K. and Hurwich, B. J. (1966). Chronic haemodialysis using venipuncture and a surgically created arteriovenous fistula. *N. Engl. J. Med.*, 275, 1089

14 Haimov, M. (1975). Vascular access for haemodialysis. *Surg. Gynaecol. Obstet.*, 141, 619

15 Haimov, M., Burrows, L., Baez, A., Neff, M. and Slifkin, R. (1974). Alternatives for vascular access for haemodialysis. Experience with autogenous saphenous vein autografts and bovine heterografts. *Surgery*, 75, 447

16 Burbridge, G. E., Biggers, J. A., Remmers, A. R. Jr., Lindley, J. D., Sarles, H. E. and Fish, J. C. (1976). Late complications and results of bovine xenografts. *Trans. Am. Soc. Artif. Intern. Organs*, 12, 418

17 Ota, K., Ara, R., Takahashi, K., Toma, H. and Agishi, T. (1977). Clinical experience with circumferentially reinforced expanded polytetrafluoroethylene graft as a vascular access for haemodialysis. In Robinson, B. H. B. (ed.) *Dialysis Transplantation Nephrology. Proceedings of the Fourteenth Congress of the European Dialysis and Transplant Association*, pp. 222–228. (Tunbridge Wells: Pitman Medical)

18 Beemer, R. K. and Hayes, J. F. (1973). Haemodialysis using a Mandril-Grown graft. *Trans. Am. Soc. Artif. Intern. Organs*, 19, 43

19 Mindich, B. P., Silverman, M. J., El Guezabel, A. and Levowitz, B. S. (1975). Umbilical cord vein fistula for vascular access in haemodialysis. *Trans. Am. Soc. Artif. Intern. Organs*, 21, 273

20 Flores, L., Dunn, I., Frumkin, E., Forte, R., Requina, R., Ryan, J., Knopf, M., Kirschner, J. and Levowitz, B. S. (1973). Dacron arteriovenous shunts for vascular access in haemodialysis. *Trans. Am. Soc. Artif. Intern. Organs*, 19, 33

21 Aldrete, J. A., Daniel, W., O'Higgins, J. W., Homatus, J. and Starzl, T. E. (1971). Analysis of anaesthetic-related morbidity in human recipients of renal homografts. *Anaesth. Analg.*, 50, 321

22 Bromage, P. R. and Gertel, M. (1972). Brachial plexus anaesthesia in chronic renal failure. *Anaesthesiology*, 36, 488

23 Moore, D. C. (1955). *Complications of Regional Anaesthesia*, p. 247. (Springfield, Ill.: Charles C. Thomas)

24 Seldinger, S. I. (1953). Catheter replacement of the needle in percutaneous arteriography. *Acta Radiologica*, 39, 368

25 Matalon, R., Nidus, B., Cantacuzino, D. and Eisinger, R. P. (1970). Intermittent haemodialysis with repeated femoral vein puncture. *J. Am. Med. Assoc.*, 214, 1883

26 Ramirez, O., Swartz, C., Onesti, G., Mailloux, L. and Brest, A. N. (1966). The winged in line shunt. *Trans. Am. Soc. Artif. Intern. Organs*, 12, 220

27 Lundberg, M., Erlanson, P. and Larsson, R. (1977). Quinton Scribner arteriovenous shunts for dialysis. *Scand. J. Urol. Nephrol.*, **11**, 47

28 Higgins, M. R., Grace, M., Bettcher, K. B., Silverberg, D. S. and Dossetor, J. B. (1976). Blood access in haemodialysis. *Clin. Nephrol.*, **6**, 473

29 Simonian, S. J., Stuart, P. F., Hill, J. L. and Mahajan, S. K. (1977). Conversion of a Scribner shunt to an arteriovenous fistula for chronic dialysis. *Surgery*, **82**, 448

30 Hawkins, J. B. and Robinson, B. H. B. (1967). Repeated haemodialysis with a straight silicone rubber cannula. *Br. Med. J.*, **4**, 226

31 Walls, J. and Kopp, H. (1968). Blood flow in arteriovenous shunts: observations and measurements. *Br. Med. J.*, **2**, 806

32 Robinson, P. J., Glanville, J. N., Smith, P. H. and Rosen, S. M. (1970). Management of clotting in arteriovenous cannulae in patients on regular dialysis therapy. *Br. J. Urol.*, **42**, 590

33 Berne, T. V., Turner, A. F. and Barbour, B. H. (1971). Angiographic evaluation of Quinton Scribner shunt malfunction. *Surgery*, **69**, 588

34 Schreiber, M. H. (1971). Angiographic demonstration of the causes of external arteriovenous haemodialysis shunt failure. *Clin. Radiol.*, **22**, 210

35 Wing, A. J., Curtis, J. R. and De Wardener, H. E. (1967). Reduction of clotting in Scribner shunts by long term anticoagulation. *Br. Med. J.*, **3**, 143

36 Shaldon, S. (1966). Haemodialysis in chronic renal failure. *Postgrad. Med. J.*, **42** (Suppl.), 671

37 Rees, A. J., Lockwood, C. M. and Peters, D. K. (1977). Enhanced allergic tissue damage in Goodpasture's syndrome by intercurrent bacterial infection. *Br. Med. J.*, **2**, 723

38 Roberts, W. M. and Vanzyl, J. J. W. (1968). Haemodialysis in children. Techniques of vascular shunts. *S. Afr. Med. J.*, **42** (Suppl.), 94

39 Kinnaert, P., Vereerstraetten, P., Toussaint, C. and Van Geertruyden, J. (1977). Nine years' experience with internal arteriovenous fistulae for haemodialysis: study of some factors influencing the results. *Br. J. Surg.*, **64**, 242

40 Gracz, K. C., Ign, T. S., Soung, L. S., Armbuster, K. F. W., Seim, S. K. and Merkel, F. K. (1977). Proximal forearm fistula for maintenance haemodialysis. *Kidney Int.*, **11**, 71

41 Petrella, E., Orlandini, G., Romagnoni, M., Gentile, M. G., Luciani, L. and D'Amico, G. (1976). Long term results of a new end to end anastomosis without sutures for haemodialysis A-V fistulas. *Proc. Eur. Assoc. Artif. Organs*, **3**, 200

42 Creech, O., DeBakey, M. E., Self, M. and Halpert, B. (1954). The fate of heterologous arterial grafts: an experimental study. *Surgery*, **36**, 431

43 Carrel, A. (1912). Ultimate results of aortic transplantations. *J. Exp. Med.*, **15**, 389

44 Guthrie, C. C. (1910). Survival of engrafted tissues. III. Blood vessels. *Heart*, **2**, 115

45 Chinitz, J. L., Yokoyama, T., Bower, R. and Swartz, C. (1972). Self sealing prosthesis for arteriovenous fistula in man. *Trans. Am. Soc. Artif. Intern. Organs*, **18**, 452

46 Merickel, J. H., Anderson, R. E., Knutson, R., Lipschultz, M. L. and Hitchcock, C. R. (1974). Bovine carotid artery shunts in vascular access surgery. *Arch. Surg.*, **109**, 245

47 Lefrak, E. A. and Noon, G. P. (1975). A surgical technique for creation of an arteriovenous fistula using a looped bovine graft. *Ann. Surg.*, **182**, 782

48 Rosenberg, N. (1976). The bovine arterial graft and its several applications. *Surg. Gynaecol. Obstet.*, **14**, 104

49 Butler, H. G., Baker, L. D. and Johnson, J. M. (1977). Vascular access for chronic haemodialysis. PTFE versus bovine heterograft. *Am. J. Surg.*, **134**, 791

50 Haimov, M. and Jacobson, J. H. (1974). Experience with the modified bovine arterial heterograft in peripheral vascular reconstruction and vascular access for haemodialysis. *Ann. Surg.*, **180**, 291

51 Levowitz, N. S., Flores, L., Dunn, I. and Frumkin, E. (1976). Prosthetic arteriovenous fistula for vascular access in haemodialysis. *Am. J. Surg.*, **132**, 365

52 Rubio, P. A. and Farrell, E. M. (1979). Human umbilical vein graft angio access in chronic haemodialysis. *Dial. Transplant.*, **8**, 511

53 Fujiwara, Y., Cohn, L. H., Adams, D. and Collins, J. J. (1974). Use of Gortex grafts for the replacement of the superior and inferior vena cava. *J. Thorac. Cardiovasc. Surg.*, **67**, 774

54 Matsumoto, H., Hasegawa, T., Fuse, K., Yamamoto, M. and Saigusa, M. (1973). A new vascular prosthesis for a small calibre artery. *Surgery*, **74**, 519

55 Volder, J. G. R., Kirkham, R. L. and Kolf, W. J. (1973). A-V shunts created in new ways. *Trans. Am. Soc. Artif. Intern. Organs*, **19**, 38

56 Hamlin, G. W., Rajah, S. M., Crow, M. J. and Kester, R. C. (1978). Evaluation of the thrombogenic potential of three types of arterial graft studied in an artificial circulation. *Br. J. Surg.*, **65**, 272

57 Shack, R. B., Neblett, W. W., Richie, R. E. and Dean, R. H. (1977). Expanded PTFE as dialysis access grafts: serial study of histology and fibrinolytic activity. *Am. Surg.*, **43**, 817

58 Buselmeier, T. J., Santiago, E. A., Simmons, R. L., Najarian, J. S. and Kjellstrand, C. M. (1971). Arteriovenous shunts for paediatric dialysis. *Surgery*, **70**, 638

59 Franzone, A. J., Tucker, B. L., Brennan, L. P., Fine, R. N. and Stiles, Q. R. (1971). Haemodialysis in children. *Arch. Surg.*, **102**, 592

60 Buselmeier, T. J. and Kjellstrand, C. M. (1973). A-V shunts and fistulas for haemodialysis in neonates, infants and small children. *Proc. EDTA*, **10**, 511

61 Mohaideen, A. H., Mainzer, R. A. and Avram, M. M. (1975). Comparative experience with access modalities in haemodialysis (Abstract). *Kidney Int.*, **8**, 430

62 Girardet, R. E., Hackett, R. E., Goodwin, N. J. and Friedman, E. A. (1970). Thirteen months' experience with the saphenous vein graft arteriovenous fistula for maintenance haemodialysis. *Trans. Am. Soc. Artif. Intern. Organs*, **16**, 285

63 Foran, R. F., Shore, E. H., Levin, P. M. and Treiman, R. L. (1975). Bovine heterografts for haemodialysis. *West J. Med.*, **123**, 269

64 Kaplan, M. S., Mirahmadi, K. S., Winer, R. L., Gorman, J. T., Dabirvaziri, N. and Rosen, S. M. (1976). Comparison of PTFE and bovine grafts for blood access in dialysis patients. *Trans. Am. Soc. Artif. Intern. Organs*, **22**, 388

65 Bahuth, J. J. (1977). Expanded polytetrafluoroethylene as an arteriovenous conduit for haemodialysis. *Dial. Transplant.*, **6** (11), 62

5

Hospital haemodialysis

D. N. S. Kerr

THE PLACE OF HOSPITAL DIALYSIS

Hospital haemodialysis units are built close to major renal centres in teaching or large district hospitals, sites where maintenance is expensive, building costs high and land values astronomical; they have a high staff:patient ratio. Consequently this is the most expensive major treatment for chronic renal failure. It has been adopted as the usual treatment only in countries where doctors or hospitals are reimbursed for each dialysis, usually by central government funds. In such countries the expansion of facilities has been impressive and the provision of services more comprehensive than in Britain[1]. However, the cost has been proportionately high, and in this country, where the service is provided from a fixed budget, hospital dialysis has been curtailed and used as a treatment of last resort.

This approach has apparently been justified by successive reports of the European Dialysis and Transplant Association's Registry which showed, throughout the 1970s, that survival and rehabilitation were lower on hospital than on home dialysis. However, these comparisons were unfair to hospital dialysis at a time when the best patients were selected for treatment in the home. In countries where hospital dialysis has been offered to all patients and carried out by highly professional staff the results have been excellent. One centre in Japan, treating over 100 patients, had a 5-year survival over 95% in 1978 (Terakado and Nakagawa, personal communication). In our own centre, where half the haemodialysis patients are treated in hospital, survival in hospital and home has always been identical.

Hospital dialysis has one advantage that would justify its more extensive use if resources allowed: patients prefer it. This is my impression from talking to many patients who have tried both techniques and who live close enough to a hospital that long travelling times are not a factor. It is a view confirmed by Mrs Elizabeth Ward, president of the British Kidney Patients' Association, who has had experience of both methods in her own family and who hears the uncensored comments of a large sample of British patients. For most families within easy travelling distance of a hospital unit the burdens of travel and family separation are far outweighed by the freedom from the burdens of preparation, dialysis and cleaning up. As dialysis time has shortened, but preparation time has remained much the same, the advantages of hospital dialysis have increased. However, there is no prospect of Britain being able to provide a comprehensive service based on hospital and satellite units within the next decade, so this will remain the most severely rationed form of treatment, as shown in Figure 1. Even if some technical innovation negates the economic advantage of home dialysis tight government control of new hospital building will restrict hospital dialysis for the foreseeable future.

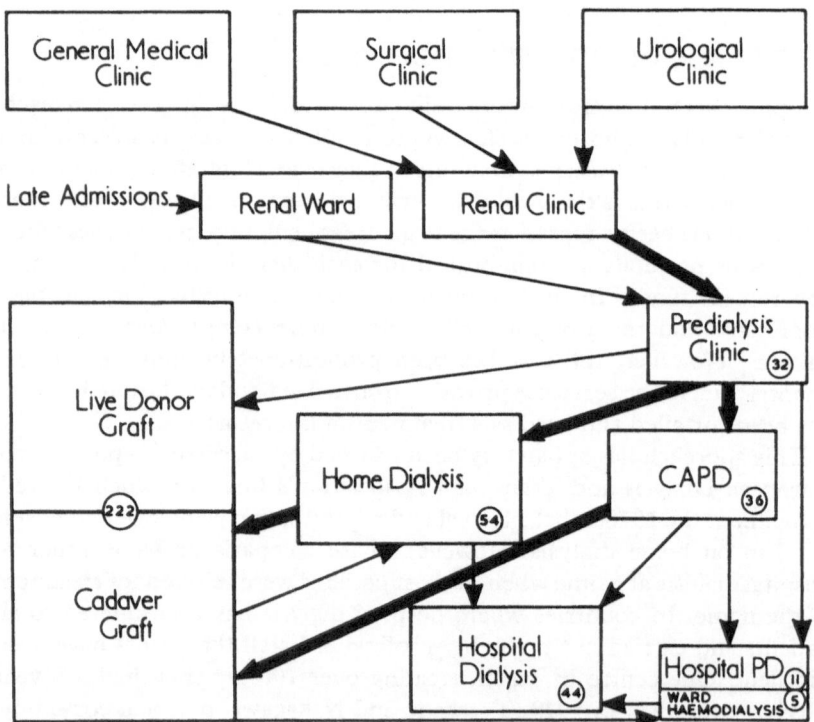

Figure 1   Major pathways of patient referral in chronic renal failure. Almost any succession of transfers between forms of treatment can be made in the lifetime of one patient; the arrows show the usual pathways. In the lower half of the diagram the sizes of boxes correspond roughly to the number of patients on that form of treatment at any one time in Newcastle. The numbers indicate exact number of patients in August 1980. The recipient pool also includes a further 90 patients on home and hospital dialysis in Sunderland and Teesside

THE PREDIALYSIS CLINIC

We have found it convenient to prepare patients for dialysis at a special clinic where they can see the doctor, dialysis administrator, dietitian and social worker at a single visit. At the first attendance, all case notes from our own and other hospitals are summarized and a *problem card* (Figure 2) is prepared by the physician. A photograph is attached to the notes to aid recall of the patient during subsequent group discussions. This card, adapted as necessary, accompanies the patient to the dialysis and renal transplant clinics and forms the basis of his entry into the unit computer.

The functions of the predialysis clinic are indicated in Table 1. A checklist is inserted in the case notes to remind staff of the formalities that must be completed during the 'dialysis work-up'. A decision is reached about the most suitable form of permanent treatment. Those who can travel easily to the predialysis clinic continue to attend, usually at monthly intervals, until dialysis is started. Those who live at a greater distance are seen in a satellite clinic or alternatively by their referring physician, who keeps the renal clinic informed by sending copies of all correspondence.

Table 1 Checklist of procedures carried out at the predialysis clinic

---

Referrals
Social worker: social report
Dialysis administrator: assessment of home circumstances and suitability for home dialysis
Dietitian: advice on phosphate, sodium, potassium and water restriction as indicated and adequate protein intake; follow-up advice as needed
Hospital dental officer: dental survey and treatment
Gynaecologist (if needed): family planning advice
Urologist/transplant surgeon: suitability for transplant if this is in doubt

Investigations
HBsAg
Blood group and tissue type
Standard laboratory tests and ECG (see text)
Radiological bone survey (if needed)
Baseline investigations if included in clinic practice: echocardiogram; bone densitometry; nerve conduction time; electroencephalogram; psychometric assessment, etc.

Decisions
Discussion with patient and family
Choice of treatment
Screening of family and choice of donor (live donor transplant)
Planning of home adaptations (home haemodialysis)
Referral for fistula (home or hospital haemodialysis)

Monitoring
Regular clinical and laboratory surveillance
Selection of time to start dialysis

Selection for type of dialysis or transplant

There are patients for whom any form of dialysis or transplant prolongs

PROFESSOR D. N. S. KERR   PROBLEMS

Name: BRANNEN, James (185731)
Address: 12 Firtree Avenue, Wallsend
Telephone No.:
Date of birth: 18.4.54
Marital state: Single   Family doctor:
Next of kin: Dr T. W. Yellowley
Religion: R/C   7 Elvaston Road
Occupation: Waiter   Ryton
Problems: Tyne & Wear NE40 3NT
                                                 (Code No.: 073)

1. Chronic glomerulonephritis   Diagnosed clinically
     Proteinuria aged 7 (see summary of Child Health notes).
     Group A streptococci isolated; ESO titre: 333
     Presentation with asymptomatic proteinuria and no history of acute attack of
       GN. Casts on urinary deposit June 1980.
2. Chronic renal failure   Found during investigation of anaemia, June 1980;
     plasma urea 26.4 mmol/l; creatinine: 750 µmol/l; creatinine clearance:
     10.0 l/24 h
3. Hypertension   BP 170/100 July 1980. Fundi: n.a.d. ECG:
4. Renal osteodystrophy   Serum calcium: 1.84 mmol/l; ionized calcium:
     0.93 mmol/l; alk. phosphatase: 87–113 iu June/July 1980
   Bone biopsy: Small sample. ?OM+OF
   Skeletal survey: Normal

Tissue Typing
   Group O Rh-positive
     HLA- A2, Aw23, Bw44, Bw49
     B locus identity   1/170
     3 Antigens incl. B. Locus match   1/290
     Any 3 antigens   1/140

MANAGEMENT

Dr T. W. Yellowley   *Mr James BRANNEN*
Ryton, Tyne & Wear   *(185731)*
(073)

Plan of Management:

1. Check serial urine micros. Renal biopsy not contemplated in view of
     smooth contracted kidneys on IVP, a marked history of proteinuria
     and prolonged nocturia before diagnosis.
2. Standard chronic renal failure follow-up.
3. Observe for the moment. Will probably need antihypertensive therapy.
4. Currently taking calcium carbonate; add 1-alpha at next visit.

Figure 2   A 'problem card' kept at the front of the case note folder at predialysis clinic and during subsequent forms of treatment

death rather than life. Diabetics are over-represented in this group. Such patients should be kept away from the predialysis clinic. We encourage colleagues to discuss doubtful candidates for dialysis over the telephone and to invite us to see them in their own wards or at a general medical clinic until a decision on suitability for definitive treatment has been reached. In a country where less than 20 patients per million were treated in 1978[2] (two-thirds of the lowest estimate of need) we have to adopt the same approach to patients of borderline suitability, such as the elderly, those who have suffered hypertensive brain damage and those who do not comply with prescribed treatments like dietary restriction and regular consumption of drugs.

Hepatitis carriers should be detected before they reach the predialysis clinic, but the tests are repeated on arrival at the clinic. It is our policy to accept hepatitis B carriers for dialysis only if they can be trained for home haemodialysis. Training takes place in a small dialysis unit attached to the infectious diseases ward and it is carried out by volunteer medical and nursing staff. Following the hepatitis epidemics in British renal units in 1969–70, several centres opened separate *'yellow units'* for hepatitis carriers, using staff who had become immune to hepatitis B during the epidemic. So far as I am aware none of these yellow units is still in operation and the supply of immune staff has ceased. I suspect, therefore, that our policy is also adopted at most other British centres.

Once the patient has been firmly accepted for some form of treatment, the procedures listed in Table 1 are carried out and the information is discussed with the patient and his family before a choice of treatment is made.

Suitability for transplantation must be assessed in all patients and a second opinion is often helpful if he suffers from obstructive uropathy; persistent reflux; chronic urinary infection; extensive atheroma, particularly involving the iliac arteries; metastatic calcification of vessels from secondary hyperparathyroidism or a disease that is likely to recur in the graft. By comparison of the patients' *blood group and HLA types* with those of the overall British population, the chances of any random kidney providing an acceptable match for the particular patient are calculated using a computer program which allows for linkage disequilibrium. This prediction is incorporated in the 'problem card' (Figure 2). Knowing the number of kidneys offered to the local transplant team annually, one can now calculate the average waiting time for a graft. For instance, the patient represented in Figure 2 has a 1:100 chance of a B locus match and is in the recipient pool at Newcastle, where a B-identical match is preferred and where about 50 kidneys are offered annually. His average waiting time for a first graft will be 2 years provided he does not develop cytotoxic antibodies. Of course, the actual waiting time may be anything from 1 day to many years, but the average waiting time gives some indication of how his future should be planned.

The choice between types of treatment is made at our centre on the following criteria.

Live donor transplant

We encourage this approach for children and young adults who have an uncommon tissue type but who have a willing and compatible parental or sibling donor. The chances of a cadaver transplant, shown on Figure 2, are still calculated on the basis of HLA A and B locus matching, since these are the basis of the National Organ Matching Service (NOMS) kidney exchange scheme. If the NOMS change to DR typing as the first criterion for exchanging kidneys between centres (as seems likely), 'uncommon tissue types' will make up a smaller proportion of the recipient pool and the indications for live donor transplant may diminish.

Live donor transplant is preceded by a short period of haemodialysis on the renal ward, or of home CAPD, so these patients do not normally join the queue for hospital dialysis.

Home haemodialysis

Other patients with uncommon tissue types (roughly those with an average waiting time of more than 2 years for a first offer of a cadaver graft) are considered for home haemodialysis. We no longer push unwilling patients into this form of treatment, since in the first 10 years of our home programme almost 15% of the patients reverted to hospital dialysis following partner's death, desertion or illness of the partner, marital breakdown, incapacity of patient (predominantly from bone disease and encephalopathy) or weariness with the effort. Strong contraindications against home dialysis are lack of a suitable partner, cramped housing conditions with no prospect of rehousing, poor intelligence or motivation. Relative contraindications include old age (particularly over 60), ischaemic heart disease and an elderly or infirm partner. Patients have been trained for the home who were completely illiterate, too deaf to hear an alarm, or nearly blind, but most patients with these disabilities are better off on hospital dialysis.

Continuous ambulatory peritoneal dialysis (CAPD) (Chapter 3)

Those judged unsuitable for home haemodialysis, and those with common tissue types who opt for transplantation (as more than 90% of our dialysis patients do) are offered CAPD, which is now our commonest form of treatment for new patients. If the initial success of this technique is maintained it will gradually replace home and hospital haemodialysis, but some patients will require haemodialysis because of previous abdominal surgery or recurrent attacks of peritonitis. In the first 20 months of our CAPD programme, three patients have been transferred to hospital haemodialysis because of obliteration of the peritoneal cavity; the number is bound to increase if the problem of peritonitis is not overcome.

The few patients who cannot master the technique of CAPD are transferred to intermittent hospital peritoneal dialysis while awaiting a place on the hospital haemodialysis unit. Hospital peritoneal dialysis is not an acceptable form of long-term treatment unless it is provided by a properly staffed unit, with suitable automated equipment.

Hospital haemodialysis

It is apparent that hospital haemodialysis is rarely the first choice of treatment because the unit is always full. As soon as a place is vacated by transplantation or death it is filled from two waiting lists: those on hospital peritoneal dialysis referred to in the preceding paragraph and patients with failed transplants who are maintained on regular haemodialysis on the ward until a new space arises on the hospital haemodialysis unit.

Table 2 Reasons for hospital haemodialysis among 44 patients in Newcastle

Relative contraindications to transplant		
Failed previous transplants		22
(one graft 11, two 8, three 1)		
Cytotoxic antibodies		20
To less than 50% of donors	7	
To 50–100% of donors	13	
Anatomical problems/chronic infection		3
Rare tissue types		
Expected wait for graft 2–5 years		22
Expected wait for graft over 5 years		8
Relative contraindications to home dialysis		
No partner available		19
Failed home dialysis		5
Medical complications (oxalosis, chronic pancreatitis,		
liver abscess, ascites, etc.)		17

The arrangements I describe are similar to those on many other British renal units. They are forced upon us by the shortage of hospital haemodialysis places and such arrangements are far from ideal. There are some patients who will obviously end up on hospital haemodialysis and who would be better treated that way from the start. It should not be necessary for them to prove their inadequacy at other techniques, to endure the misery of prolonged manual peritoneal dialysis, or to embarrass the renal ward by a prolonged period of out-patient haemodialysis before they 'earn' their places on the hospital unit.

An ever-increasing proportion of the patients on hospital haemodialysis have received one or more unsuccessful transplants, they have cytotoxic antibodies that limit their chances of future transplantation or have major contraindications to grafting such as anatomically abnormal urinary tracts (Table 2). At present a considerable proportion of our hospital haemo-dialysis patients have rare tissue types which limit their chances of a trans-plant, but this proportion should fall with the change to DR typing. The congregation of these very-long-stay patients, and those who have failed on every other form of treatment, on the hospital haemodialysis unit is bad for staff morale. A larger and more mobile hospital haemodialysis population would, in my view, be a great improvement to the care offered in Britain.

Preparation for chosen method of treatment

Most of the items in Table 1 are self-explanatory or are discussed elsewhere in this book. The *dental survey* is arranged because of the low standard of dental care in northern England. Dental extractions should be avoided by conservative dentistry, or carried out before they are complicated by thrice-weekly heparinization. The Dental Hospital undertakes much of the dental care of our dialysis and transplant patients because of reluctance by dental practitioners to treat patients with such complicated illness or to expose themselves to the supposed risk of hepatitis. Our patients, who are regularly screened for HBsAg, are probably a smaller risk to dentists than are the unscreened 'normal' population. The hysteria which once surrounded this subject is subsiding and it should soon be possible to restore the proper place of the local dentist.

Family planning advice is important for women who are still of child-bearing age. The fertility of women in late renal failure and on haemodialysis is very low; the Registry of the European Dialysis and Transplant Associ-ation (EDTA) could trace only 14 successful pregnancies among 25 000 women on dialysis and all these mothers still had some residual renal function[3]. Our experience suggests that abortion and still-birth are several times commoner than successful pregnancy, but even so the conception rate must be exceptionally low. Nonetheless, it is probably worth while taking precautions against pregnancy. Few families with the burden of regular haemodialysis wish to take on another child. Furthermore, menstrual periods are irregular or absent, giving rise to false scares about pregnancy which may be compounded by false–positive pregnancy tests on the urine (if any) of women with renal disease. If pregnancy is suspected it should be confirmed by measurement of blood gonadotrophins, but it is best to avoid the anxiety by good contraceptive advice.

This is easier said than given. Oral oestrogen–progestagen contraceptives may aggravate hypertension and intrauterine devices may exacerbate men-orrhagia caused by heparinization for dialysis. If a woman has completed her family the best solution may be tubal ligation, or even hysterectomy if menorrhagia is troublesome. Vasectomy for her husband is an attractive alternative, but, in my view, it should not be used unless the doctor is willing to tell him honestly his wife's prognosis on modern treatment (which is still far below normal life expectation) so that he can weigh up the possibility of remarriage in the event of her death. Personally, I prefer to avoid this awkward discussion if I can.

A gynaecologist willing to take a special interest in this group of patients, to give contraceptive advice, discuss the common sexual difficulties that they encounter and to undertake their gynaecological surgery, is a great asset to a renal unit.

Laboratory investigations at the predialysis clinic are dictated partly by local tradition and research interest and they differ considerably from centre to centre. I shall list those which we perform and attempt to justify them. Plasma creatinine, urea and electrolytes are measured at each visit and plasma creatinine is plotted on reciprocal paper to show a graph (usually roughly linear) of declining renal function. This is helpful in anticipating problems before they arise. Serum calcium, magnesium, phosphate and alkaline phosphatase are measured monthly; ideally the bone isoenzyme of alkaline phosphatase should be measured, since other isoenzymes are often present in renal failure[4] and the bone isoenzyme gives a much better reflection of bone disease[5]. Serum calcium samples should be handled promptly, since artifactual hypocalcaemia may be diagnosed if they are left to stand, probably due to the formation of calcium soaps in renal failure serum. Serum calcium and phosphate are guides to the adjustment of doses of calcium carbonate, aluminium hydroxide and vitamin D analogues. Serum magnesium results seldom influence treatment, but in renal failure a few patients have hypomagnesaemia which perpetuates hypocalcaemia[6,7]. We measure serum ionized calcium each month and find that this uncovers more cases of hypercalcaemia than measurement of total serum calcium alone[8]. Serum PTH should be measured every month or two if a suitable and reliable C-terminal assay is available. A Coulter count is carried out at each monthly visit; the absolute indices give a good guide to the presence of superimposed iron deficiency anaemia, so we do not measure serum iron or transferrin routinely. Serum ferritin is measured as a guide to iron stores once the patient starts haemodialysis[9,10], but is probably unnecessary at the predialysis clinic.

HBsAg should be rechecked monthly if the patient undergoes surgery (e.g. for fistula) and especially if there is a unit policy of routine transfusion in anticipation of transplantion. Otherwise a 6-monthly check is sufficient until the start of haemodialysis.

One of the most difficult problems is when to carry out a first radiological skeletal survey or/and a bone biopsy. In this centre, with its long history of severe bone disease, these tests are done almost routinely at predialysis clinic, but bone disease requiring treatment is rarely found if serum bone alkaline phosphatase is normal and serum PTH only modestly raised (up to three times the upper limit of normal in our assay which is not C- or N-terminal specific). In centres where bone disease is not a major problem it would be reasonable to postpone skeletal survey until these tests are clearly abnormal. Nerve conduction time, and quantitative electroencephalography, are used by those who believe they are important guides to the adequacy of dialysis and who want baseline figures. Since clinical neuropathy is rare in our haemodialysis population, and since we are not convinced of the value of these tests in adjusting dialysis time, we have abandoned their routine use. We use echocardiography and bone densitometry because cardiomyopathy and bone disease are important local problems, but would not recommend their use in all centres.

Discussions with the patient and family have been sorely neglected in the past. This is a deficiency in management that has been revealed by having nursing observers in the clinic. They have gained the confidence of patients who have revealed how little they absorb from initial conversations with doctors. The world of haemodialysis and CAPD, so familiar to the doctor, is totally strange to the patient. He requires repeated explanation of what is involved, preferably reinforced by well-illustrated, simply written literature which he can read at leisure, but this cannot be a substitute for painstaking explanation by the doctor. Articulate patients have proved very helpful in building the confidence of newcomers.

Clinical and laboratory surveillance often concentrates too much attention on the laboratory tests. The decision to start dialysis is still largely clinical, although the plasma creatinine plot is a very useful adjunct, and a plasma phosphate which will not fall on tolerable doses of calcium carbonate and aluminium hydroxide may be an indication for starting early. I have found it helpful to have a checklist of symptoms that should be sought at each visit. Symptoms and signs that call for an urgent start to dialysis (and indicate that the optimum time has been missed) include pericarditis, peripheral neuropathy, notable mental symptoms or fits. The earlier symptoms and signs which should lead one to start dialysis include troublesome muscular twitching, restlessness, weakness, fatigue, pruritus, progressive pigmentation and especially excoriation of the skin, irregular periods, impotence or severe loss of libido (not explained by drug therapy).

Bonomini and his colleagues in Bologna[11] have produced impressive evidence that it is better to start dialysis early than late. They begin treatment at a GFR of 20 ml/min or more, which may involve the patient receiving (and the state paying for) haemodialysis a year or more before he would do so in this country. That would be difficult to justify in the UK, where treatment is still offered to only half the potential patients, but it would be very reasonable to start almost asymptomatic patients at an arbitrary plasma creatinine level such as 1000 μmol/l in men and 800 μmol/l in women.

Referral for fistula insertion calls for fine judgement. A fistula should be inserted well in advance of the anticipated time when it will be needed. This is particularly true of fistulas constructed with artificial materials, heterografts or umbilical cord, since these are most likely to bleed or become infected if needled in the first few weeks after creation[12]. Even conventional fistulas are better left for a few weeks, so that veins can arterialize and blood flow increase before they are first used. Moreover, patients close to the start of dialysis tolerate general anaesthesia and even minor surgery very badly. For all these reasons, we aim to arrange fistula insertion at least 6 months before the start of dialysis in all patients with sufficiently slow progression, and early enough referral to the clinic, to make this possible.

I am a patient with

CHRONIC RENAL FAILURE

If in doubt please contact:

The Renal Unit,
Royal Victoria Infirmary,
Newcastle upon Tyne.

Telephone: Newcastle 25131

Because of this, certain drugs are potentially harmful to me and should be avoided in any treatment I receive.

Please see overleaf for details.

DRUGS TO BE AVOIDED

(1) Tetracycline and related antibiotics*

(2) Nitrofurantoin

(3) Clofibrate...........

(4) ....

(5) ....

*Doxycycline is the exception amongst the Tetracyclines. If indicated, it may be prescribed to patients with renal failure.

Known sensitivities

(1) ....

(2) ....

(3) ....

(4) ....

Figure 3   Outside and inside of drug card issued to patients with renal failure

On the other hand too early insertion of the fistula has disadvantages. The patient cannot be asked to consent to the operation without a thorough explanation of the need for it. This commits the medical team to a decision in favour of haemodialysis, which they may later regret if the patient develops complications like myocardial infarction or stroke over the next year at pre-dialysis clinic. It also imposes a longer period of worry about the future on the patient and his family. It imposes an unnecessarily prolonged burden on the heart and it may result in the loss of a fistula site; one of my patients whose function stabilized unexpectedly bore an unnecessary fistula for 3 years before it thrombosed spontaneously – she is now maintained on CAPD!

Until 1980 we referred all patients destined for CAPD for a fistula, so that access for haemodialysis was available if CAPD failed. We have now abandoned this policy because so few of the fistulas have been required. We now rely on an indwelling subclavian cannula[13] to tide us over the period between abandoning CAPD and using a newly inserted fistula.

A *drug card* (Figure 3) is issued to all patients at predialysis clinic and carried throughout their period of dialysis. They are taught to produce this card at any consultation with a doctor other than a member of the renal team.

THE DESIGN OF A HOSPITAL DIALYSIS UNIT

Many dialysis centres have been improvised from available facilities. The first British unit at the Royal Free Hospital was made up of several small rooms, with open gas fires on the walls. The first three areas utilized at our own unit in Newcastle were a basement store ('The Black Hole'), a urological side room and an ENT theatre. Even the recently opened St Thomas's Hospital unit is unmistakably derived from an operating theatre suite.

The purpose-built units that have followed have often been severely constrained by the limited sites available; our home training unit was built on stilts over a flimsy ground-floor building and has had no room to expand as work-load has increased and techniques have changed. A 'grand tour' of British dialysis centres provides a quick education in improvisation and ingenious space-saving design, and even at today's transport and hotel prices such a tour is a lot cheaper than making your own mistakes from inexperience.

Those who wish to see dialysis centres as they should be designed when money is no object should travel to selected centres abroad. The Japanese centre referred to above (Terakago and Nakagawa, personal communication) has one complete floor for dialysis and a ground floor with its own out-patient suite, laboratories, radiology and radioisotope department. A brief description of the ideal unit, as seen from Belgium, is provided by

Table 3 Essential components of a hospital haemodialysis unit

Entry facilities
Reception area
Washing and changing area for visitors
Patient changing rooms and toilets
Staff changing rooms and toilets
Patients' and visitors' waiting area

Dialysis facilities
Dialysing space
Nurses' station
Drug cupboard

Preparation facilities
Water treatment room
Dialyser preparation/re-use room
Technicians' workshop

Office space
Sister's office
Filing space for notes and X-rays

Catering facilities
Beverage bay and standing room for food trolleys
Staff eating room

Storage space for
Disposables
Prepared/re-used dialysers
Laundry
Chemicals for water treatment

Table 4 Desirable additional features of a hospital haemodialysis unit

Seminar room(s)
For staff training and patient discussion
For patient training (if home training undertaken)

Offices for
Doctor
Dialysis administrator and secretary
Dietitian/social worker

Out-patient space
Examination room
Small out-patient clinic

Operating space
Declotting room/small procedures room
Room for fistula insertion, etc.

Laboratory space
Sample preparation room
Small laboratory for emergency estimations
For research

Separate dialysis facilities
For hepatitis carriers
For other infected patients
For children

Ringoir[14]; it includes attractive interior design and air-conditioning among its essentials. In the following description I shall assume that I am writing for readers who suffer similar financial constraints to those in Britain, who must choose between priorities and must sometimes sacrifice desirable features to remain within a limited building site. I shall take it for granted that the hospital provides such essential services as radiology, medical physics, biochemistry, microbiology, etc., and that these need not be supplemented because of the addition of a hospital dialysis centre. This is an assumption that the nephrologist cannot afford to make without checking his facts. At one time our dialysis unit provided 15% of the hospital's biochemical workload. Dialysis units are heavy consumers of many other services, so it is essential, when designing one, to consult the directors of all laboratory services to confirm that they can handle the additional work.

The essentials in a hospital unit are listed in Table 3. Desirable additional facilities, some of which must be supplied somewhere but not necessarily on the dialysis unit itself, are listed in Table 4. The subheadings below correspond to the items in those tables. A sketch of one possible design (modified from one of our own hospital dialysis units) is shown in Figure 4.

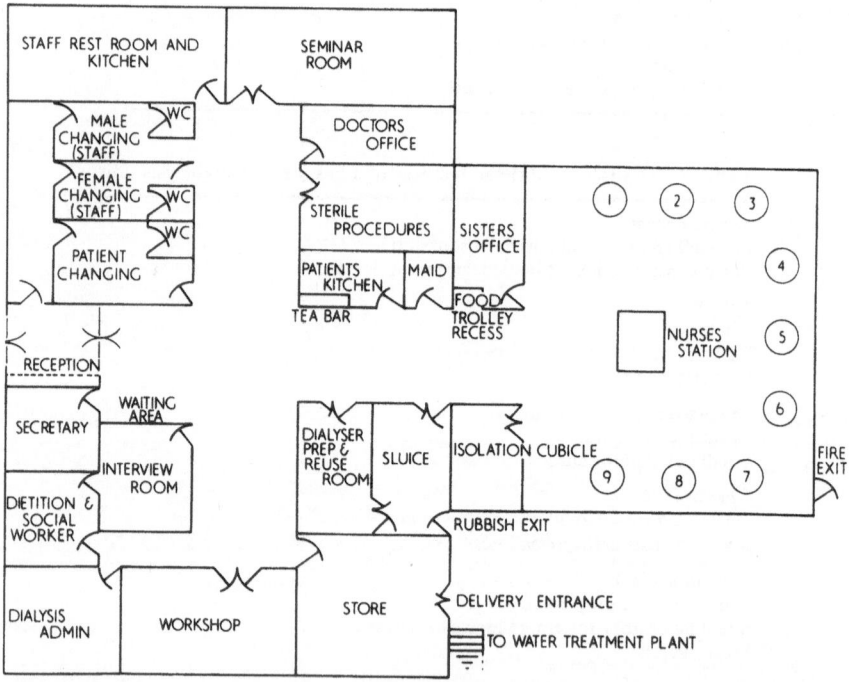

Figure 4 Schematic diagram of a hospital dialysis unit. The rooms shown correspond roughly to those provided at the Freeman Hospital dialysis unit, Newcastle, though the layout is closer to what our nursing staff would have wished if not confined to their roof-top site

Although the Rosenheim Report on precautions against hepatitis[15] is now well out of date it has not been superseded by any new document and those designing a hospital unit should consult it and discuss arrangements with the Health and Safety Executive or their equivalent in other countries.

Entry facilities

Reception area

This area should lie outside the entry barrier which marks the start of anti-hepatitis precautions. Ideally there should be a secretary or ward clerk in an office or bay, who answers telephone calls, directs visitors, receives supplies, passes on specimens, etc.

Washing and changing area for visitors

The extent to which visitors (including visiting medical staff who are not proposing to engage in activities like fistula needling) are expected to change and wash before entering a dialysis unit varies considerably and owes more to habit or prejudice than science. However, it is important that there should be facilities for handwashing (elbow-operated taps and soap dispensers), disposable towels and disposal bins, dispensers for sterilized laundered gowns (or disposable paper gowns) and disposable masks and shoe covers, in case these are needed during a 'hepatitis scare'. There should be adequate coat-hooks for hanging white coats or outside clothing. Sadly, it is necessary in British hospitals to erect a notice warning visitors not to leave valuables in their clothing.

Patient changing rooms and toilets

Many patients undergo hospital haemodialysis in indoor clothing, sitting in chairs. However, there should be facilities for them to change into separate clothing if they wish to and this should be strongly encouraged during any hepatitis quarantine period, since there is a considerable risk of clothing being spattered with blood during a haemodialysis. There should be sufficient locking lockers to hold the personal effects of two shifts of patients simultaneously. Changing rooms should be provided for the two sexes separately, and it is required in Britain that separate toilets should be provided for the two sexes. This is a considerable expense in a small dialysis unit and it is a regulation that is not universally observed. However, few hospital units are now built with less than ten stations and, with the fast turnover permitted by short dialysis, separate changing and toilet facilities are efficient as well as aesthetically pleasing.

Showers for patients (again separate for the two sexes) are recommended fixtures, but in our experience they are seldom used (except in hepatitis epidemics) and I regard them as among the least essential features of a dialysis unit.

Staff changing room and toilets

Staff who work continuously in the dialysis unit normally change into special clothing; it is mandatory that nurses or other staff who are at high risk of being contaminated with blood should do so. In many British units such staff are nearly all female. Nonetheless, British practice demands the provision of separate changing and toilet facilities for the two sexes. We do not possess such separate facilities on one of our units and have not found that the need for staff to visit the changing rooms or toilets sequentially is a major problem. One locker with secure lock should be provided for each member of staff, to hold outdoor clothing, handbags, etc., during the working day.

Patients' and visitors' waiting areas

Ideally there should be a comfortable waiting area with easy chairs, tables, magazines and a beverage dispenser outside the entry barrier, adjacent to the reception area. This is used by relatives waiting to collect patients and casual visitors. Dialysis units attract a surprising number of these, including schoolgirls, who have completed sponsored swims in aid of the kidney unit, reporters, television cameramen, mayors on Christmas visits, etc. They need somewhere to wait before being instructed how to change and being escorted through the entry barrier.

A patient waiting area is needed inside the barrier for those who attend the unit for extra procedures (shunt declotting, transfusion, iron injections, etc.) or follow-up visits. It is also popular with those who have to wait for transport home.

Dialysis facilities

Dialysing space

Cross-infection, particularly with hepatitis, is a serious problem in hospital haemodialysis units so subdivision of the dialysing space into cubicles or small rooms has obvious attractions. However, it requires large numbers of nursing staff. Ringoir[14] found that the subdivision of his dialysis unit raised the nurse:station ratio from 1.1:1 to 1.33:1, an extra seven full-time staff in his 30-bed unit. Consequently, nearly all hospital dialysis units are designed with a single main dialysing area. Ideally, this should form most of a circle around a central nursing station to give maximum nursing observation from one position. However, circular rooms do not form a convenient part of most architectural plans and are usually impracticable at any but ground-floor level. There are several acceptable alternatives; wide rectangular rooms with a central station, L-shaped rooms with the nursing station on the angle of the L, and oblong rooms with the nursing station protruding from one of the long sides, to form a ⊏- shaped dialysing area are the most popular.

Centres which combine hospital dialysis with home training (a combination to be avoided if possible, since it saps the determination of prospective home patients) need smaller rooms in which patients can complete their home training in relative isolation to simulate conditions at home.

Satellite dialysis centres, for the use of self-sufficient patients who are prevented from dialysing at home by lack of a partner, etc., need not conform to this pattern. They are designed for self-dialysis with nursing help available at the push of a button, but not for continuous nursing supervision. Some very successful satellite units are in converted dwelling houses, the patients dialysing two or three to a room.

For the main hospital unit, about 100 ft^2 (9 m^2) are needed per patient to provide comfortable, airy conditions with free circulation of staff. Ringoir[14] recommended 6–12 m^2 per patient according to choice of equipment, but I regard the lower figure as inadequate for anything except satellite dialysis and the higher figure is well beyond the budget one is likely to receive in this country.

Nurses' station

This provides a writing desk, a telephone and often an intercom to other parts of the renal unit, storage space for patients' current records and either the main drug cupboard or a smaller ready-use cupboard. In centres equipped for electronic monitoring, oscilloscopes are sited at the nurses' station.

Drug cupboard

A resuscitation trolley should be sited in or near the dialysing space; it should hold supplies of the most vital drugs for immediate resuscitation (intravenous sodium bicarbonate; drugs for the treatment of cardiac arrest; dextran and plasma products for immediate restoration of blood volume after haemorrhage; muscle relaxants and sedatives to assist artificial respiration; diazepam and other anticonvulsants for the treatment of uraemic fits, etc.), a laryngoscope, a set of intratracheal tubes, an Ambu bag, a mouth gag, connecting pieces for the oxygen supply and other standard equipment. A cardiac monitor and defibrillator should also be in, or immediately adjacent to, the dialysing space.

   Additional supplies of these drugs for emergencies should be in the ready-use drug cupboard, along with supplies of heparin, protamine and remedies for the more minor emergencies of dialysis: calcium gluconate, hypertonic saline or glucose for muscle cramps, analgesics of varied strength, sedatives, intravenous and oral antihypertensives and the most frequently used anti-biotics. Consumption of other drugs in the dialysis unit is low and there is no need to keep large or varied stocks if wards or the dispensary are in easy reach. However, it is cheaper to buy some supplies, like multivitamin tablets, in bulk and dispense them to patients on the unit, rather than issuing individual prescriptions. It also gives the staff a check on how regularly the drugs are consumed. Not all pharmaceutical committees in hospital will allow this practice.

Preparation facilities

Water treatment room

In the early years of regular haemodialysis, about half the British centres and many overseas used raw tap water to prepare dialysate. It was usually passed through a $25\,\mu M$ or similar fabric filter to remove particulate matter and a finer filter of 3 or $5\,\mu M$, which had some effect in reducing bacterial count. True bacterial filters, with a pore size less than $1\,\mu M$, have a high resistance to flow and were seldom employed. In most of southern England water had to be softened because its calcium content was above the optimum for dialysis fluid. Some other centres used softened water because of a lower, but variable, calcium and magnesium content.

   The theoretical argument for better purification has always been strong. In 1973 I drew the attention of a British audience, including representatives of the Department of Health, to the long list of contaminants in tap water, most of which are unaffected by water softeners and which are added to dialysis fluid unmonitored[16]. There was general acceptance of the proposition that such contaminants should be removed, if only for medicolegal reasons, but no action resulted; water treatment was expensive and money was short. The epidemics of dialysis encephalopathy and fracturing osteo-dystrophy, referred to in the section on the absorption of trace contaminants, changed the situation completely. It became mandatory for units supplied with water containing aluminium to remove it. Deionizers do this efficiently in some water areas, or at some times of the year, but are not always reliable; the variations probably reflect the amount of aluminium in colloidal form which escapes chemical reaction with the ion-exchange resins[17]. Reverse osmosis has been consistently successful in removing aluminium in our experience and in all other published studies so it is the treatment of choice in high-aluminium areas. However, there are a few troublesome solutes which are not well removed by reverse osmosis, such as chloramines[18]. The best policy is, therefore, to treat water by initial filtration, pH adjustment and softening (to reduce its damaging effects on reverse osmosis membranes), then by reverse osmosis and finally by deionization. Since the solute content of the water entering the deionizer is very low the cartridge has a long life and adds little to the running costs.

To use this combination of water treatments in every home would be prohibitively expensive; it would negate most of the cost advantage of home haemodialysis. Selective use of different forms of treatment is necessary, based on regular analysis of the water supply. This involves some risk for the patient, but compared with the other hazards of life on dialysis it is a small one and only one life is at stake. In a hospital dialysis unit many lives are at stake and the capital cost per patient of good water treatment is lower, although still considerable (about £2000 per station). It is my strong personal view, not yet shared by all directors of dialysis units, that all hospital units merit full water treatment. Aluminium appeared unannounced in water supplies from which it was previously absent and was recognized only after lives had been lost from encephalopathy[19]. The same may happen with other contaminants or additives, so a long history of freedom from trouble is not a guarantee for the future.

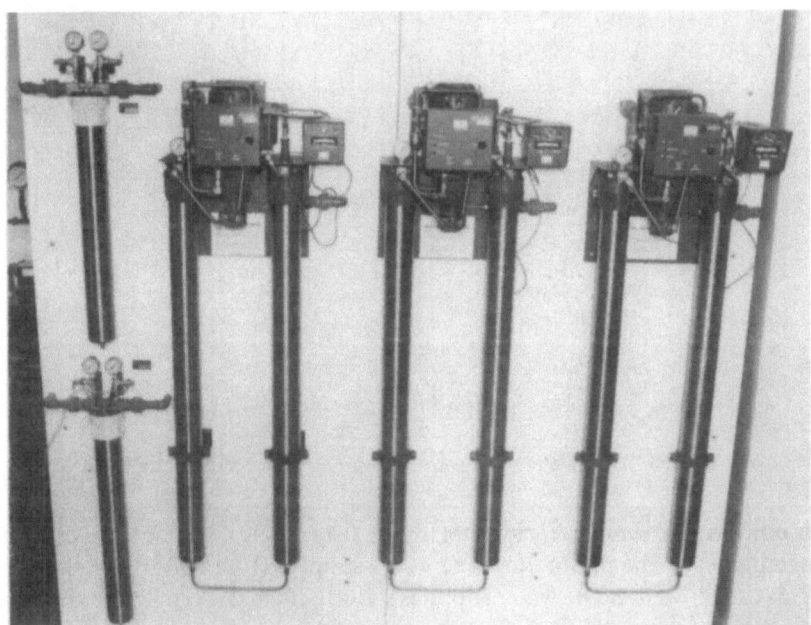

Figure 5 Water treatment system at Newcastle, Royal Victoria Infirmary. Shown are the reverse osmosis (RO) units and the final filters (left). Behind the screen are the storage tank, deionizer, circulating pumps and filter. The pretreatment plant (which needs little attention) is in the roof space

The water treatment system at one Newcastle unit is illustrated in Figure 5 and, diagrammatically, in Figure 6. Water is filtered through three grades of membrane filter (typically 25, 5 and 2 mM pore), the last of which is illustrated at the left of Figure 5. The filter is duplicated so that operation of the system is not interrupted while a filter is changed. Between the second and third filters water passes through a base-exchange softener, since high-calcium water is more damaging to reverse osmosis membranes than softened water. The pH meter and automatic acid-dosing unit will be added

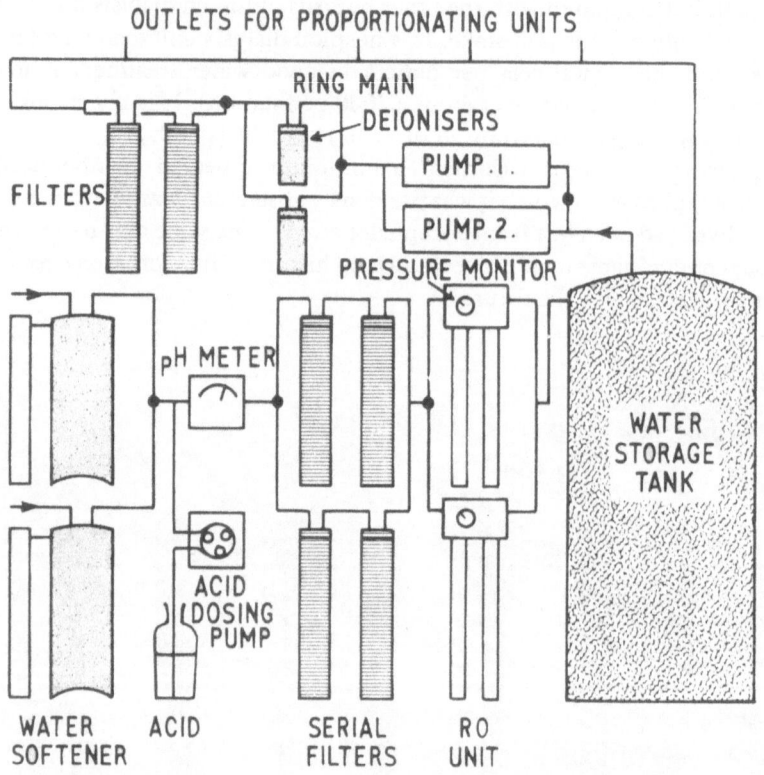

Figure 6 Diagram of water treatment system, Royal Victoria Infirmary

to our system shortly because of rapid deterioration of reverse osmosis membranes at the pH of our local water supply. Hydrochloric or ascorbic acids can be used. Some water supplies require alkali dosing. There are three reverse osmosis units because one does not have sufficient output for our unit; more recent models will provide sufficient output for a ten-bed dialysis centre so that only two reverse osmosis units would be required (one in use and one on standby).

The importance of good pretreatment of the water cannot be overemphasized. Some water supplies in the UK (e.g. Newcastle and Oxford) destroy a reverse osmosis membrane within 3 months, whereas their expected life is about 2 years in other geographical areas. It may prove necessary to use pre-filters finer than $2\,\mu M$ and to pressurize the water supply in order to do so if particulate matter is particularly prevalent in the water supply. The system illustrated is a Millipore spiral-wound membrane. Several other firms supply similar equipment and there are at least two suppliers of hollow-fibre reverse osmosis apparatus. A choice between systems should be based on thorough study of the water supply.

The reverse osmosis unit incorporates a water pump which generates the high pressures needed to force water through a membrane which is virtually impermeable even to small molecules. Recent equipment is acceptably quiet but is still better housed in a separate room which is not continuously occupied by staff.

Water emerging from the reverse osmosis apparatus passes to a storage tank, from which it is circulated continuously around the dialysis unit, passing through a deionizer cartridge on the way. This ensures a high flow through the deionizer, avoiding channelling. Deionized water readily dissolves metals and is particularly liable to do so when the deionizer is approaching exhaustion, at which point the pH of effluent water falls. Consequently all parts of the circuit are made of materials approved by the Department of Health and Social Security (DHSS) for this purpose – approved plastics and high-grade stainless steel. Advice on the choice of materials can be obtained from the DHSS[20].

Reverse osmosis membranes are impermeable to bacteria and bacterial pyrogens. Consequently the water in our circuit starts off sterile, but bacteria can build up with surprising ease in such solute-free and apparently non-sustaining fluid. The reverse osmosis membrane is automatically flushed with a fast flow of chlorinated tap water every hour and this has so far prevented more than occasional trace contamination of our circuit with saprophytes. In a warmer climate we might not be so fortunate; a bacterial filter might then be inserted in the circuit, as shown in Figure 6, and the reverse osmosis membranes would be sterilized regularly with formalin or iodine.

Rapid technological advances in water treatment spring from the needs of the pharmaceutical and microchip industries for very pure water; information on the subject is hard to find in the medical literature. Those needing advice on the subject are welcome to phone Dr Michael Ward on 0632 25131 for an informal discussion.

Dialyser preparation/re-use room

In 1976 over 60% of British patients were dialysed with non-disposable (Kiil-type) haemodialysers[21]. Most of our hospital haemodialysis patients still use them, but we have changed to re-used disposables in home haemo-dialysis and the trend to disposables, already apparent in 1976[21], has prob-ably continued nationally. All the non-disposables in use in Newcastle, and I suspect all those in use nationally, are Meltec multipoint dialysers.

In the heyday of the Kiil dialyser, every dialysis unit had a large building area and an equally large, preferably separate, stripping area. The former was equipped with easily washed benches holding soaking trays for mem-branes, ports, scalpel blades, etc., shelves to hold containers of 2% formalin for filling dialysers, and a wash-down floor with a floor drain. Exhaust ventilation was essential to remove formalin vapour. The stripping area had a similar impermeable floor and a supply of deep sinks, large enough to hold Kiil boards while they were scrubbed down. There were tanks of formalin in which the boards were periodically soaked. Exhaust ventilation was again essential.

Re-use of disposables is now so widely accepted[21] that I doubt whether anyone designing a new dialysis centre would incorporate the facilities just described and I have not shown them in detail in Figure 4. Dialyser re-use takes place conveniently in the former 'building space'. Re-use is discussed later in this chapter. Both hospital-built non-disposables and re-used dis-posables are sterilized with formalin which must be washed out before re-use. Safe levels of residual formalin can only be achieved by prolonged washing, which is most economically carried out by attaching the dialysate pathway to a tap water supply. An area in the building space may therefore be equipped with a row of taps and corresponding small sinks or drip cups for rinsing.

Although a 'stripping area' is not required when disposables are re-used there is still a need for what Ringoir calls a 'garbage room': a space where the dialyser and its circuit are tidied up, attached haemostats retrieved, the dialyser preserved for re-use and other items discarded into impermeable bags, securely fastened. An adjoining space can be used for bagging soiled linen. This is placed in alginate-stitched nylon bags which can be inserted unopened into a foul-washer; the alginate stitches dissolve, spilling the bag's content into the wash-water. However, foul-washers do not usually sterilize foul linen so a preliminary autoclaving step is necessary if the unit is in quarantine for hepatitis.

Technicians' workshop

Round-the-clock working in hospital haemodialysis has deprived tech-nicians of the opportunity to service proportionating units and similar equipment on idle days. It has therefore become necessary to keep several machines in reserve and to rotate them regularly for routine servicing. At least one machine must be ready at all times to substitute for any which break down. The workshop must be large enough to store these surplus machines, to permit storage of a wide range of accessories and servicing records and still leave adequate working space for technicians repairing two or more machines. An extra-large workshop is required if it also services machines for the home dialysis programme.

Office space

The nurses' station is too public a place for giving nursing reports or discussing patients, so a sister's room is essential. I have listed all other offices as desirable rather than essential. It makes for a happier and more efficient unit if the doctor in charge has an office in the unit in which he is accessible for a good part of his working week. If he and the dialysis administrator are usually some distance away from the unit it is helpful if they can be linked to the unit by intercom.

Catering facilities

If the hospital has a central food supply system, arrangements for keeping food warm on trolleys until it is convenient to serve it are essential. A day space in which patients can eat meals before or after dialysis is a useful adjunct if many travel from a distance; with dialysis times of 3 or 4 h some patients prefer not to eat during the procedure.

Staff are strongly encouraged to change their clothes and leave the unit for main meals, but one can hardly expect them to do so for morning coffee or afternoon tea. Consequently a beverage bay (which also serves the patients) is needed adjacent to a staff eating area. Handwashing facilities must be available between the dialysing space and the coffee room. Smoking should be prohibited in the dialysing space but has to be permitted in the coffee room as nearly half Britain's nurses still smoke cigarettes – a sad and inexplicable exception to the general trend among professional workers of all kinds.

Storage space

The invariable comment of the nurse in charge of any new dialysis unit is 'we did not plan enough storage space'. Disposables and linen are surprisingly bulky and large stocks have to be held.

Seminar rooms

It is valuable if a seminar room for staff training and discussion meetings can be located inside the cross-infection barrier; it is less bother for one lecturer to put on a gown than for all of his audience to change their clothes.

Patients learn home haemodialysis mainly by repeated oral instruction and practice. However, learning can be accelerated by formal teaching, tape slides, videotapes and examinations. A room, or rooms, should be set aside for these activities if home training is undertaken on the hospital unit.

Out-patient space

Full examination of a patient in the dialysing space is very difficult. There should be a separate examination and interview room for dealing with complaints that arise at routine dialysis visits. It is also very convenient for the patient if his formal follow-up assessments can be carried out in a clinic attached to the dialysis centre. However, we have had to arrange such out-patient surveillance in the main out-patient department and have not found it an excessive burden.

Operating space

When arteriovenous shunts were the main means of access to the circulation, and renal physicians had to insert most of them personally, a 'shunt room' equipped to small operating theatre standards was a great asset on a dialysis unit. Now that fistulas are used, most access procedures can be carried out on cold operating lists by vascular surgeons. A mini-theatre is no longer required, but the few patients who still bear shunts do need a space in which declotting can be carried out and minor revisions performed. Our mini-theatre is now used for bone biopsy and similar procedures that do not call for general anaesthesia or full theatre precautions.

Laboratory space

We have been fortunate in having a service laboratory a few yards from our dialysis unit since it was erected on its present site. Those who have to transport samples over longer distances may need a small laboratory for spinning and separating blood samples and carrying out a few emergency tests like microhaematocrit. A refrigerator can be used to store samples, but long delays should be avoided if possible, particularly for calcium estimation.

Separate dialysis facilities

It is British policy to segregate hepatitis carriers completely from the main dialysis unit, but in other countries, where hepatitis carriers are commoner in the general population or where the problem was tackled too late to prevent infection of many patients, this is not practicable. In such centres it may be necessary to treat carriers and susceptible patients in the same unit, but they should be segregated physically and their equipment kept separate.

Some dialysis centres have an isolation room in which a regular dialysis patient with a severely infected shunt, influenza or some other infection can be treated with a reduced risk of infecting his fellow-patients. Lacking this facility in one of our two units we admit such patients to a cubicle in the general ward for dialysis.

Paediatric nephrologists advise separate dialysis facilities for children, staffed by nurses trained in paediatric nursing. This ideal is not attainable in centres serving only a small paediatric population, but it may be possible to congregate the children on a single shift in an adult dialysis unit.

EQUIPMENT OF A HOSPITAL DIALYSIS UNIT

Beds and chairs

Reclining chairs (Parker Knoll recliner type) have largely displaced beds for routine regular haemodialysis (Figure 7). For a time they had the disadvantage that they precluded continuous weighing during dialysis, but with electronic bed-weighers this is no longer a problem. Continuous weighing is in any case only required for a minority of patients starting dialysis or suffering complications.

However, beds are more suitable for seriously ill patients and any who suffer from hypotension. Some warning of impending hypotension and

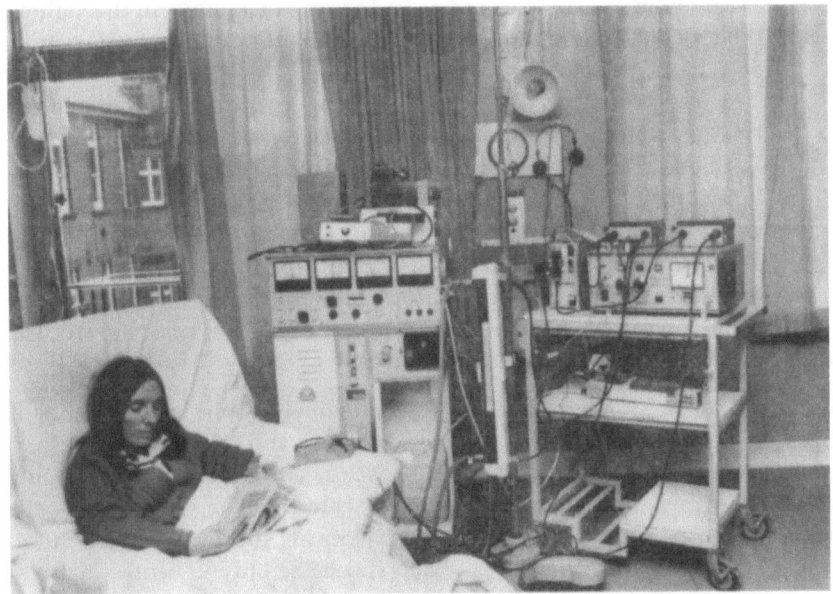

Figure 7   Patient undergoing hospital dialysis in a reclining chair, covered by a sheet

sufficient muscle power to operate the reclining chair are necessary to avert fainting if the patient is dialysed in the sitting position.

Bed-weighers

Two electronic bed- or chair-weighers are sufficient for a ten-bed unit employed solely for regular dialysis of chronic patients. More are required if the unit is also responsible for acute renal failure (an uncommon arrangement in Britain and one that is not recommended in the Rosenheim Report). We have found the Datex weigher eminently suitable; baseline drift is difficult to eliminate altogether but is not a serious problem during a 4 h dialysis. There are several other makes available.

Proportionating units

A hospital dialysis centre has a choice of two main systems: a central supply system for dialysis fluid with bed-head monitors or single-patient proportionating units at each bed. Each has its advocates. Single-patient proportionating units are clearly preferable if the centre combines hospital dialysis and home training in a single dialysing space; patients learn on the machinery they will use at home. We have chosen to use single-patient units, even though hospital dialysis and home training are segregated in Newcastle, for the following reasons:

(1) It has allowed us to standardize on one type of equipment throughout the city and surrounding region. This simplifies technician training and the stocking of spare parts.
(2) The few patients on the hospital unit who eventually switch to home training already know the machinery well.
(3) Each station can be closed down and prepared for the next dialysis individually, which allows a rolling change of shifts. This facility is not always available on central supply systems.
(4) The problems of controlling bacterial growth in dialysis fluid are diminished; each proportionating unit has its own sterilizing equipment and can be taken out of service for repair if it ceases to sterilize the dialysis fluid pathway satisfactorily.

On the other hand, the capital cost of individual proportionating units is higher than that of some central supply systems and the maintenance and replacement costs are also higher. They occupy more room in the dialysing space and this is not compensated by the extra storage space for a well-designed central supply system. In general, central supply systems are used in large hospital dialysis centres which specialize only in centre dialysis; there are virtually no such centres in the United Kingdom and our pattern in Newcastle reflects current British practice.

Choice of individual proportionating units

There is a bewildering variety of units on the market; at any large congress, like the European Dialysis and Transplant Association or the International Society of Nephrology, 20 such machines will be displayed by rival manufacturers. A visit to such a commercial exhibition is the best way of surveying the market. Having heard the manufacturers' accounts of their wares, the prospective buyer should then seek an independent opinion and he is unlikely to find it in the medical literature. In Britain the Supplies Branch of the Department of Health and Social Security runs two testing programmes for dialysis equipment:

(1) A study of electrical safety, suitability of materials, safe separation of electronic and plumbing components, design logic, fail-safe monitoring, ease of maintenance and reliability during prolonged bench running, which is conducted at Aldermaston. The problem of electrical safety is discussed by Whelpton[23].

(2) A user's appreciation carried out on two or three British dialysis units, where records are kept of mechanical failure, problems with staff handling the machine, etc.

This information is fed back to manufacturers who often modify their machines as a result. Consequently the reports are not currently circulated or published, but information can be obtained by enquiry from the Supplies Branch[22].

The Lucas Mark 2, the standard machine used at Newcastle, is illustrated in Figure 8. We have purchased Lucas equipment for the last 14 years in spite of being a test centre for other equipment. This is partly due to the inertia produced by a large investment; a decision to change manufacturer results in a long period when technicians must train on two machines and keep two sets of spares. However, it also reflects general satisfaction with this robust and easily maintained machine. Illustrated features in Figure 8 include:

(A) The concentrate tank, holding 35 × concentrate for manufacturing dialysis fluid. This is diluted with water in a fixed-ratio double-cylinder pump controlled by a rotating valve. Some of the alternative proportionating units have variable-ratio double-cylinder pumps or twin peristaltic pumps which allow a change in the dilution over a fairly narrow (and therefore safe) range. They will be preferred by those who like to vary the sodium concentration of dialysis fluid for each individual patient. The usual concentrate contains acetate, but the Lucas can be modified to use a mixture of about two-thirds bicarbonate and one-third acetate. Some rival machines, notably the Drake Willock, can be used with all the acetate replaced by bicarbonate.

(B) The dialysis fluid flow monitor. The Lucas produces a fixed dialysis fluid flow rate of about 530 ml/min, so the rotameter is provided solely as a visual confirmation that the effluent pump is working normally. Some alternative machines have a variable dialysis fluid flow rate, but the great majority of clinicians (guided by habit more than scientific evidence) use a flow rate of about 500 ml/min.

(C) The dialysis fluid negative pressure control. This knob controls a needle valve upstream of the dialyser. A similar device is standard on almost all proportionating units.

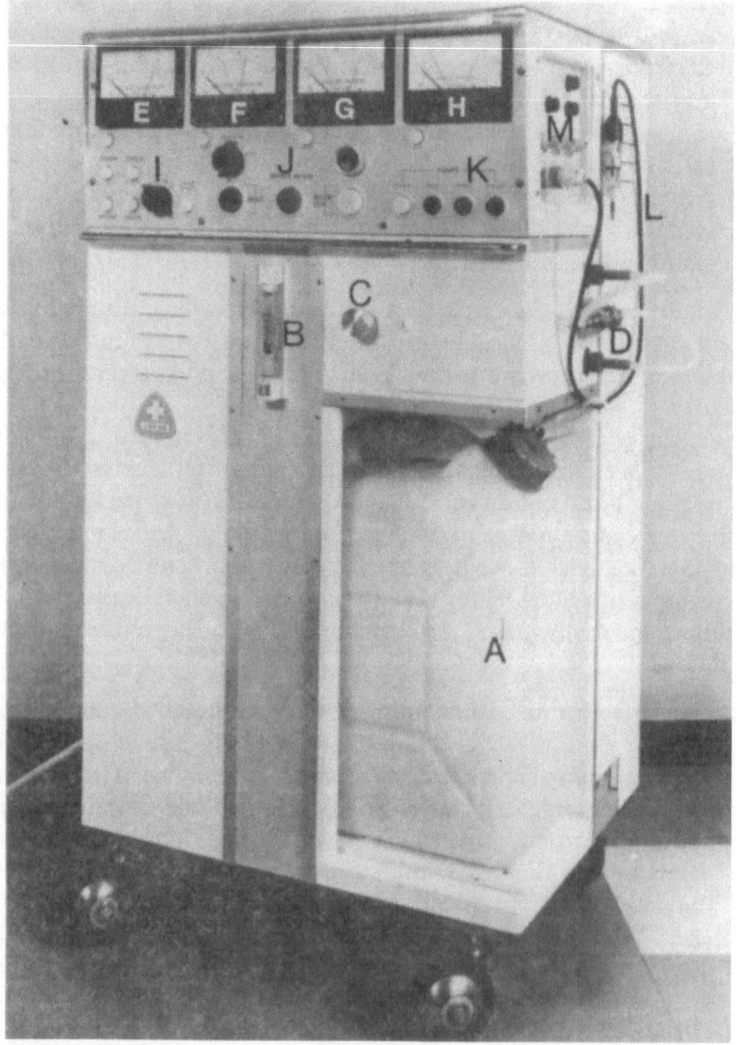

Figure 8 Lucas Mark 2 proportionating unit. The letters are explained in the text

(D) Dialysis fluid output and return connections. These are connected to the dialyser by Quick-fit stainless steel connectors, which are shown joined over a short stainless steel bar, to allow circulation of fluid during the sterilization cycle.

(E) Conductivity monitor, which detects changes in dialysis fluid electrolyte content and therefore reveals any malfunction of the mixing unit. The two red alarm pointers (grey in this black and white photograph) are set with the aid of small black buttons immediately below the dial (not clearly visible). The 'window' is usually set at $\pm 2\%$ of the desired conductivity. The controls for adjusting the desired conductivity are not accessible to the patient or nurse; they must be set by the technician. An earlier proportionating unit had the controls too accessible and this led to a fatality on our unit when a patient chose to adjust his monitor rather than report an alarm.

(F) Dialysis fluid temperature monitor with alarm pointers which are usually set at about $\pm 2\,°C$ from the desired temperature of 37–$39\,°C$, which depends on the ambient temperature and therefore the cooling of blood that occurs in the return lines. The thermostat is set by the knob below this dial.

(G) Dialysis fluid negative pressure monitor with alarm pointers which are typically set about 50 mmHg above and below the negative pressure chosen to achieve the necessary fluid removal.

(H) Venous pressure monitor which records pressure in the air space of the bubble trap on the venous blood line (see Figure 11). The alarm pointers can be set wide for start-up and take-off but should be narrowed to about 50 mmHg above and below the desired pressure as soon as dialysis is stable. If the venous pressure is below 50 mmHg, the lower alarm limit should be closer to the actual pressure – it should never be below zero during dialysis.

The option of running the machine with the venous pressure alarm limits too wide is sometimes chosen by nurses either because they forget to adjust the limits after completing start-up or because they are bothered by too-frequent alarms in a patient with unstable blood flow. This is a hazard which applies to all machines with adjustable alarm limits, which has led some manufacturers to apply electronically imposed fixed alarm limits, e.g. $\pm 15\%$ of the recorded pressure. Although theoretically safer, this arrangement is very inconvenient during start-up, take-off and, especially, after any temporary interruption of blood flow caused by an alarm. Consequently we prefer the adjustable alarm limits.

(I) Control switch for setting operational phase and indicator lights telling at a glance in which phase the machine is operating. It will only work in one sequence: 'standby', 'sterilize', 'dialyse', 'sterilize'. 'Sterilize' is strictly a misnomer; the circuit is pasteurized with $85\,°C$

water. With an input of low bacterial count this system has given us remarkably little trouble from bacterial build-up. We prefer it to formalin sterilization (in which the 'sterilization' is again a misnomer), since it is difficult to eliminate all smells and exposure of staff to liquid and vapour. However, in the Lucas it has the disadvantage that the electricity consumption during the heating phase is just above 13 A. It must therefore be attached to a 30 A circuit. This is an added expense in the home and a nuisance when the machine is moved to non-renal wards, but is no great problem in hospital dialysis; heavy wiring is necessary in a unit where many machines may be drawing current simultaneously.

(J) Visual and auditory alarms. The buzzer can be muted temporarily while a fault is corrected. Individual lights beside the meters indicate the source of an alarm.

(K) Pump-on indicator lights for effluent, blood and heparin pumps.

(L) Lead for connection to venous bubble trap. It should be connected through a disposable isolator to prevent contamination of any part of the sensing device with blood, which readily creeps up the tube during fluctuations in venous pressure.

Figure 9 shows the Nycrotron ADPAC, an alternative proportionating unit which we have used less extensively. Its advantages are that it is small

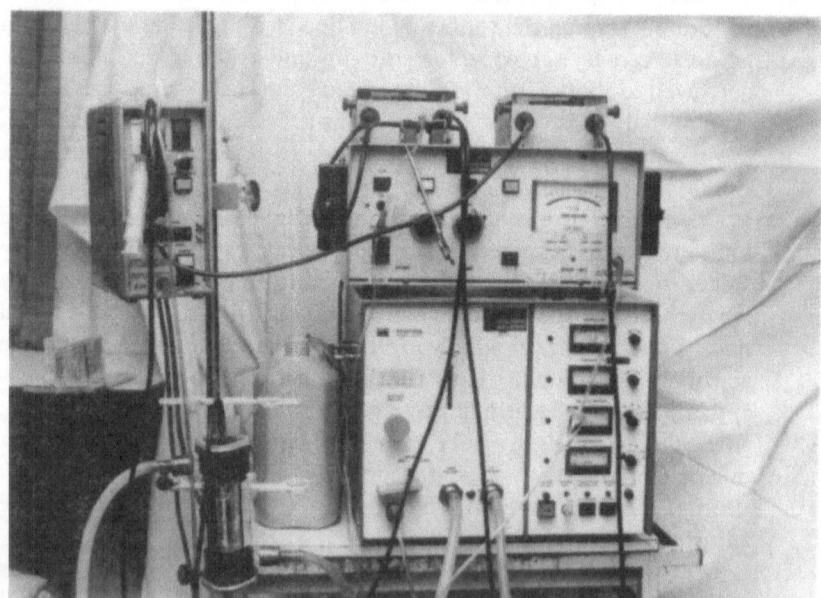

Figure 9 Nycotron ADPAC proportionating unit with Bellco double-headed pump and air embolism monitor

and compact, it runs off 13 A power plugs and it can be discharged into any sink, whereas the Lucas requires a low-level drain. These differences make it easier to install in the home without major alterations. It is truly sterilized by superheated water in a pressurized circuit, which is an added reassurance against spread of hepatitis between patients. Because of this feature, and the ease with which it can be plugged into almost any location in hospital, we have adopted it for in-patient treatment of acute renal failure, postoperative transplant recipients and patients on regular dialysis with complications.

The Achilles heel of the Nycotron is its effluent pump which has been ingeniously designed to avoid breaching the pressurized circuit. However, it wears out more quickly than conventional pumps. It cannot be run at a negative pressure closer to zero than − 70 mmHg, which limits the choice of dialyser if the patient is prone to hypotension; on the other hand it has a very efficient de-aeration system which permits the use of dialysers like the Travenol Hoeltzenbeim, which are susceptible to air-trapping. It has preset alarm limits which give rise to the problems mentioned above under (H).

Of the present generation of proportionating units, several others deserve brief mention. The Drake Willock 7000 is easy to service, robust and the product of more experience than any competitor; it is equipped with an ultrafiltration predictor which computes the expected fluid loss from measured transmembrane pressure and a figure for the ultrafiltration capacity of the dialyser in use, supplied by the operator.

The Bellco Unimat has one valuable, unique feature − a disposable dialysate pathway. This can be changed within a few minutes and eliminates the need for a sterilization cycle. It speeds up the changeover between shifts by the best part of an hour. It can be used with the dialysate pressure at zero or positive for sequential ultrafiltration haemodialysis, though this procedure is not currently approved by the Department of Health.

The Cobe Centry 2 is a popular unit internationally because of three desirable features: easy layout for maintenance; a predetermined arrangement of dialysis lines, which speeds setting-up, provided the appropriate lines are bought; and the presence of an ultrafiltration monitor. This monitor only operates on demand by temporary diversion of the dialysis fluid flow, so it cannot be used for continuous read-out of ultrafiltration and automatic control.

A new generation of proportionating units is now coming on to the market which will probably displace the older types described above. The pumping, plumbing and monitoring parts are little different from those of present machines, but the microprocessor will take over some of the supervisory functions of the nurse. The first such machine to be approved in Britain was the Gambro AK10. It will automatically control transmembrane pressure, which determines ultrafiltration rate. Some versions of the AK10 can be used for sequential ultrafiltration haemodialysis, but the machine will be modified for the British market to ensure that it cannot operate with dialysis fluid pressure above that in blood, which will limit its use in sequential ultrafiltration dialysis.

Fresenius–Dylade are in the process of introducing the first British-made machine of this type: the Dylade Series E. Initial impressions of those conducting pilot trials are favourable. Several other manufacturers have microprocessor-controlled machines at the trial stage.

Blood pumps

The Watson Marlow MHRE is the pump in general use in Britain; it is cheap, robust and effective. It does not have accurate control of occlusion, and, because it operates on smaller-bore tubing than some of its competitors, it produces a little more haemolysis[24]; however, haemolysis contributes so little to the anaemia of renal failure that it need not influence the choice of pump. The Bellco 760 N twin-headed pump shown in Figures 7 and 9 was designed for single-needle dialysis but can also be used for conventional dialysis. We use it with all machines employed in the wards, intensive therapy unit, etc., since it allows us to preserve vessels by using a single access point, e.g. in the subclavian vein. It is about five times as expensive as a Watson Marlow pump but extremely reliable and well engineered. Of the wide choice of other pumps available, the Rhone Poulenc deserves special mention. It uses rollers pressing against a stretched silicone rubber tube, without an opposing surface. Consequently it will not pump against very high resistances and it has the unusual feature of failing to pump air forwards in the circuit. It therefore reduces the risk of membrane rupture and air embolism.

Heparin pumps

In Britain a slow-running Watson Marlow pump is widely used to infuse heparin. Some centres, including my own, prefer syringe pumps, such as Sage, Dasco or Scientifica and Cook. The syringe pump should be equipped with a flashing light that operates when it is functioning normally, since it is virtually silent and its slow progress is not visible to the unaided eye.

Additional monitors

In addition to the monitors incorporated in the proportionating unit, one is mandatory and another desirable.

Air embolism monitor

Fatal air embolism has nearly always been due to a portal of entry upstream of the blood pump: an arterial needle that has slipped out of the fistula, an infusion bottle, with an air inlet, that has emptied unnoticed, a broken heparin line or a split blood pump insert (which causes a combination of rapid blood loss and air embolism). Rarer sources of embolism – which have not, to my knowledge, caused a recorded fatality – include frothing in the bubble trap when dialysate is poorly de-aerated (Chapter 6), air creeping past the barrel of a syringe pump inserted into a low-pressure segment of the arterial line[26], cracks in needle hubs and syringes, and re-expansion of the air in the bubble trap when venous pressure is suddenly released. The now obsolete practice of returning the dialyser contents with an 'air rinse' carried an obvious risk of air embolism.

The most important precaution against air embolism is the avoidance of these hazards. Heparin should be infused downstream of the blood pump (blood will creep back into the heparin line and syringe but does no harm), and if there is an infusion point for saline upstream of the blood pump it should be attached only to plastic bags of saline with no air inlet. However, it is impossible to avoid all risk of air embolism, particularly the risk of a needle falling out when the patient turns in his sleep. A monitor should therefore be fitted as an extra precaution.

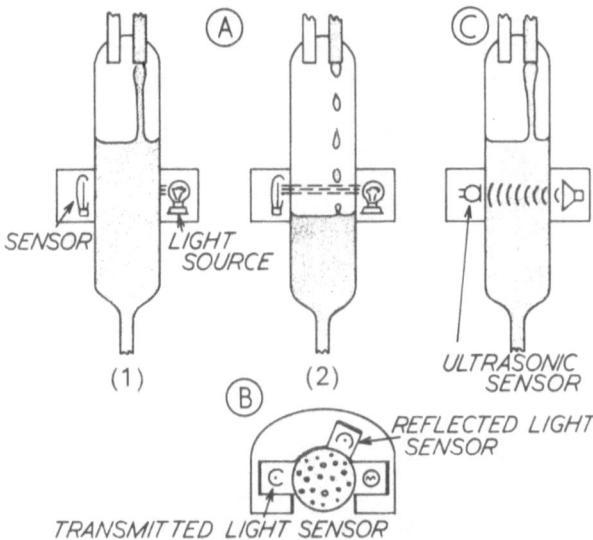

Figure 10   Three types of air embolism monitor: (A) transmitted light sensor in alarm (1) and operational (2) modes; (B) reflected light monitor detecting froth; (C) ultrasonic detector with beam interrupted by froth. Modified from von Hartitzsch[27]

The oldest style of monitor uses transmitted light (Figure 10A): a light source and photoelectric light detector are on opposite sides of the venous bubble trap. The system sounds an alarm if light falls on the sensor. False alarms are caused by bright ambient light if the 'collar' is badly adjusted, but the main objection to this cheapest monitor is that it fails to detect froth[27].

A more recent modification uses reflected light (Figure 10B): a second sensor is activated if light scattered by bubbles falls upon it. This variety reliably detected froth in von Hartitzsch and Medlock's experiments[27], but is not widely used in Britain.

Capacitance monitors (Figure 11) react to the varying quantity of blood in the bubble trap, rather than its level, so they are sensitive to froth if it

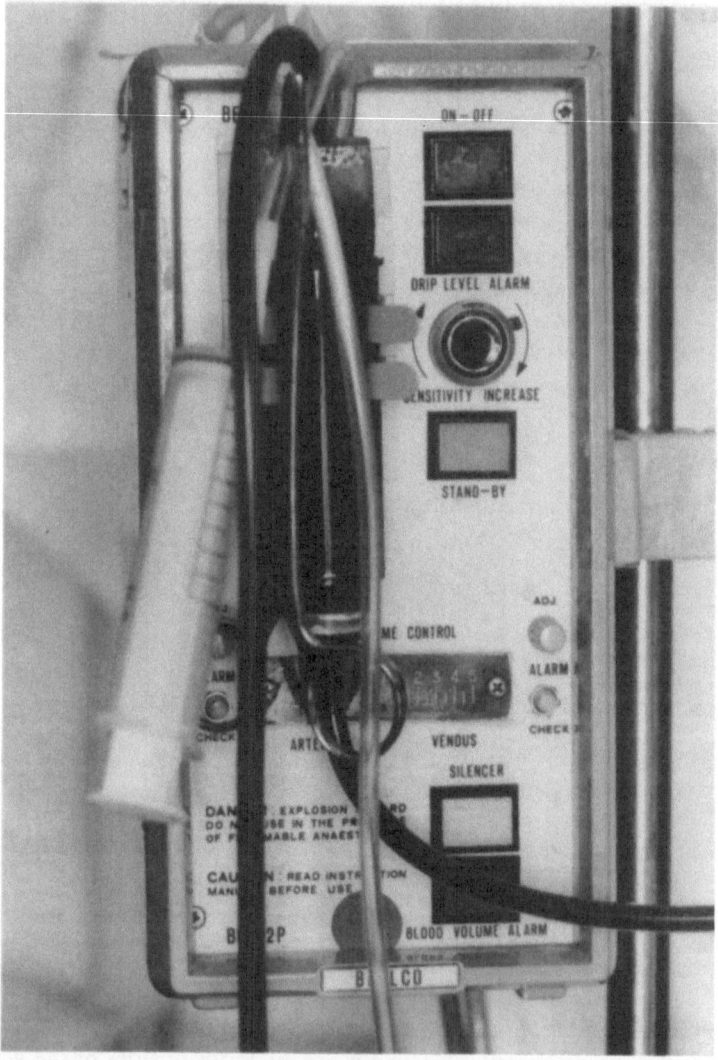

Figure 11   A fourth type of air embolism monitor, measuring the capacitance of the partially filled bubble trap

displaces sufficient blood. They do not detect a small trickle of froth, but are probably the most popular monitors in Britain.

The most reliable, and most expensive, monitors use ultrasound in place of a light beam (Figure 10C). The sensor is continuously stimulated while blood is in the bubble trap, since ultrasound (like sound) travels well through fluid. The beam is interrupted by air or froth. This system is easier to make fail-safe than transmitted light monitors.

Arterial line pressure monitors

A collapsible sac on the arterial line, attached to a pressure switch, detects a fall in pressure upstream of the pump and switches off the blood pump until the sac has refilled. This is useful as an extra precaution against air embolism and it prevents excessive suction on the arterial wall.

Single-needle apparatus

The original (Vital Assists) single-needle system used a Y-connector followed by a lever which flicked rapidly from side to side, occluding the arterial and venous line alternately. The blood pump ran continuously, sucking on an empty blood line when the arterial line was occluded, and blood returned to the patient under venous pressure alone. High blood flow rate could only be achieved by maintaining a high pressure in the dialyser, to force blood out rapidly during the venous phase, and by switching from arterial to venous phase at short intervals. The latter procedure led to a high rate of recirculation at high blood flows – up to $60 + \%$ in the studies of Ogden[28]. The Gambro, Rhone Poulenc, Mossley and Royal Free devices use two clamps, one each for arterial and venous lines, and these are both closed momentarily at the time of switch-over to limit recirculation. Their function, and probably that of the Vital Assists machine, can be considerably improved by the introduction of a collapsible reservoir between the arterial clamp and the blood pump[29]. However, the problem of high pressure in the dialyser remains, since blood is still returned by venous pressure alone.

The Bellco twin-headed pump (Figure 12) permits high blood flow with a recirculation rate of less than 10%, provided the fistula can deliver this flow rate[30]. The pressure in the dialyser can be varied at will to determine ultrafiltration over a wide range and this system has even been used with the very permeable RP6 Dialyser in open circuit[31]. We have encountered two extra hazards with this ingenious system. The presence of a venous pump must increase the risk of air embolism and it is mandatory that a high-quality air embolism detector be attached to the venous bubble trap. The segment of line between the venous pump and the venous needle contains no pressure monitor; if the venous return is occluded (e.g. by bending the elbow) the pump will generate a pressure over 1000 mmHg in that segment of line. This could blow the venous needle out of the vein, and on one occasion in our unit it blew the venous line apart. However, we have encountered this problem only once in a long experience with the Bellco pump. In compensation, there is an extra safety precaution – a revolution counter which switches off the blood pump after a predetermined number of revolutions if it is not switched off by a rise in pressure in the venous bubble trap. This helps to detect the rare hazard of a blood leak downstream of the blood pump (other than a membrane rupture, which should be detected anyway by the blood leak detector).

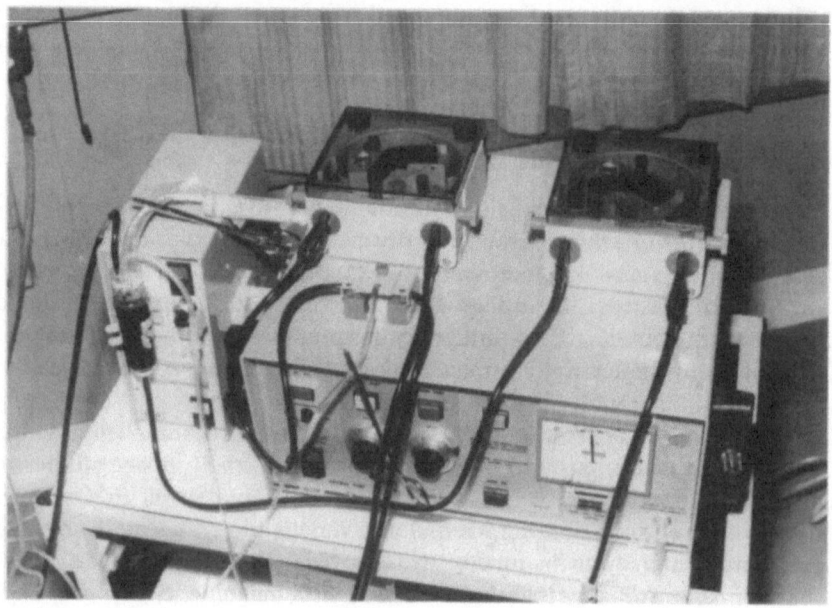

Figure 12   The Bellco double-headed pump

The main usefulness of the Bellco system is in running dialysis from a single access point like a subclavian catheter when a fistula has failed. The commoner problem of the difficult fistula with only one good needling site is more easily tackled by using a double-lumen needle[32], of which the coaxial varieties, like the Duo-cath, are probably best[33].

Dialysers

The choice of dialysers is even more bewildering than the variety of pro-portionating units. Promising new dialysers that are to be sold in Britain are sent to Newcastle for testing, and reports on their performance are submitted to the Department of Health, Supplies Branch, who distribute them to all British dialysis centres. Other interested medical, nursing and technical staff in the NHS can obtain copies from the Supplies Branch[22]; commercial organizations and colleagues overseas can obtain them from the author at cost. About 20 new dialysers and membranes are submitted for study each year, so some guidance is needed by the purchaser, who should ask himself three questions:

Which type of dialyser?

There are four major types available:

(1) *Non-disposable parallel-flow (Kiil-type) dialysers* are built by technicians or by patients in the home training unit. They are often re-used several times[21]. They are still the cheapest dialysers if the boards are kept for longer than 2 or 3 years; most of ours have been in service for about 7 years. The Meltec multipoint gives a high and consistent performance which has made it our standard of comparison for all other dialysers[34]. Existing centres which have the necessary building and stripping space and technicians skilled in building Meltecs will probably wish to keep them in service for several more years. Some development in membrane technology in that time could well prolong their lives. However, new centres starting now are more likely to adopt disposables, with re-use if necessary for economy.

(2) *Disposable parallel flow dialysers* have similar characteristics to the Meltec and some now rival it in performance at the same membrane area. They have a low resistance to blood flow so they can be operated at low transmembrane pressure, which is useful in patients who are susceptible to hypotension or have a low interdialytic weight gain because of residual renal function. Their residual blood volume after a standard saline wash-back is a little higher, on average, than that of the other types of dialyser, but the difference is small and not of clinical significance; it does not prevent the re-use of several of these dialysers.

(3) *Hollow fibre dialysers* are made from several different cellulose products – Cuprophan, cellulose and cellulose acetate – giving considerable differences in ultrafiltration rate and middle molecular clearance but fairly small differences in small molecular clearance. Hollow fibre kidneys (HFAKs) have the lowest priming volume and smallest compliance, per unit of membrane area or performance, of all dialysers. They are also small and compact to store, often an important consideration in a hospital dialysis unit. They have a low resistance to blood flow so they can be run at low ultrafiltration rates if necessary. Many can be re-used and they are easy to inspect after re-use for signs

of residual clot. However, they are the most expensive dialysers. There is a wide choice of conventional shaped dialysers from Cordis, Travenol, Organon, Asahi and Terumo, flat ones from Nipro, baffled cylinders from Bentley, triple bundles from Extracorporeal, knitted webs from Fresenius and so forth – varied designs to overcome the problem of maldistribution of dialysis fluid, leading to non-perfusion of part of the fibre bundle, to which HFAKs are prone. In spite of this problem, their performance is excellent and, when related to priming volume, superior to that of all other designs.

(4) *Coils* are the cheapest disposables. They provide a good and consistent performance and clean wash-out and most can be re-used. The problem that dogged them for many years – an unacceptably high burst rate – has now been overcome. Modern designs with wide pathways are also less troubled by another traditional problem – high resistance to blood flow, causing a high ultrafiltration rate even under basal conditions. Several designs are available as open coils for use in a recirculating machine or enclosed coils for use in single pass. The latter can be used with the proportionating machines described above, but at a dialysate flow rate of 500 ml/min they usually have a performance below that of parallel plate dialysers and appreciably below that of HFAKs. Travenol – the original makers of coil dialysers – Dasco, Bentley and several other firms offer a variety of sizes and shapes.

What size of dialyser?

Having chosen a design, should one go for large surface area to maximize performance? Should the dialyser's size be tailored to the patient's? The latter approach seems logical to me. Dialysis patients come in varied sizes, from less than 40 to more than 80 kg, but it is convenient in a hospital unit to treat them all for the same length of time. They should therefore be given dialysers roughly proportional to their size. If a $1.3\,m^2$ HFAK is used for the smaller patients, a $1.6\,m^2$ for the middle-sized ones and a 1.8 or $2.1\,m^2$ for the largest, the majority will receive a roughly standard amount of dialysis per hour. Large surface area dialysers lose some performance per square metre in scaling up[35] and their indiscriminate use causes an undesirably high ultrafiltration rate leading to an unacceptable incidence of hypotension and cramps.

Which manufacturer?

The answer to this question will depend on many factors, including price, regular deliveries, back-up services at weekends and bank holidays, willingness to replace defective dialysers, etc. One of the important factors will be the performance of the dialyser compared with its competitors, and it is this information that our reports provide. A comparison of many dialysers is published in the standard textbook on haemodialysis[36].

Dialysis circuits

Several firms compete in this market so it is worthwhile 'shopping around'. However, there is a considerable advantage in using the lines designed to fit a particular dialyser and proportionating unit, particularly if it has a closely planned pathway, as has the Cobe Centry 2.

TREATMENT POLICIES

Choice of dialysis fluid concentrate

Although there is only one supplier of dialysis fluid concentrate in Britain there are many different formulae which must reflect habit and prejudice rather than deliberate choice.

Sodium concentration was originally fixed at around 130 to aid control of hypertension, but this results in a high incidence of cramps and hypotension[37]. Since Stewart in Dundee introduced 'isonatric' haemodialysis there has been a general tendency to adopt a more physiological sodium concentration. However, even a return to the normal range can result in a rise in blood pressure[38], and an increase to 143 mmol/l caused pulmonary oedema in one centre[39]. Isonatric dialysis fluid produces hypernatraemia in the patients post-dialysis[40]. A reasonable compromise for general use is 136 mmol/l.

Potassium concentration needs to be varied for individual patients more often than sodium. Plasma concentrations on arrival at the dialysis unit vary considerably and some patients habitually arrive with plasma levels over 6 mmol/l. They need adequate potassium removal, which calls for a low dialysis fluid concentration, e.g. 1.5 mmol/l. Patients with ischaemic heart disease, particularly those taking cardiac glycosides, have a high incidence of arrythmias when dialysed against low potassium fluid; for them a concentration of 3.5 mmol/l is safer and may abolish the arrythmias[41]. If they need more potassium removed it should be achieved by prolonging dialysis or administering Calcium Resonium between dialyses. For a hospital dialysis unit a standard concentration of 2.0 mmol/l, boosted by addition of extra potassium to the concentration of patients who need a higher level, is a sensible compromise.

Acetate is used as sole source of bicarbonate in most dialysis units, and for most patients using dialysers appropriate to their size it presents no problems. When it is used with excessively large or very efficient dialysers, at high blood flow or with ill patients, acetate overload can occur and lower the blood pressure. Although there is general agreement about the rise in plasma acetate in a minority of patients[42–45], there is more dispute about its importance as a cause of hypotension. Some authors believe it to be very important in stable dialysis patients[44,46], whereas others consider it important only in the seriously ill[47], and yet others believe it has little effect[37,45]. It is, therefore, difficult to decide whether a hospital dialysis unit should continue to use acetate alone, particularly if it adopts short dialysis and has to raise the acetate concentration to 40 + mmol/l to maintain acid–base balance. We are currently comparing acetate alone with a 2 : 1 bicarbonate acetate mix before deciding whether to go to the bother and slight expense of changing over to the mixture routinely.

Dextrose can be omitted from dialysis fluid and most patients will tolerate dialysis without it. It has been omitted partly to control bacterial growth in dialysis fluid, which is not a major problem with modern equipment, and partly in the hope of preventing hyperlipidaemia in patients on dialysis. There are conflicting reports on its effect: plasma lipids falling modestly in one study[48] and remaining unchanged in another[49]. To me it seems logical to include dextrose in the dialysis fluid at about the physiological level, i.e. about 100 mg/dl (5.6 mmol/l) until there is strong evidence that some other course is superior.

Calcium concentration in dialysis fluid was studied in the 1960s with balance techniques; a concentration of about 1.5 mmol/l was found to produce zero calcium transfer[50,51]. Since then most nephrologists in Britain have used a concentration at, or just above, 1.5 mmol/l and we have confirmed that a concentration of 1.6 mmol/l raises serum ionized calcium during dialysis[52]. Others have argued that patients are in negative calcium balance between dialyses so a positive balance should be established during dialysis by raising dialysis fluid calcium to 1.75 or 2.0 mmol/l. Such dialysate calcium concentrations certainly produce positive calcium balance during dialysis, often provoking hypercalcaemia[53], but in general this has not caused prolonged amelioration of secondary hyperparathyroidism[54–57] or osteomalacia[58]. It carries the risk of provoking acute hypertension, which was probably responsible for one fatal stroke on our unit during a prospective trial of 2.0 mmol/l calcium in dialysis fluid, and if plasma phosphate is not rigidly controlled it is liable to produce vascular and myocardial metastatic calcification. Apart from the brief, ill-fated study referred to above, we have maintained our dialysis fluid calcium at 1.55–1.6 mmol/l, since 1964, and have relied on oral calcium supplements and vitamin D analogues to restore calcium balance.

Magnesium concentration varies considerably between centres. Many still use a magnesium concentration of 1.0 mmol/l or above, which maintains hypermagnesaemia throughout the dialysis cycle. This was once thought to be beneficial in protecting against metastatic calcification and helping to suppress parathyroid secretion. The latter effect is negligible compared with the suppressive effect of calcium. Reducing serum magnesium to normal by the use of a low (less than 0.5 mmol/l) magnesium dialysis fluid improves intracellular biochemistry[59] and nerve conduction time[60], and in one case report it relieved uraemic pruritus[61]. Pruritus is a characteristic feature of the 'hard water syndrome' of hypercalcaemia and hypermagnesaemia caused by failure of a water softener or other water treatment plant. It is described as a burning sensation in the skin[62] and can be attributed to the hypermagnesaemia, since it has also occurred when an excess of magnesium was added accidentally to dialysate[63]. These complications are not a hazard of the mild hypermagnesaemia produced by commercial dialysis fluid and the benefits from restoring serum magnesium to normal so far described are tenuous. Nonetheless it seems reasonable to maintain serum magnesium in the normal range until someone shows that an alternative course is better; this suggests a dialysate concentration of 0.2–0.5 mmol/l.

Choice of dialysis time

In the early 1970s nearly all British renal units used the Kiil dialyser for 24–36 h per week. Dialysis time was reduced in proportion to the improved efficiency of newer dialysers, but schedules of 6–8 h three times a week remained standard even after the introduction of the Meltec multipoint. Short dialysis came in almost by mistake when Cambi and his colleagues used it to test the importance of middle molecules. The effectiveness of thrice-weekly dialysis for 3–4 h, using 1 m² dialysers at highest attainable blood flow, was dramatically confirmed in several North Italian centres[64]. The experience has been confirmed in Britain[65–67] and elsewhere[68]. However, there are a few problems. The time available for fluid removal is shortened, so some patients may fail to lose their interdialytic weight gain and develop hypertension or pulmonary oedema[69]. Potassium removal can also be critical, calling for low potassium dialysis fluid, with the problems discussed above. Often the most difficult problem is phosphate removal. This can be achieved between dialyses by increasing the dose of aluminium hydroxide, but patients often find this unacceptable and it increases the risk of aluminium overload (only a significant problem in those areas already at risk from their water supply). Probably the best policy is a tailored dialysis time varying from 3 to 5 h and depending on the patient's dietary intake and residual renal function. It is essential that dialysis time be increased if blood flow through the dialyser is sub-optimal (less than 200 ml/min).

Hepatitis policy

Reference has been made to this subject under the heading 'The design of a hospital dialysis unit', and the continuing importance of the Rosenheim report[15] has been mentioned. This report was written just as the techniques for detecting carriers and excluding infected blood from transfusion services became available. It is clear, with hindsight, that the ability to recognize and isolate hepatitis carriers was the crucial factor in control of hepatitis and I am doubtful how large a part the very expensive and time-consuming hygienic precautions actually played. Today's nephrologist has to choose a policy which will not waste money but will also not offend staff long accustomed to the Rosenheim precautions. That policy should certainly take account of the measures used in controlling the epidemics in British dialysis units[70,71]. From the extensive literature on this topic (see references 72–76 for a small sample) I conclude:

(1) Hepatitis carriers are the main source of infection; they must be detected early, so regular screening of all dialysis patients, at least monthly, is mandatory. It should be continued for the first 6 months after successful transplant.

(2) Hepatitis carriers with high titre of HBsAg or detectable HBeAg after the acute phase of the illness are particularly dangerous sources of infection. They are more likely to have chronic hepatic disease than other carriers, but this association is less pronounced than in the general population.

(3) Patients with HLA antigen B8 are particularly liable to become carriers and deserve special attention during an epidemic.

(4) Transfused blood cannot be guaranteed free of hepatitis B, but at least it should be negative for HBsAg by a sensitive test – haemagglutination or radioimmunoassay.

(5) Blood is the main vehicle of infection between patients and every effort should be made to prevent it contaminating equipment. The venous pressure gauge has already been mentioned as a vulnerable spot for contamination. Recirculating tanks are readily contaminated by a blood leak and difficult to sterilize; hepatitis carriers and patients in quarantine should be treated with disposable dialysers, which are discarded after single use, and preferably with a machine like the Bellco Unimat, in which the dialysate pathway is disposable.

(6) However, other modes of transmission cannot be ruled out; HbsAg can be detected in unexplained spots around the unit during an epidemic, so physical separation of hepatitis from other patients is highly desirable.

(7) High-titre anti-HBsAg immunoglobulin is of some value in preventing spread between patients. It should be given in a dose such as 750 mg i.m. every 2 months during a quarantine period.

(8) Staff who contract hepatitis B nearly always develop a febrile illness which carries a 2% mortality rate. It is therefore unnecessary to screen them for HBsAg except on joining the unit (mainly for

medicolegal and compensation purposes) and during an epidemic. However, they should be warned to report all illness that could conceivably be hepatitis.

(9) Anti-HBsAg immunoglobulin has a protective effect if given soon after an inoculation accident involving HBsAg-positive material. It is uncertain whether its regular administration to staff protects them, but many staff take comfort from its administration during a hepatitis B epidemic, so it is reasonable to administer in a dose of 750 mg every 2–3 months to the staff at highest risk – nurses and technicians and doctors responsible for needling and similar invasive procedures.

(10) Active immunization against hepatitis has been shown to be effective on dialysis centres in pilot trials, but no vaccine has yet been made available for general use.

(11) Epidemics of hepatitis, other than hepatitis B, also occur on dialysis units. Hepatitis A is no more common than among the general population. Viruses resembling EB virus have been held responsible, but the unidentified organism is usually classified as 'non A, non B'. The modes of transmission are similar to those of hepatitis B and the precautions the same.

(12) Patients with chronic hepatitis B or 'C' who are transplanted often tolerate the graft well but have an increased mortality from chronic liver disease. The excess mortality is not high enough to preclude this form of treatment, particularly in view of the great difficulties of continuing dialysis. These include an increased risk for immediate family members (particularly the dialysis helper in home dialysis) who merit protection with anti-HBsAg in the same way as dialysis staff.

(13) After a case of hepatitis has been identified on the hospital dialysis unit, it should be declared 'in quarantine' for 6 months. If possible, new patients should not be accepted on the unit but should be transferred to another centre from the predialysis clinic. The carrier should be isolated and given separate treatment. Full hygienic precautions should be enforced, including the wearing of gowns, disposable gloves, masks and eyeshields during procedures like needling fistulas. Holiday exchanges should be cancelled and transfer of patients to other centres halted. Anti-HBsAg should be offered to patients and staff as outlined above. All blood samples and excreta sent to laboratories should carry a prominent warning. There should be full discussion with pathologists before an autopsy is requested on any patient who dies during quarantine.

Holiday facilities

Holiday facilities were first provided for home dialysis patients (Chapter 6). Most regions of Britain now have attractive holiday homes supported partly or wholly by charitable funds. Rotary and Lions clubs have played a prominent part in buying and maintaining these homes. Movement of patients between regions has been severely restricted by hepatitis precautions but is now becoming freer. The Northern Region has attractive facilities fully equipped for home dialysis. Facilities for hospital dialysis patients are in much shorter supply. Our house at Whitley Bay was chosen partly to allow hospital patients to travel back to Newcastle for dialysis – or the home sister to travel out from Newcastle to supervise dialysis in the house. The British Kidney Patients Association (BKPA)[77] has recently opened a national holiday centre (Figures 13 and 14) which can be used by hospital dialysis patients and their families. Staff are provided to conduct the dialysis and take care of the equipment. The centre is part of a holiday village providing company for the rest of the family. The BKPA also helps to fund holidays abroad at approved centres like those in Spain and at Glyfada, Greece. To take part in such holidays away from his home region a patient must be free of hepatitis, in a unit which is not in quarantine, and all arrangements must be approved by the director of his dialysis centre. Portable dialysis machines of several designs are now available[78] and some have been bought by BKPA and other charities for patients to take on independent holidays. A group of patients from my own centre have gone on holiday to Spain using portable machines in hotel bedrooms. In my view, the hotel ought to be warned in advance!

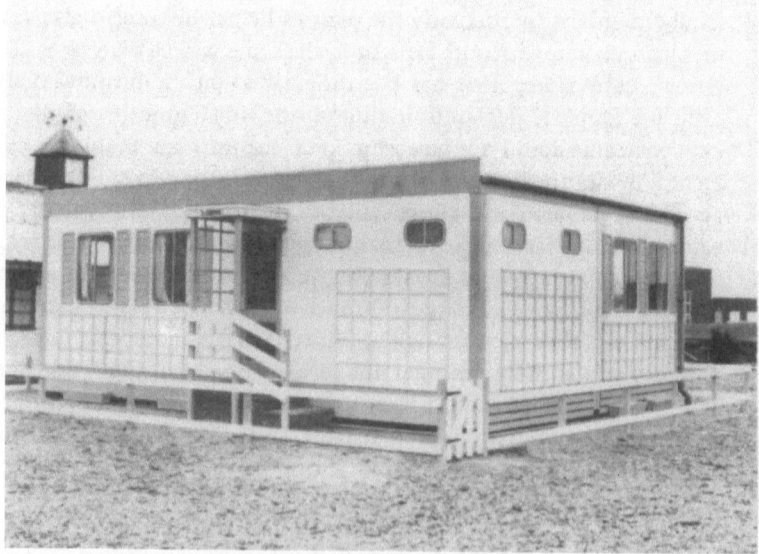

Figure 13 The Grove, Earnley, Bracklesham Bay, the BKPA's new holiday centre for dialysis patients. Here treatment is carried out by trained staff while the family are free to enjoy the amenities of the Sussex Beach Holiday Village

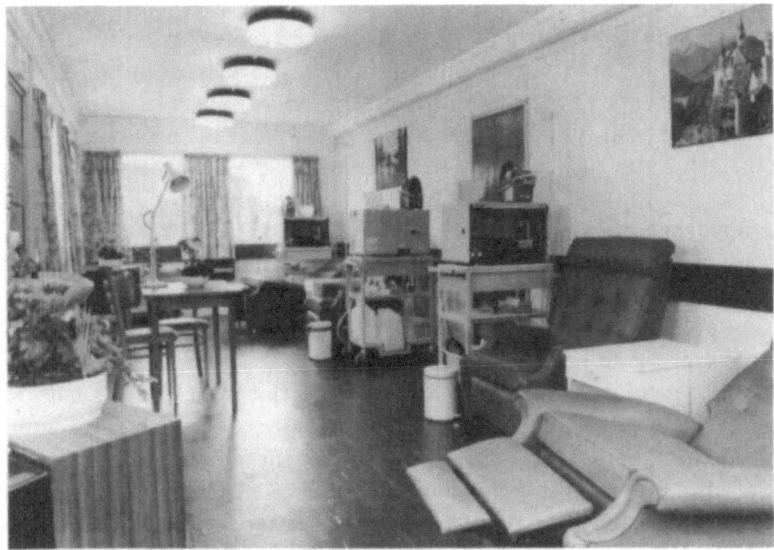

Figure 14   Interior of the Grove

Re-use of dialysers

Re-use of haemodialysers has been practised since the very start of regular haemodialysis, but the attitudes of manufacturers and governmental authorities have been cautious, to say the least. Our reports on the re-use of dialysers are issued separate from the main report and sometimes under a 'confidential' label because manufacturers are anxious not to be associated with recommendations for re-use. Their anxiety is understandable; they produce the original dialyser under very strictly controlled conditions of sterility and exclusion of pyrogens and do not want their reputation besmirched by the re-use of dialysers under far less ideal conditions in hospital. It has been hard to get official approval from governments for re-use. As recently as January 1980 the US Department of Health, Education and Welfare took the view that it would never *require* re-use of dialysers though it does approve the practice[79]. Nonetheless, many US physicians have undertaken re-use on their own responsibility[80]. In Britain there has been a similar widespread adoption of the technique[21] despite an eerie silence from the Department of Health. The physician who undertakes re-use of dialysers, therefore, does it on his own responsibility, but can at least take comfort in the company of many colleagues.

Several automated or semi-automated systems for rinsing have been described[81-85], but only one of these is now commercially available. It is convenient to use but, as currently programmed, it does not adequately rinse out formalin before dialysis[86]. The problems of manual re-use of dialysers have been discussed in a recent symposium[87], which also contains practical advice on how to do it, from a very experienced centre[88]. Some of the techniques described in that article (disassembly of the dialyser and scrubbing of the blood inlet and outlet compartments) are only applicable to a minority of HFAKs. For coils, parallel-flow dialysers and most HFAKs one must rely upon rinsing the dialyser only. Many centres have used tap water for this purpose, passing it through the blood compartment without an unacceptable incidence of pyrogen reactions, but I find it hard to recommend this procedure. We use reverse osmosis (RO) water which is sterile and pyrogenfree and we sterilize chemically all lines connecting the RO unit to the rinsing point between rinsing sessions. It is best to use a dialyser with a transparent casing so that it can be at least partially inspected from the outside for residual clot. Removal of stubborn clot from HFAKs can sometimes be achieved by applying tap water pressure to the dialysate compartment and inducing 'reverse ultrafiltration' into the blood compartment. The loss of fibre bundles can be estimated in HFAKs by draining them into a measuring cylinder, but this technique is not readily applicable to other dialysers.

Five per cent formalin (formaldehyde 2%) has been almost universally used as a sterilizing agent between uses of cellulose-based dialysers. There has been little recent work on the use of alternative sterilizing agents, but in the past hypochlorite appeared to result in a high incidence of blood leaks from etching of the membrane. One report described satisfactory use of 27% sodium chloride solution[89], but there has been no follow-on to this report.

One of the biggest worries about re-use has been loss of performance[90]. One dialyser has performed consistently well when re-used; the RP6, having polyacrylonitrile membrane, can be cleansed with sodium hypochlorite. Its performance is maintained or even improved after four or six uses[91] and showed little fall aften ten uses[85]. Results with cellulose dialysers which have not been cleansed with hypochlorite are less consistent and probably depend on the individual dialyser and local heparinization regimen amongst other factors. A very small minority of patients produce a lot of clot in dialysers, regardless of heparinization regimen, and are unsuitable for re-use[87]. Anyone re-using cellulose dialysers should check that his method does not result in unacceptable fall-off in the clearance of small molecules over the range of re-uses in practice. Although there have been fears that middle molecular clearance might be more affected by fibrin deposition in dialysers published data do not give much support to this fear so the more difficult task of studying the effect of re-use on middle molecular clearance can be left to a few research units.

One of the difficult problems of re-use and of hospital-built dialysers is the complete washout of formalin. Approximately 1 h rinsing of the dialysate compartment with water or dialysis fluid at 500 ml/min, the passage of

1500 ml of saline through the blood compartment during this procedure and a final 500 ml of saline just before needle connection reduce formalin concentrations to an accepted low level, though there is still some residual formalin in the dialyser membrane[86,92]. Thorough washout of formalin is essential to prevent the formation of anti-N antibodies[92-94].

There should be a regular routine of sampling re-used dialysers for bacteriological study at the completion of formalin washout. Any outbreak of pyrogen reactions in the unit calls for a thorough review of all re-use procedures.

Heparinization

The majority of dialysis units employ a very simple rule-of-thumb method of heparinization. A few hundred units of heparin are left in the dialyser by adding 1000–2000 units of heparin to the saline which is last washed through the blood compartment. A loading dose, typically 3000–5000 units, is given into the venous line at the time of connection of dialyser to patient (or through the venous needle if the dialyser is to be drained) and then an infusion is run into the arterial circuit which is switched off just before or just after the end of dialysis. The infusion rate is found by trial and error for each patient during the first few dialyses. A typical total dose of heparin for a 4 h dialysis is about 10 000 or 12 000 units. Several studies have shown that this method results in the excessive heparinization of some patients, particularly towards the end of dialysis, contributing to the problem of haemostasis after withdrawal of the fistula needles, and therefore to chronic blood loss. The half-life of heparin varies considerably between patients so it is worth while 'modelling' each patient by injecting heparin and carrying out serial measurements of whole-blood partial thromboplastin time as a measure of heparin level; the required loading dose, infusion rate and duration of infusion can then be calculated from nomograms[95]. We have used this method and found it effective, but the work of modelling a large throughput of patients is considerable and we have not found it easy to maintain enthusiasm amongst medical and nursing staff.

An unexplained increase in the incidence of clotting episodes during dialysis should lead to review of the activity of the heparin batch in use and of dialysis fluid pH, since a fall in this pH can inactivate heparin[96]. Excessive clotting in dialysers may be countered by increasing the heparin dose or by administering an anti-platelet agent such as sulphinpyrazone[97]. The opposite problem of bleeding tendency in patients who have undergone recent surgery or have bleeding lesions like active ulcers can be tackled by reducing the dose of heparin and monitoring it carefully by a suitable clotting test[98], or by substituting prostacyclin partially or wholly for heparin[99]. Prostacyclin is at the clinical trial stage and has to be obtained on a named-patient basis from the manufacturers (the Wellcome Foundation). It may cause a fall in blood pressure if given in excessive dosage, but in our hands has produced few side-effects and has permitted dialysis in the total absence of heparinization without recurrence of major bleeding. Dosage schedules are being found by trial and error and the advice of the manufacturer should be sought.

COMPLICATIONS OF HAEMODIALYSIS

Patients receiving regular haemodialysis are subject to a very wide variety of complications, many originating from their primary illness, from past or present hypertension and hyperparathyroidism, or from incomplete control of their chronic renal failure. For discussion of such complications the reader is referred to larger textbooks of haemodialysis[100] or nephrology. In this closing section I mention only a few complications of the dialysis procedure itself which have not been dealt with in preceding sections.

Electrocution

Dialysis equipment is specifically designed to avoid this complication and there is only one recorded fatality from it[101]. However, it may well be underdiagnosed because it leaves no diagnostic signs, is rarely thought of, and can only be diagnosed retrospectively by a thorough study of the equipment. Any unexplained sudden death during dialysis calls for an inspection of the equipment, including a test for current leakage[102].

Overheating

Simultaneous failure of the thermostat and the warning device (or incorrect setting of the alarm pointers) is usually detected by the patient complaining that the return blood feels warm. However, if he misses this physical sign, e.g. because he is asleep, heating of the blood beyond about 42 °C results in severe haemolysis[103,104], which has caused fatalities[105].

Acute hyponatraemia and hypernatraemia

These were fairly common accidents in the early days of haemodialysis when the solution was mixed up in batches by medical, nursing and technical staff and when laboratory checks on the concentration were not always available. It was not difficult during night dialysis for a tired member of staff to forget to insert the salts or concentrate, or to insert them twice over. Several patients in our own unit were dialysed accidentally against tap water. The accident was readily recognized because the patient always complained of pain up the return arm and it was then noticed that the blood in the venous line looked like port wine. No serious harm resulted. A more serious accident was the insertion of only part of the solute. This caused prolonged haemolysis without the same dramatic changes and therefore was detected later. Again, however, recovery was uneventful. Today the more likely accident is mild hyponatraemia due to malfunction of a mixing unit, and this is likely to be detected by increasing muscle cramps or some other symptom rather than haemolysis.

An outbreak of hypernatraemia occurred at Lyon[106] and resulted in headache, hot flushes, nausea, vomiting, weakness, disorientation and, in some cases, low-back pain, abdominal pain, dyspnoea and hypoacousia. The less severe hypernatraemia that is likely to occur from malfunction of a mixing unit will probably be detected by rising blood pressure or increasing dyspnoea.

Because these accidents are now rare they are easily forgotten; any unexplained illness of a patient during the course of dialysis calls for a full analysis of dialysis fluid.

Pyrogen reactions

These were a very common problem in the early days of haemodialysis. The reactions typically occurred about 1 h after the start of dialysis and were manifest by *angor animi*, chest pain, malaise, shivering, rapid rise in temperature, followed by sweating, muscle pains, exhaustion and, the following day, outbreak of facial herpes. They closely resembled the pyrogen reactions that were familiar to physicians obliged to re-use rubber tubing for transfusion or gum elastic catheters for cardiac catheterization in the days before disposable products. It was therefore natural to assume that they were due to contamination of the blood pathway by blood products. Many of the early reactions on our unit, in the days when lines, connectors and other equipment were re-used after autoclaving, were traced to this source. Nylon connectors seemed to be a particularly potent source of pyrogen reactions. The problem has not arisen in recent years with the re-use of p.v.c. and Silastic lines chemically sterilized with formalin.

When a single patient in a dialysis unit develops a fever one should first look for an individual cause, such as infection of the shunt or fistula. Pyrogenic reactions due to a failure in dialysis technique should be considered when there is an increasing incidence of febrile illness affecting several patients or, particularly, numerous patients develop febrile reactions simultaneously. When this has happened the instinct of most nephrologists in recent years has been to blame the dialysis fluid[107-110]. This approach has never appealed to me because the pattern of the attacks does not suggest an origin in dialysis fluid. They occur early in the procedure when bacterial counts in dialysis fluid are still low and one would not expect bacteria or pyrogens to cross the dialysis membranes; indeed, they have been shown not to do so[111]. In the days when we used recirculation tanks for a very prolonged dialysis, bacterial counts rose to astronomical levels, even producing murky bathwater with a strong smell of pseudomonas; yet patients treated with single-use disposable dialysers had no pyrogen reactions. Even in the study of Rosenbaum et al.[112], when such bacterial soup produced severe acidosis in patients on prolonged dialysis for poisoning, there was no mention of pyrogen reactions. Though there are some studies in which the elimination of bacteria from dialysis fluid has appeared to eliminate outbreaks of pyrogen reactions[113], such reports are difficult to evaluate. In my own unit, on two occasions, a severe pyrogen outbreak ceased dramatically when the dialysis fluid system was changed to reduce bacterial counts. However, the temporary recurrence of the problem showed us that the true cause of the epidemic on both occasions had been contamination of the membrane soaking tray and that the improvement was due to technicians returning to prescribed procedures when a strong interest was being taken in the unit.

Pyrogen outbreaks have been caused by bacteraemia from incomplete sterilization of the Kiil dialyser[114], or contamination of re-used coils[115], so blood cultures during the attack should be a routine part of the investigation of any pyrogen outbreak. The second step should be a re-examination of all techniques on the unit to see whether there is any possibility of bacterial pyrogen entering the blood pathway. Only when these sources of reactions have been eliminated should one consider blaming the dialysis fluid. However, in spite of the objections I have listed above, the possibility that dialysis fluid does sometimes cause pyrogen reactions must be entertained; there are some patients, who are reliable observers, who are convinced they have their pyrogen reactions only in response to dialysis fluid made from certain contaminated water supplies (Dr Robert Eady, personal communication, 1980). It is in any case good hygienic practice to keep the dialysis fluid as close to sterile as possible.

Absorption of trace contaminants from dialysis fluid

Much the most important of these, aluminium poisoning from water supplies to which aluminium has been added in the purification process, has been referred to above. It causes two syndromes:

(1) Dialysis encephalopathy: a progressive form of brain damage leading to change in personality, speech disorder, myoclonic jerks, convulsions, spike and slow-wave discharges on the EEG and eventual global dementia leading to death.
(2) Fracturing renal osteodystrophy: a progressive form of osteomalacia typically developing 2–4 years after the start of dialysis leading to bone pain, myopathy and spontaneous fractures.

These topics have recently been reviewed elsewhere[115,116]. They are problems which should not recur if the recommendations for water treatment given in a previous section are followed. Several other trace elements have caused morbidity or mortality.

Copper is contained in most dialysis membranes, since they are made from cellulose by the cuprammonium process. In the past accumulation of copper in the patient from this source was regularly detected biochemically, though it did not appear to give rise to any clinical symptoms[118]. There have been no very recent studies to see whether this is still happening in spite of better quality control in the production of membranes. Acute copper poisoning has resulted from two main sources. Softened water which lies in copper pipes dissolves considerable copper overnight[119-121]. Since most hospitals have copper pipes in their plumbing system it is good practice to flush through the piping for a few minutes before starting to make dialysis fluid if a complete water treatment system has not been installed. An episode of 'copper fever' has been described from this source. The patient had a febrile reaction whenever she was exposed to copper through haemodialysis, the symptoms resembling the industrial copper fever that occurs on Monday mornings[121]. More severe, sometimes fatal, poisoning producing severe intravascular haemolysis, has resulted only from the dissolution of copper parts in a dialysis system on contact with acidic water or dialysis fluid[121,122]. Copper parts have now been eliminated from dialysis fluid circuits of all machines sold in the last few years, but some of the older machines with copper parts may still be in use. There are many causes of a rapid drop in the haemoglobin of dialysis patients; when this happens to several simultaneously it should alert the clinician to the possibility of contamination of the dialysis fluid by copper, zinc or chloramines.

Zinc metabolism is abnormal in chronic renal failure. Plasma levels are typically low before and during haemodialysis though red cell and perhaps tissue levels are normal. Zinc deficiency causes loss of taste and sexual dysfunction and there have been recent suggestions that restoration of normal plasma zinc in dialysis patients restores normal taste and potency[123-125]. More recent studies do not support these suggestions[126,127], the usual policy of ignoring the patient's plasma zinc seems sensible until more evidence in favour of correcting it is adduced. Acute hyperzincaemia has been produced by leakage of zinc oxide plaster from coils[128] which, however, no longer contain this contaminant, and elution of zinc from galvanized iron piping[129]. In the latter outbreak anaemia was blamed on the hyperzincaemia and was corrected when a carbon filter was installed to remove the zinc. However, chloramines were present in the water supply of Brisbane at the time and are effectively removed by carbon filters, so the case against zinc contamination is unproven. These problems should not occur in a properly designed water system as described above.

Nickel has been leached from nickel-plated stainless steel components in the dialysis circuit and caused nausea, vomiting, weakness and headache[130].

This newly-described accident occurred in spite of the installation of approved materials throughout the dialysis circuit. It was traced to an incorrect procedure in the manufacture of the nickel-plated stainless steel tank. It is a further reminder that any unexplained symptoms in a dialysis centre, particularly affecting several patients, calls for a thorough investigation of the dialysis fluid supply.

Leaching of plasticizers

Many of the components of dialysers, dialysis circuits and infusion bags contain plasticizers which are leached out and infused into the patient. Even in subjects with normal renal function, who excrete most of the plasticizer in the first 24 h in their urine[131], some is lodged in tissues, such as lung, for longer periods of time[132]. Prolonged administration of plasticizers to primates, in the doses readily absorbed by haemodialysis patients, cause changes in hepatic function[133]. Since many patients now survive more than 10 years of such plasticizer infusion on haemodialysis it is unlikely that it commonly causes serious problems, but the amount released by different plastics varies and some instances of hepatitis have been attributed to excessive leaching of diethylphthalate or other unidentified substances[134, 135].

Disequilibrium syndrome

A syndrome of headache, confusion, drowsiness, fits and coma coming on in the first 2 or 3 h of haemodialysis for acute renal failure was common in the days when that condition was treated at a very high plasma urea level with high-efficiency, large surface area dialysers[136]. The pathogenesis of the syndrome has been reviewed elsewhere[115]; it is probably due to disequilibrium between intra- and extracellular fluid in osmotically active solutes including urea and sodium. The full syndrome should not be encountered on a hospital Regular Dialysis Unit where patients are treated three times a week and encouraged to restrict their sodium intake. Patients with intercurrent illness, and those who go on sodium or protein binges, are at some risk of developing at least a modified form of the syndrome. This can be reduced by matching the dialysis fluid sodium to that of plasma, reducing blood flow and prolonging dialysis time. Sophisticated tests of cerebral function showed defective performances in some dialysis patients; these probably reflect their chronic uraemia which may improve after dialysis[137, 138]. It is likely, though unproven, that such finer cerebral functions deteriorate after dialysis in patients with mild dialysis disequilibrium. Until this problem has been more thoroughly studied it seems sensible to discourage patients driving home when they are at high risk of disequilibrium syndrome.

Hypotension during dialysis

This topic has received intensive study since a demonstration by Bergstrom[139] that fluid could be removed by isolated ultrafiltration without hypotension while a similar removal of fluid during haemodialysis caused a substantial fall in blood pressure. It is now generally agreed that during isolated ultrafiltration cardiac output falls as plasma volume contracts, but there is a compensatory rise in peripheral resistance, whereas during haemodialysis the same fall in cardiac output is not compensated by vasoconstriction[140]. What aspect of dialysis prevents vasoconstriction is still uncertain, but there is considerable evidence that the fall in plasma osmolality, which is an inevitable concomitant of the removal of urea, plays an important part[141]. The great majority of regular dialysis patients who practise prudent restriction of fluid intake can lose the necessary weight during dialysis without trouble from hypotension. However, a minority suffer repeated episodes of hypotension with even small fluid loss. Some of these may be helped by sequential ultrafiltration dialysis in which the fluid is removed during the first hour, then dialysis takes place without further fluid loss[141-144]. This procedure is not recommended for routine use in dialysis units, since it curtails the time for dialysis and results in no improvement in symptoms if overall time in the dialysis unit is kept constant[145]. When it is used for patients with problematic hypotension, sequential ultrafiltration haemodialysis should occupy more time than was previously devoted to haemodialysis alone.

References

1 Kerr, D. N. S. (1973). Provision of services to patients with chronic uremia. *Kidney Int.*, 3, 197

2 Brunner, F. P., Brynger, H., Chantler, C., Donckerwolcke, R. A., Hathway, R. A., Jacobs, C., Selwood, N. H. and Wing, A. J. (1979). Combined report on regular dialysis and transplantation in Europe, IX, 1978. *Proc. Eur. Dial. Transplant. Assoc.*, 16, 2 (relevant data on page 12)

3 Wing, A. J., Brunner, F. P., Brynger, H., Chantler, C., Donckerwolcke, R. A., Jacobs, C., Gurland, H. J. and Mansell, M. (1980). Successful pregnancies in women treated by dialysis and transplantation in Europe. *Br. J. Obstet. Gynaecol.*, 87, 839

4 Pierides, A. M., Skillen, A. W. and Ellis, H. A. (1979). Serum alkaline phosphatase in azotemic and hemodialysis osteodystrophy: a study of isoenzyme patterns, their correlation with bone histology, and their changes in response to treatment with 1-alpha OHD$_3$ and 1,25 (OH)$_2$D$_3$. *J. Lab. Clin. Med.*, 93, 899

5 Siede, W. H., Seiffert, U. B., Bundschuh, F., Malluche, H. H. and Schoeppe, W. (1980). Alkaline phosphatase bone isoenzyme activity in serum various degrees of micromorphometrically assessed renal osteopathy. *Clin. Nephrol.*, 13, 277

6 Mennes, P., Rosenbaum, R., Martin, K. and Slatopolsky, E. (1978). Hypomagnesemia and impaired parathyroid hormone secretion in chronic renal disease. *Ann. Intern. Med.*, 88, 206

7 Rude, R. K., Oldham, S. B. and Singer, F. R. (1976). Functional hypoparathyroidism and parathyroid hormone end-organ resistance in human magnesium deficiency. *Clin. Endocrinol.*, **5**, 209

8 Conceicao, S. C., Weightman, D., Smith, P. A., Luno, J., Ward, M. K. and Kerr, D. N. S. (1978). Serum ionised calcium concentration: measurement versus calculation. *Br. Med. J.*, **1**, 1103

9 Aljama, P., Ward, M. K., Pierides, A. M., Eastham, E. J., Ellis, H. A., Feest, T. G., Conceicao, S. and Kerr, D. N. S. (1978). Serum ferritin concentration: a reliable guide to iron overload in uremic and hemodialyzed patients. *Clin. Nephrol.*, **10**, 101

10 Bell, J. D., Kincaid, W. R., Morgan, R. G., Bunce III, H., Alperin, J. B., Sarles, H. E. and Remmers, A. R. Jr. (1980). Serum ferritin assay and bone-marrow iron stores in patients on maintenance hemodialysis. *Kidney Int.*, **17**, 237

11 Bonomini, V., Albertazzi, A., Vangelista, A., Bortolotti, G. C., Stefoni, S. and Scolari, M. P. (1976). Residual renal function and effective rehabilitation in chronic dialysis. *Nephron*, **16**, 89

12 Akhondzadeh, L., Wilson, S. E., Williams, R. and Owens, M. L. (1980). Infection of materials used in vascular access surgery: an evaluation of dacron, bovine heterograft, teflon and human umbilical vein grafts. *Dial. Transplant.*, **9**, 697

13 Friedman, E. A., Butt, K. M. H., Pascua, L. J., Hardy, M. A., Lawton, R. L. and Uldall, P. R. (1979). Panel Conference Vascular Access Update. *Trans. Am. Soc. Artif. Organs*, **15**, 526

14 Ringoir, S. (1980). Design and function of a hospital artificial kidney centre. *Int. J. Artif. Organs*, **3**, 134

15 Hepatitis and the Treatment of Chronic Renal Failure: Report of the Advisory Group 1970-1972: Chairman Lord Rosenheim. (London: Department of Health and Social Security)

16 Kerr, D. and Hill, A. V. L. (1973). *Water Contaminants and their Effects on Dialysed Patients*. (Elga Products Ltd)

17 Marsden, S. N. E., Parkinson, I. S., Ward, M. K., Ellis, H. A. and Kerr, D. N. S. (1979). Evidence for aluminium accumulation in renal failure. *Proc. Eur. Dial. Transplant. Assoc.*, **15**, 587

18 Kjellstrand, C. M., Eaton, J. W., Yawata, Y., Swofford, H., Kolpin, C. F., Buselmeier, T. J., von Hartitzsch, B. and Jacob, H. S. (1974). Hemolysis in dialized patients caused by chloramines. *Nephron*, **13**, 427

19 Rozas, V. V., Port, F. K. and Easterling, R. E. (1978). An outbreak of dialysis dementia due to aluminium in the dialysate. *J. Dial.*, **2**, 459

20 Dr G. Pincherle, Department of Health and Social Security, Hannibal House, Elephant and Castle, London SE1

21 Wing, A. J., Brunner, F. P., Brynger, H. O. A., Chantler, C., Donckerwolcke, R. A., Gurland, H. J., Jacobs, C. and Selwood, N. H. (1978). Mortality and morbidity of reusing dialysers. *Br. Med. J.*, **2**, 853

22 Dr H. Robinson, Scientific and Technical Division, Department of Health and Social Security, 14 Russell Square, London WC1B 5EP

23 Whelpton, D. (1978). National and International electrical safety requirements in dialysers. In Frost, T. H. (ed.) *Technical Aspects of Renal Dialysis*, p. 235. (Tunbridge Wells: Pitman Medical)

24 Veitch, P., Hawkins, F., Frost, T. H., Jolly, D. and Kerr, D. N. S. (1978). Factors affecting haemolysis in extracorporeal dialysis circuits. In Frost, T. H. (ed.) *Technical Aspects of Renal Dialysis*, p. 218. (Tunbridge Wells: Pitman Medical)

25 Ward, M. K., Shadforth, M., Hill, A. V. L. and Kerr, D. N. S. (1971). Air embolism during haemodialysis. *Br. Med. J.*, **3**, 74

26 Weseley, S. A. (1972). Air embolism during hemodialysis. *Dial. Transplant.*, **1**, 14

27 von Hartitzsch, B. and Medlock, T. R. (1979). New devices to prevent air foam emboli. *Dial. Transplant.*, **8**, 514

28 Ogden, D. A. (1979). *In vivo* measurement of blood recirculation during 'Y' type single needle dialysis. *J. Dial.*, **3**, 265

29 Ahmad, R., Large, B. and Redman, D. (1979). A simplified method of single needle dialysis. *Dial. Transplant.*, **8**, 260

30 Piron, M., Becaus, I., Lameire, N., Bleyn, J. and Ringoir, S. (1978). An *in vitro* study of recirculation in single needle dialysis with the double headpump. In Frost, T. H. (ed.) *Technical Aspects of Renal Dialysis*, p. 169. (Tunbridge Wells: Pitman Medical)

31 Hilderson, J., Singoir, S., van Waeleghem, J., van Egmond, J., van Haelst, J. P. and Schelstraete, K. (1975). Short dialysis with a polyacrylonitrile-membrane (RP6) without the use of a closed recirculating dialyzate delivery system. *Clin. Nephrol.*, **4**, 18

32 Vereerstraeten, P., Dehout, F., Vanherweghem, J.-L., Thaysc, J.-P., Hautekiet, P., Delaruelle, M. and Kinnaert, P. (1979). Comparison of three hemodialysis procedures with unipuncture. *Int. J. Artif. Organs*, **2**, 23

33 Ogden, D. A. and Cohen, I. M. (1980). Hemodialysis with a coaxial counterflow single-needle blood access catheter. *Am. Soc. Artif. Intern. Organs*, **3**, 33

34 von Hartitzsch, B., Hoenich, N. A., Samson, P., Erickson, J., Ashcroft, R. A. and Kerr, D. N. S. (1973). A clinical evaluation of the new dialysers. *Kidney Int.*, **3**, 35

35 Hoenich, N. A., Conceicao, S., White, T., Ward, M. K. and Kerr, D. N. S. (1976). Large surface area dialysers—a question of performance. *Proc. III Meeting of the European Society of Artificial Organs*, p. 185. (London)

36 Hoenich, N. A., Frost, T. H. and Kerr, D. N. S. (1978). Dialysers. In Drukker, W., Parsons, F. M. and Maher, J. F. (eds.) *Replacement of Renal Function by Dialysis*, p. 80. (The Hague: Martinus Nijhoff) (2nd Edn. due 1981)

37 Wehle, B., Asaba, H., Castenfors, J., Furst, P., Grahn, A., Gunnarsson, B., Shaldon, S. and Bergstrom, J. (1978). The influence of dialysis fluid composition on the blood pressure response during dialysis. *Clin. Nephrol.*, **10**, 62

38 Wilkinson, R., Barber, S. G. and Robson, V. (1977). Cramps, thirst and hypertension in hemodialysis patients—the influence of dialyzate sodium concentration. *Clin. Nephrol.*, **7**, 101

39 Robson, M., Oren, A. and Ravid, M. (1978). Dialysate sodium concentration, hypertension, and pulmonary edema in hemodialysis patients. *Dial. Transplant.*, **7**, 678

40 Redaelli, B., Sforzini, S., Bonoldi, G., Dadone, C., Di Filippo, G., Filoramo, F., Limido, D., Mimmo, R., Pincella, G. and Vigano, M. R. (1979). Hemodialysis with 'adequate' sodium concentration in dialysate. *Int. J. Artif. Organs*, **2**, 133

41 Morrison, G., Michelson, E. L., Brown, S. and Morganroth, J. (1980). Mechanism and prevention of cardiac arrhythmias in chronic hemodialysis patients. *Kidney Int.*, **17**, 811

42 Tolchin, N., Roberts, J. L., Hayashi, J. and Lewis, E. J. (1977). Metabolic consequences of high mass-transfer hemodialysis. *Kidney Int.*, **11**, 366

43 Desch, G., Oules, R., Mion, C., Descomps, B. and Crastes de Paulet, A. (1978). Plasma acetate levels during hemodialysis. *Clin. Chim. Acta*, **85**, 231

44 Graefe, U., Milutinovich, J., Follette, W. C., Vizzo, J. E., Babb, A. L. and Scribner, B. H. (1978). Less dialysis-induced morbidity and vascular instability with bicarbonate in dialysate. *Ann. Intern. Med.*, **88**, 332

45 Mansell, M. A., Nunan, T. O., Laker, M. F., Boon, N. A. and Wing, A. J. (1979). Incidence and significance of rising blood acetate levels during hemodialysis. *Clin. Nephrol.*, **12**, 22

46 Raja, R. M., Kramer, M. S. and Rosenbaum, J. L. (1980). Prevention of intradialytic hypotension using bicarbonate dialysate and mannitol. *Dial. Transplant.*, **9**, 234

47 Viljoen, M. and Gold, C. H. (1979). Danger of haemodialysis using acetate dialysate in combination with a large surface area dialyser. *S. Afr. Med. J.*, **56**, 170

48 Swamy, A. P., Cestero, R. V. M., Campbell, R. G. and Freeman, R. B. (1976). Long-term effect of dialysate glucose on the lipid levels of maintenance hemodialysis patients. *Trans. Am. Soc. Artif. Intern. Organs*, **11**, 54

49 Hubner, W., Sieberth, H. G., Diemer, A., Finke, K. and Prange, E. (1971). Effects of regular haemodialysis with glucose and glucose free dialysate on hyperlipaemia. *Proc. Eur. Dial. Transplant. Assoc.*, **8**, 174

50 Kaye, M., Mangel, R. and Neubauer, E. (1966). Studies in calcium metabolism in patients on chronic haemodialysis. *Proc. Eur. Dial. Transplant. Assoc.*, **3**, 17

51 Wing, A. J. (1968). Optimum calcium concentration of dialysis fluid for maintenance haemodialysis. *Br. Med. J.*, **4**, 145

52 Conceicao, S., Hoenich, N. A., Ward, M. K., White, T., Aljama, P., Dewar, J. and Kerr, D. N. S. (1977). Ionised calcium during haemodialysis. *Proc. Eur. Dial. Transplant. Assoc.*, **14**, 229

53 Raman, A., Chong, Y. K. and Sreenevasan, G. A. (1976). Effects of varying dialysate calcium concentrations on the plasma calcium fractions in patients on dialysis. *Nephron*, **16**, 181

54 Bouillon, R., Verberckmoes, R. and de Moor, P. (1975). Influence of dialysate calcium concentration and vitamin D on serum parathyroid hormone during repetitive dialysis. *Kidney Int.*, **7**, 422

55 Malluche, H. H., Ritz, E., Lange, H. P. and Schoeppe, W. (1976). Changes of bone histology during maintenance hemodialysis at various levels of dialyzate Ca concentration. *Clin. Nephrol.*, **6**, 440

56 Regan, R. J., Peacock, M., Rosen, S. M., Robinson, P. J. and Horsman, A. (1976). Effect of dialysate calcium concentration on bone disease in patients on hemodialysis. *Kidney Int.*, **10**, 246

57 Drueke, T., Bordier, P. J., Man, N. K., Jungers, P. and Marie, P. (1977). Effects of high dialysate calcium concentration on bone remodelling, serum biochemistry and parathyroid hormone in patients with renal osteodystrophy. *Kidney Int.*, **11**, 267

58 Evans, R. A. and Somerville, P. J. (1976). The use of high calcium dialysate in the treatment of renal osteomalacia. *Aust. NZ J. Med.*, **6**, 10

59 Stewart, W. K. and Fleming, L. W. (1973). The effect of dialysate magnesium on plasma and erythrocyte magnesium and potassium concentrations during maintenance haemodialysis. *Nephron*, **10**, 222

60 Fleming, L. W., Lenman, J. A. R. and Stewart, W. K. (1972). Effect of magnesium on nerve conduction velocity during regular dialysis treatment. *J. Neurol. Neurosurg. Psychiat.*, **35**, 342

61 Graf, H., Kovarik, J., Stummvoll, H. K. and Wolf, A. (1979). Disappearance of uraemic pruritus after lowering dialysate magnesium concentration. *Br. Med. J.*, **2**, 1478

62 Freeman, R. M., Lawton, R. L. and Chamberlain, M. A. (1967). Hard-water syndrome. *N. Engl. J. Med.*, **276**, 1113

63 Govan, J. R., Porter, C. A., Cook, J. G. H., Dixon, B. and Trafford, J. A. P. (1968). Acute magnesium poisoning as a complication of chronic intermittent haemodialysis. *Br. Med. J.*, **2**, 278

64 D'Amico, G., Petrella, E., Orlandini, G., Cambi, V., Savazzi, G., Migone, L., Castellani, A., Mioni, G. and Maiorca, R. (1976). Long-term multicentric experience with short dialysis treatment. In Giovannetti, S., Bonomini, V. and D'Amico, G. (eds.) *Proceedings of the VIth International Congress on Nephrology, Florence, 1975*, p. 629. (Basel: Karger)

65 Martin, A. M., Oduro-Dominah, A., Gibbins, J. K., Devapal, D. and Mitchell, D. C. (1975). Regular short haemodialysis in end-stage renal failure. *Br. Med. J.*, **3**, 758

66 Aljama, P., Conceicae, S., Ward, M. K., Feest, T. G., Martin, A. M., Craig, H., Bird, P. A. E., Sussman, M. and Kerr, D. N. S. (1978). Comparison of three short dialysis schedules. *Dial. Transplant.*, **7**, 334

67 Trafford, J. A. P., Sharpstone, P., Evans, R. and Ireland, R. (1979). Evaluation of ultra-short dialysis. *Br. Med. J.*, 1, 518

68 Chapman, G. V., Mahony, J. F. and Farrell, P. C. (1980). A crossover study of short time dialysis. *Clin. Nephrol.*, 13, 78

69 Sellars, L., Robson, V. and Wilkinson, R. (1979). Sodium retention and hypertension with short dialysis. *Br. Med. J.*, 1. 520

70 Public Health Laboratory Service Survey (1976). Hepatitis B in retreat from dialysis units in United Kingdom in 1973. *Br. Med. J.*, 1, 1579

71 Public Health Laboratory Service Survey (1974). Decrease in the incidence of hepatitis in dialysis units associated with prevention programme. *Br. Med. J.*, 4, 751

72 Corey, L., Stamm, W. E., Feorino, P. M., Bryan, J. A., Weseley, S., Gregg, M. B. and Solangi, K. (1975). HB$_s$Ag-negative hepatitis in a hemodialysis unit: relation to Epstein–Barr virus. *N. Engl. J. Med.*, 293, 1273

73 Sengar, D. P. S., McLeish, W. A., Sutherland, M., Couture, R. A. and Rashid, A. (1975). Hepatitis B antigen (HBAg) infection in a hemodialysis unit. I. HL-A8 and immune response to HBAg. *CMA Journal*, 112, 968

74 Dankert, J., Uitentuis, J., Houwen, B., Tegzess, A. M. and van der Hem, G. K. (1976). Hepatitis B surface antigen in environmental samples from hemodialysis units. *J. Infect. Dis.*, 134, 123

75 Snydman, D. R., Bryan, J. A., London, W. T., Werner, B., Bregman, D., Blumberg, B. S. and Gregg, M. B. (1976). Transmission of hepatitis B associated with hemodialysis: role of malfunction (blood leaks) in dialysis machines. *J. Infect. Dis.*, 134, 562

76 London, W. T., Drew, J. S., Lustbader, E. D., Werner, B. G. and Blumberg, B. S. (1977). Host responses to hepatitis B infection in patients in a chronic hemodialysis unit. *Kidney Int.*, 12, 51

77 Mrs Elizabeth Ward, British Kidney Patients Association, Bordon, Hants.

78 Kendal, A. P., Smith, C. E. and Branch, K. W. (1980). Make-it-yourself carry-on kidney machine. *Dial. Transplant.*, 9, 333

79 Crystal, R. C. (1980). The health care financing administration's position on re-use. *Dial. Transplant.*, 9, 23

80 Deane, N., Blagg, C., Bower, J., De Palma, J., Gutch, C., Kanter, A., Ogden, D., Sadler, J., Siemsen, A., Teehan, B. and Sosin, A. (1978). A survey of dialyzer reuse practice in the United States. *Dial. Transplant.*, 7, 1128

81 Albertazzi, A., Ruggeri, G., Ardizzoia, B., Franchini, L. and Burzi, L. (1974). Automatic machine for dialysers re-use. *Proc. Eur. Dial. Transplant. Assoc.*, 11, 187

82 Man, N. K., Glace, M., Becker, A., Di Giulio, S., Zingraff, J. and Funck-Brentano, J. L. (1978). A new dialyser re-use machine. In Frost, T. H. (ed.) *Technical Aspects of Renal Dialysis*, p. 73. (Tunbridge Wells: Pitman Medical)

83 Ahmad, R. and Goldsmith, H. J. (1975). Automated dialyser rinsing machine. *Dial. Transplant.*, 3, 29

84 Hardy, D. W., Higgins, M. R., McFarlane, D. F. and Hughes, R. V. (1976). An automated cleaning device for dialyzers; machine design and technology. *Clin. Nephrol.*, 5, 275

85 Vandenbroucke, J. M., Stragier, A. and de Strihou, C. van Y. (1977). Efficiency of automated reuse of disposable dialysers. *Proc. Eur. Dial. Transplant. Assoc.*, 14, 598

86 Lewis, K. J., Dewar, P. J., Ward, M. K. and Kerr, D. N. S. (1981). Formation of anti-N like antibodies in dialysis patients; effect of different methods of dialyser rinsing to remove formaldehyde. *Clin. Nephrol.*, 15, 39

87 Lanning, J. T., Winterich, C. and Zuanaich, N. (1980). Multiple use of hollow fiber dialyzers in a free-standing center. *Dial. Transplant.*, 9, 36

88 Levin, N. (1980). Dialyzer re-use in a hospital. *Dial. Transplant.*, 9, 40

89 Bilinsky, R. T. and Morris, A. J. (1971). Hemodialysis coil reuse; a safe and economical new method. *J. Am. Med. Assoc.*, 218, 1806

90 Balter, P. (1979). Reusing the dialyzer. *Int. J. Artif. Organs*, 2, 112

91 Aljama, P., Ward, M. K., Feest, T. G., Martin, A. M., Alvarez-Ude, F., Hoenich, N. A., Marcen, R. and Kerr, D. N. S. (1978). Prospective long term comparation of short and conventional haemodialysis. In Frost, T. H. (ed.) *Technical Aspects of Renal Dialysis*, p. 310. (Tunbridge Wells: Pitman Medical)

92 Lewis, K. J., Dewar, P. J., Ward, M. K. and Kerr, D. N. S. (1981). Residual formaldeyhyde in dialyzers: quantity, location and the effect of different methods of rinsing. *Artif. Organs* (submitted for publication)

93 Koch, K. M., Frei, U. and Fassbinder, W. (1978). Hemolysis and anaemia in anti-N-like antibody positive hemodialysis patients. *Trans. Am. Soc. Artif. Intern. Organs*, 24, 709

94 Sandler, S. G., Sharon, R., Bush, M., Stroup, M. and Sabo, B. (1979). Formaldehyde-related antibodies in hemodialysis patients. *Transfusion*, 19, 682

95 Ward, R. A. and Farrell, P. C. (1978). Precise anticoagulation for routine hemodialysis using nomograms. *Trans. Am. Soc. Artif. Organs*, 24, 439

96 Schwarzbeck, A., Wagner, L., Squarr, H.-U. and Strauch, M. (1978). pH-dependent heparin inactivation during hemodialysis. *Dial. Transplant.*, 7, 740

97 Woods, H. F., Ash, G., Parsons, V. and Weston, M. J. (1979). Reduction of dialyzer fibrin deposition with sulphinpyrazone. *Clin. Nephrol.*, 12, 122

98 Shapiro, W. B., Faubert, P. F., Porush, J. G. and Chou, S-Y. (1979). Low-dose heparin in routine hemodialysis monitored by activated partial thromboplastin time. *Artif. Organs*, 3, 73

99 Turney, J. H., Fewell, M. R., Williams, L. C., Parsons, V. and Weston, M. J. (1980). Platelet protection and heparin sparing with prostacyclin during regular dialysis therapy. *Lancet*, 2, 219

100 Drukker, W., Parsons, F. M. and Maher, J. F. (1978). *Replacement of Renal Function by Dialysis*. (The Hague: Martinus Nijhoff)

101 Minetti, L., di Belgiojoso, G. B., Civati, G., Durante, A., Scatizzi, A. and Surian, M. (1975). Acute renal failure due to Rifampicin (R-ARF). *Proc. Eur. Dial. Transplant. Assoc.*, 12, 210

102 Gotloib, L. and Tuchman, I. (1978). A new device for continuous monitoring of grounding and of current leakage in the microampere range for artificial kidneys. In Frost, T. H. (ed.) *Technical Aspects of Renal Dialysis*, p. 242 (Tunbridge Wells: Pitman Medical)

103 Berkes, S. L., Kahn, S. I., Chazan, J. A. and Garella, S. (1975). Prolonged hemolysis from overheated dialysate. *Ann. Intern. Med.*, 83, 363

104 Tielemans, C., Herbaut, C., Geurts, J. and Dratwa, M. (1980). Hemolysis and consumption coagulopathy due to overheated dialysate. *Kidney Int.*, 17, 706

105 Fortner, R. W., Nowakowski, A., Carter, C. B., King, L. H. Jr. and Knepshield, J. H. (1970). Death due to overheated dialysate during dialysis. *Ann. Intern. Med.*, 73, 443

106 Linder, A., Moskovtchenko, J. F. and Traeger, J. (1972). Accidental mass hypernatremia during hemodialysis. *Nephron*, 9, 99

107 Robinson, P. J. A. and Rosen, S. M. (1971). Pyrexial reactions during haemodialysis. *Br. Med. J.*, 1, 528

108 Favero, M. S., Petersen, N. J., Boyer, K. M., Carson, L. A. and Bond, W. W. (1974). Micro bial contamination of renal dialysis systems and associated health risks. *Trans. Am. Soc. Artif. Organs*, 20, 175

109 Hindman, S. H., Carson, L. A., Favero, M. S., Petersen, N. J., Schonberger, L. B. and Solano, J. T. (1975). Pyrogenic reactions during haemodialysis caused by extramural endotoxin. *Lancet*, 2, 732

110 Petersen, N. J., Carson, L. A., Favero, M. S., Marshall, J. H. Jr. and Aguero, S. M. (1980). Removal of bacteria and bacterial endotoxin from dialysis fluids by sorbents. *Am. Soc. Artif. Intern. Organs*, 3, 6

111 Bernick, J. J. and Port, F. K. (1980). Absence of bacteremia and endotoxaemia despite contaminated dialyzate. *Clin. Nephrol.*, **14**, 13

112 Rosenbaum, B. J., Alfrey, A. C. and Holmes, J. H. (1969). Dialysis acidosis. *Arch. Intern. Med.*, **124**, 184

113 Dawids, S. G. and Vejlsgaard, R. (1976). Bateriological and clinical evaluation of different dialysate delivery systems. *Acta Med. Scand.*, **199**, 151

114 Curtis, J. R., Wing, A. J. and Coleman, J. C. (1967). Bacillus cereus bacteraemia: a complication of intermittent haemodialysis. *Lancet*, **1**, 136

115 Kuehnel, E. and Lundh, H. (1976). Outbreak of pseudomonas cepacia bacteremia related to contaminated reused coils. *Dial. Transplant.*, **5**, 44

116 Kerr, D. N. S. (1980). Clinical and pathophysiologic changes in patients on chronic dialysis: the central nervous system. In *Advances in Nephrology*, **9**, 109. (Year Book Medical Publishers, Inc.)

117 Pierides, A. M., Edwards, W. G. Jr., Cullum, U. X. Jr., McCall, J. T. and Ellis, H. A. (1980). Hemodialysis encephalopathy with osteomalacic fractures and muscle weakness. *Kidney Int.*, **18**, 115

118 Bustamante, J., Mateo, M. C. M., de Pedro, A. DeP. and Manchado, O. O. (1978). Changes in copper and ceruloplasmin in chronic renal insufficiency treated by hemodialysis and peritoneal dialysis. *Nephron*, **22**, 312

119 Blomfield, J., Dixon, S. R. and McCredie, D. A. (1971). Potential hepatotoxicity of copper in recurrent hemodialysis. *Arch. Intern. Med.*, **128**, 555

120 Manzler, A. D. and Schreiner, A. W. (1970). Copper-induced acute hemolytic anemia; a new complication of hemodialysis. *Ann. Intern. Med.*, **73**, 409

121 Lyle, W. H., Payton, J. E. and Hui, M. (1976). Haemodialysis and copper fever. *Lancet*, **1**, 1324

122 Klein, W. J., Metz, E. N. and Price, A. R. (1972). Acute copper intoxication: a hazard of hemodialysis. *Arch. Intern. Med.*, **129**, 578

123 O'Nion, J. V., Atkin-Thor, E., Rothert, S. W., Stephen, R. L., Goddard, B. W. and Ogilvie, S. (1978). Effect of zinc supplementation on red blood cell zinc, serum zinc, taste acuity, and dietary intake in zinc deficient dialysis patients. *Dial. Transplant.*, **7**, 1208

124 Mahajan, S. K., Prasad, A. S., Lambujon, J., Abbasi, A. A., Briggs, W. A. and McDonald, F. D. (1979). Improvement of uremic hypogeusia by zinc. *Trans. Am. Soc. Artif. Intern. Organs*, **15**, 443

125 Antoniou, L. D., Sudhakar, T., Shalhoub, R. J. and Smith, J. C. Jr. (1977). Reversal of uraemic impotence by zinc. *Lancet*, **2**, 895

126 Zetin, M. and Stone, R. A. (1980). Effects of zinc in chronic hemodialysis. *Clin. Nephrol.*, **13**, 20

127 Brook, A. C., Johnston, D. G., Ward, M. K., Watson, M. J., Cook, D. B. and Kerr, D. N. S. (1980). Absence of a therapeutic effect of zinc in the sexual dysfunction of haemodialysed patients. *Lancet* (In press)

128 Blomfield, J., McPherson, J. and George, C. R. P. (1969). Active uptake of copper and zinc during haemodialysis. *Br. Med. J.*, **2**, 141

129 Petrie, J. J. B. and Row, P. G. (1977). Dialysis anaemia caused by subacute zinc toxicity. *Lancet*, **1**, 1178

130 Webster, J. D., Parker, T. F., Alfrey, Al. C., Smythe, W. R., Kubo, H., Neal, G. and Hull, A. R. (1980). Acute nickel intoxication by dialysis. *Ann. Intern. Med.*, **92**, 631

131 Rubin, R. J. and Schiffer, C. A. (1976). Fate in humans of the plasticizer, di-2-ethylhexyl phthalate, arising from transfusion of platelets stored in vinyl plastic bags. *Transfusion*, **16**, 330

132 Jaeger, R. J. and Rubin, R. J. (1972). Migration of a phthalate ester plasticizer from polyvinyl chloride blood bags into stored human blood and its localization in human tissues. *N. Engl. J. Med.*, **287**, 1114

133 Jacobson, M. S., Kevy, S. V. and Grand, R. J. (1977). Effects of a plasticizer leached from polyvinyl chloride on the subhuman primate: a consequence of chronic transfusion therapy. *J. Lab. Clin. Med.*, **89**, 1066

134 Neergaard, J., Nielsen, B., Faurby, V., Christensen, D. H. and Nielsen, O. F. (1971). Plasticizers in P.V.C. and the occurrence of hepatitis in a haemodialysis unit. *Scand. J. Urol. Nephrol.*, **5**, 141

135 Neergaard, J., Nielsen, B., Faurby, V., Christensen, D. H. and Nielsen, O. F. (1975). On the exudation of plasticizers from PVC haemodialysis tubings. *Nephron*, **14**, 263

136 Kennedy, A. C., Linton, A. L., Luke, R. G. and Renfrew, S. (1963). Electroencephalographic changes during haemodialysis. *Lancet*, **1**, 408

137 Teschan, P. E., Ginn, H. E., Bourne, J. R., Walker, P. J. and Ward, J. W. (1975). Quantitative neurobehavioural responses to renal failure and maintenance dialysis. *Trans. Am. Soc. Intern. Organs*, **21**, 488

138 Edwards, A. E., Kopple, J. D., Miller, J. M., Fields, L. G. and Der, DuF. (1977). Time perception and hemodialysis. *Nephron*, **19**, 140

139 Bergstrom, J. (1978). Ultrafiltration without dialysis for removal of fluid and solutes in uremia. *Clin. Nephrol.*, **9**, 156

140 Rouby, J. J., Rottembourg, J., Durande, J-P., Basset, J-Y., Degoulet, P., Glaser, P. and Legrain, M. (1980). Hemodynamic changes induced by regular hemodialysis and sequential ultrafiltration hemodialysis: a comparative study. *Kidney Int.*, **17**, 801

141 Kjellstrand, C. M., Rosa, A. A. and Shideman, J. R. (1979). Hypotension during hemodialysis: osmolality fall is an important pathogenetic factor. *Am. Soc. Artif. Intern. Organs*, **3**, 11

142 Hampl, H. (1978). Hemodynamic studies during hemodialysis, sequential ultrafiltration, and hemofiltration. *Dial. Transplant.*, **7**, 1095

143 Ivanovich, P. (1978). Sequential ultrafiltration–hemodialysis: 18 months' experience. *Dial. Transplant.*, **7**, 1077

144 Lynggaard, F. (1978). One year's experience with sequential filtration/hemodialysis. *Dial. Transplant.*, **7**, 1106

145 Jones, E. O., Ward, M. K., Hoenich, N. A. and Kerr, D. N. S. (1977). Separation of dialysis and ultrafiltration – does it really help? *Proc. Eur. Dial. Transplant. Assoc.*, **14**, 160

6

Home haemodialysis

B. H. B. Robinson

THE DEVELOPMENT AND OBJECTIVES OF HOME DIALYSIS

The successful application of regular dialysis treatment (RDT) to the maintenance of patients with end-stage renal failure offered the chance of survival and rehabilitation from this previously fatal condition, but presented the problems of finding the cost and resources for medical care in a particularly acute and dramatic (not to say newsworthy) form, and committed the patients themselves to a life of frequent and unending visits to hospital for treatment. The rapid improvement in patient well-being following the initiation of RDT abolished the need for the intensive care environment required for dialysis in acute renal failure. Professional supervision could be reduced and several patients treated together in the same dialysis area with minimal nursing supervision. But dialysis places in the hospital centre for new patients remained limited because of the continuing commitment to patients already undergoing treatment and the high cost of providing staff for the preparation and supervision of dialysis. As experience with RDT increased, it was found possible to train the patients themselves to undertake many of the routine tasks in the preparation of dialysis equipment and the supervision of their own dialyses, thereby reducing the staffing requirements relative to the numbers being treated. The patient still had to attend hospital for treatment several times each week. The logical, but courageous, step was to transfer the dialysis from hospital to the patient's own home, either with professional supervision[1] or, more significantly, unattended by hospital personnel[2]. The success of Shaldon's group with unsupervised home haemodialysis was confirmed by Scribner and co-workers in Seattle[3]. Home dialysis increased the potential number of patients who could receive treatment based on one hospital centre and reduced the staffing requirement, and thereby the cost per patient treated. In addition it freed the patient from incessant visits to hospital and offered a solution to the problem of treating patients who lived remote from a hospital with dialysis facilities.

Although much of the pressure for the development of home dialysis came from considerations of cost, staffing and convenience, the place of treatment in relation to the patient's life-style is another important factor. Most other forms of new therapy may first of all be administered in hospital, but are soon translated to the patient's home and the patient's own control. RDT for renal failure has been compared with insulin for the diabetic. Just as most diabetics administer their own injections, it would seem appropriate that we should try to make it possible for patients with end-stage renal failure to manage their own treatment. Haemodialysis remains a relatively cumbersome and demanding technique with bulky hardware and a host of problems for management within the family. But this does not detract from the need to try to make most dialysis patients independent of the hospital centre and responsible for their own treatment.

The objectives of home dialysis are summarized in Table 1. The order of priority of these objectives has varied from time to time and place to place. The early incentive was the need to free hospital dialysis places to increase

Table 1   Objectives of home dialysis

1. Making patient independent of hospital with improved understanding and control of his treatment
2. Freeing hospital centre dialysis places for new patients, hence increasing potential size of dialysis programme
3. Reducing staffing requirements, hence cost of treatment
4. Treatment of patients living far from the dialysis centre, and reducing travelling for those living nearer
5. Improved rehabilitation and flexibility in dialysis times to suit work and family requirements
6. Avoidance of cross-infection (e.g. hepatitis)

the patient load, and to provide treatment for patients remote from dialysis centres. In most developed countries these needs have been met by increasing the number of dialysis centres, and the major motivation for home dialysis has been to give the patient independence from the hospital centre, a greater understanding and control of his treatment and the convenience of choosing his dialysis times to fit his work and recreation plans. In many areas home dialysis has been adopted little or not at all, or the reduction in professional staff and the nearness of dialysis to the patient's home has been achieved by the development of 'minimal' or 'self-care' dialysis units – an alternative discussed in more detail later in this chapter.

The objectives of home dialysis which influence the dialysis centres have a great deal of bearing upon the selection of patients, equipping of the home and organization of the programme. The requirements for a programme designed to expand limited treatment facilities or deal with patients remote from the hospital centre may well differ from a programme purely concerned with patient convenience and well-being. The availability of renal transplantation provides a further dimension to planning.

These variations in philosophy between centres, and within centres at different times in their evolution, mean that there are few dogmatic rules for home dialysis planning. Dialysis centre directors and staff must preserve a flexible and innovative approach to this treatment.

VASCULAR ACCESS FOR HOME DIALYSIS

Fundamental to treatment by regular haemodialysis is easy but reliable access to the circulation. The Silastic–Teflon arteriovenous shunt[4] provided this for many patients during the early years of haemodialysis. Such shunts are easily connected and disconnected from the dialyser and have the advantage that low resistance dialysers, such as the Kiil, can often be adequately perfused direct from the arterial cannula without the need for a blood pump. This simplifies and increases the safety of dialysis at home. The two main disadvantages of this type of external prosthesis are clotting and infection. Patients can be taught to declot their own cannulae using fine plastic cannulae of the type often used for intravenous infusions. The importance of a safe 'no-touch' technique when dealing with direct access to the circulation must be taught to the patient and assisting relatives. For some patients it is probably safer not to encourage them to attempt clot removal, although this will increase their dependence upon trained professional help. Nevertheless, most of our patients have successfully declotted cannulae, although we discourage attempts to clear clot from the arterial cannula by direct injection of saline under pressure because of the hazards of retrograde embolization.

The risk of infection of the external prosthesis may actually be less at home than in hospital, although this is difficult to prove. The cross-infection risk is reduced and the patient has a vested interest in handling his shunt carefully. Training is important here. Over-enthusiastic and obsessional shunt toilet may actually loosen the cannula or damage the skin exit site leading to erosion or infection. On the other hand, some patients can never achieve acceptable standards of hygiene, and the unfortunates who are chronic staphylococcal carriers may have difficulty preserving the integrity of their shunts, no matter how careful they are. For any patients remote from immediate medical care we have provided a stock of an antistaphylococcal agent, such as flucloxacillin, which can be taken at the first signs of cannula infection, such as pain, redness or pus appearing at the exit hole of the cannula, pending medical consultation and bacteriological examination. The advantages of early treatment have outweighed the drawbacks of this rather indiscriminate use of chemotherapy. We have chosen to select *Staphylococcus* on the grounds that it is the commonest infecting agent and that most Gram-negative infections will prove impossible to eliminate without replacing the cannula anyway.

These drawbacks of the Silastic–Teflon cannula, as well as the inconvenience of an external prosthesis, were greatly reduced by the introduction of the Brescia–Cimino subcutaneous arteriovenous fistula for regular dialysis[5]. The training of patients or their relatives to needle these fistulae with large bore needles at home seemed, at first, a daunting prospect, but in practice proved quite feasible[6]. Motivation of the patient is important if he is to achieve competence at inserting fistula needles, and for some patients this has proved a handicap to home dialysis training, so that a spouse or other relative has had to be trained instead. Assistance is also required if the fistula is relatively inaccessible to the patient himself. Clearly it is an advantage if the fistula is created in the non-dominant limb. Occasionally it is necessary to revert to an external Silastic–Teflon shunt if self-dialysis is to be practised at home. There is no doubt that learning the technique of dialysis through a subcutaneous fistula is more difficult for the patient than learning to dialyse through an external arteriovenous shunt and has increased the time and difficulty of training for home dialysis.

Satisfactory and trouble-free access to the circulation is essential to home dialysis. Repeated failures or difficulties with cannulation seriously undermine the patient's confidence and morale and the need to call in professional help or return to the hospital centre negates the objectives of home dialysis. The surgeon creating the access site needs to be familiar with the special requirements of home dialysis and if necessary be prepared to refashion a 'difficult' fistula or insert a suitable vein graft or a prosthetic graft of materials such as bovine carotid or woven Teflon[7,8]. The aim is to have a suitable length of accessible vessel in a site where it is easily needled, preferably by the patient himself. The non-dominant arm is preferable because leg fistulae are usually rather more difficult to needle, whereas if a Silastic–Teflon shunt is necessary the leg is a convenient site for self-dialysis.

For patients with fistulae with few convenient needling sites, or who have difficulty with repeated needling, single-needle dialysis[9] can be a real help. But the patient must be aware that the reduced efficiency of single-needle dialysis necessitates longer dialysis times. In large patients we have found a tendency for single-needle dialysis to lead to an under-dialysis syndrome or fluid overload because, away from supervision, the patient may disregard the need for more dialysis.

The selection of needles for access to fistulae is a matter of individual choice within centres. For self-insertion it is preferable to use a very sharp needle with a short bevel and to aim for the smallest bore that is compatible with the required blood flow rate. This is usually about 14-gauge. The needle design should allow easy manipulation and positioning by an operator using one hand.

EQUIPMENT FOR HOME DIALYSIS

Equipment requirements

It is easy to draw up a list of requirements for home dialysis equipment (Table 2). It is more difficult to reconcile these requirements or to allot an order of priority. The requirements are essentially similar to those for hospital equipment, although the emphasis is sometimes different. Reliability and ease of operation have high priority ratings for the home, where unobtrusive compact design is also more valued by the family. Some of the requirements tend to be incompatible. Thus, increasing safety by additional monitoring and a series of fail-safe devices increase complexity, size and cost and may well decrease overall reliability and ease of operation and servicing.

Table 2   Requirements for home dialysis equipment

Safety – including fail-safe provision and electrical safety
Reliability – with minimal service requirement
Simplicity in operation
Without unusual water supply, drainage or power needs
Compact and light weight of unobtrusive design
Quiet operation
Low cost
'Patient-proof'

On the other hand, simple easily set-up equipment may be relatively less safe, not only for lack of monitors or fail-safe devices but also because the components are readily accessible for inappropriate and dangerous adjustments by the patient. This risk is one aspect included in our term 'patient-proof'. This requirement also applies to the robustness of equipment which may be exposed to unusual stresses or knocks. The multipoint pattern of the Kiil dialyser, for example, has great advantages as a dialyser over the previous grooved pattern but is easily damaged when scrubbed in the bath tub at home. However, most patients take great care of their dialysis equipment, and accidental damage is probably more likely to take place in hospital. The other and more serious aspect of 'patient-proofing', to which we alluded above, is the need to eliminate, both by training and by equipment design, the risk that patients could make adjustments or take short cuts which might be dangerous. One example of this was a type of dialysate proportioning machine allowing easy access to the adjustment of the gain on the amplifier concerned with the conductivity meter. Although this facility was intended only for use by trained renal technicians, an enterprising patient was able to eliminate the monitor alarm signal related to a faulty valve by turning down the gain on the amplifier and thus allowing the production of a hypotonic dialysate with serious consequences. Somehow equipment design should make it impossible to override warnings of potentially dangerous situations and for the equipment still to function.

Electrical safety should be a self-evident requirement, both for home and hospital, yet dialysis equipment has been marketed which is not free from hazard to patients and other operators. Standards have been proposed for electromedical equipment covering earthing and insulation. Even when the major equipment is adequately earthed, faults may be present in ancillary equipment, such as pumps or additional monitors. The home patient has the extra hazard of domestic appliances for which standards are lower and which may in any case be faulty[10]. An earth leakage trip device would then be necessary to ensure safety[11]. With dialysis, there is the added hazard that dialysate as well as some cleaning and sterilizing agents are corrosive and may render faulty otherwise safe connections or earthing devices.

Reliability is especially pertinent to home dialysis because repeated equipment failures undermine the patient's confidence and may cause panic or attempts at dangerous 'short-cuts'. Repeated visits by technical staff for repairs or obligatory return to the hospital centre because of equipment failures make home dialysis impossible. Clearly, if patients of widely varying intelligence are to operate dialysis equipment at home, the control layout must be plain and easily understood. Indicators and gauges should be explicit and alarm systems should clearly indicate the source of the fault. Setting up and fault connection should be simple. With the proviso above, that complexity may run counter to reliability, a simple-to-operate machine may actually be complex behind the facia, but, as with cars, televisions or washing machines, may be used very successfully by individuals with no idea of how the underlying machinery or electronics function. Elegance of design does not always make for easy understanding, and some equipment on the market has gauges or controls which are difficult to comprehend. Enthusiastic engineers are not always the best people to design controls for the layman, often overlooking simple sources of confusion in favour of convenient technical design.

One example is the provision of a monitor attachment, such as a venous pressure line, adjacent to a gauge indicating some other function.

Choice of dialyser

The types of dialyser most commonly used for hospital dialysis are equally suitable for home use and can be selected according to the patient's needs with regard to surface area and ultrafiltration potential. There are several features of particular importance for home dialysis, although applicable to hospital dialysis as well. A low priming volume is desirable to minimize the amount of blood in the extracorporeal circuit in case of mishaps, and to reduce the potential disturbance at the commencement of dialysis due to sudden changes in circulating blood volume. A low internal resistance to blood flow is a great advantage if the dialyser is to be perfused from the arterial limb via a Silastic–Teflon shunt, as discussed in the previous section, and is still desirable when used with a blood pump in order to avoid high pressures in the extracorporeal circulation. Such high pressures increase the risk of membrane rupture, increase the rate of blood loss in the event of leaks or disconnections, probably increase damage to cellular components of blood and create the potential risk that if air accidentally enters the system it may reach the return cannula too rapidly for the patient or observers to take avoiding action. Disasters have happened from this cause.

The major requirement for a dialyser used at home is a predictable ultrafiltration rate. For successful home dialysis the patient must have some grasp of the rudiments of fluid balance and understand how this can be corrected by ultrafiltration during dialysis. It is therefore important that he can predict from his pressure settings the rate of fluid removal and be able to spread this through the dialysis rather than cause sudden periods of rapid ultrafiltration leading to blood volume depletion and faintness or actual loss of consciousness, which would be hazardous in an unsupervised dialysis. Dialysers with excessively high ultrafiltration rates should normally be avoided for home dialysis unless the patient has been specially trained and is employing special equipment. With the wide choice of dialysers now on the market it is usually possible to select a dialyser with an ultrafiltration rate suitable for the particular patient, defined in terms of size, residual urine volumes, control of blood pressure and mean weight gain between dialyses.

During home dialysis one naturally wishes to keep the dosage of heparin as low as is compatible with trouble-free dialysis. In practice there is probably more difference between individual patients in heparin requirement during the dialysis than between the types of dialyser with which they are treated. The question of fibrin formation in the dialyser becomes more important if one is contemplating re-use of dialysers. It was inherent in the use of the Kiil dialyser, with which most home programmes started, that the dialyser was 're-built' for each dialysis by the patient and his relatives. A chemical sterilizing agent, usually formalin, was then run in and the dialyser left to stand until ready for use. The time taken in preparation for the dialysis could be considerably reduced by re-using the individual 'build' of the Kiil several times. This required the patient to wash-back the blood efficiently into his circulation at the end of dialysis and soon after disconnection to rinse the dialyser through with clean water until there was no visible trace of blood. It could then be re-sterilized with formalin. Even further economy could be effected by re-using the blood lines as well, although this required specially designed lines without inserts which might react with formalin. The running cost of a dialysis programme using disposable dialysers is a great deal higher than that of a programme using the Kiil type of dialyser. This difference in cost can be reduced by using the same type of re-use technique on 'disposable' dialysers. In practice this has been possible with nearly all types of dialysers currently on the market, although there are a few types of flat-bed and hollow-fibre artificial kidneys which are more difficult to wash clear of blood than others. Naturally, manufacturers are loath to recommend this procedure, not only for the cynical reason that it might reduce dialyser sales but from the real reason that they could be held legally responsible for mishaps were they to recommend re-use. Government and hospital authorities have been equally reluctant to condemn or recommend re-use because, whilst their bacteriological experts would suggest that it is potentially dangerous, re-use of dialysers does save a great deal of money. A recent survey on the practice of re-using dialysers does not suggest that it affects patient survival, and statistically at least it would seem that re-use is acceptable[12]. We have encountered problems in home dialysis from the re-use and sterilization of Kiil dialysers. These have usually arisen when the technique has been faulty, either because the patient has left the dialyser full of traces of blood for a while after dialysis, before washing through and re-sterilizing, or the patient has used water stored for some time in a container which has permitted the growth of organisms such as *Pseudomonas* species. One of our patients undoubtedly developed *Pseudomonas* endocarditis from a mishap of this type. More usually they are lucky enough to have little more than troublesome pyrogen reactions.

Although in the hands of well-trained patients the Kiil type of dialyser has proved very efficient, safe to use and relatively less expensive than other types of dialyser, there is no doubt that patients find preparation for dialysis much quicker and simpler with one of the disposable dialysers now available. Even in terms of cost it takes several months of use of disposable dialysers to exceed the initial high capital cost of the Kiil boards. Increasingly in our own home dialysis programme we have changed from the Kiil dialyser to capillary or flat-bed dialysers, to the great satisfaction of our patients, even though we have usually persuaded them to re-use dialysers on grounds of cost.

Preparation of dialysate

The composition of dialysate used for home and for centre dialysis is similar. Home dialysis does make it easier to provide a dialysate composition selected for the individual patient. Most dialysers currently in use require a dialysate flow of 300–500 ml/min to give optimal clearance and ultrafiltration values. To provide dialysate in this quantity for a dialysis of several hours, the solution can be (i) provided before dialysis in a large tank, (ii) produced continuously from tap water and a concentrated electrolytes solution or (iii) prepared in small volumes and regenerated during dialysis with the use of an adsorbent column.

The bulk preparation of dialysate in a tank requires less expensive and simpler equipment than the other two techniques but has the disadvantages that preparation time is increased and that the bulk and weight of the tank of dialysate is inconveniently large. For a 12-hour dialysis a tank holding up to 400 litres is required, the weight of which when full could well prove too much for the floor of the average domestic bedroom. With the shorter dialysis hours which are now more popular, bulk is less of a problem, but even a 4-hour dialysis requires a reservoir of over 120 litres, which is heavy, bulky and takes some time to prepare and mix. Despite these drawbacks the use of a pre-prepared tank of dialysate provides a simple and cheap approach to home dialysis where unit cost is very important. The solution can be adequately mixed with a simple paddle, providing the stirring is thorough, or by recirculation through a small header tank in which the heating element can be placed. Recirculation of dialysate from a reservoir was used in the early years of dialysis employing 100-litre or up to 300-litre tanks. With shorter dialysis hours smaller reservoirs could be used, but the drawbacks of recirculation are the progressive lowering of the gradient for various solutes between plasma and dialysate, with resulting reduction in the efficiency of dialysis and bacterial growth. Heavy bacterial growth may alter the composition of dialysate and present an infection hazard. There is less certainty as to the extent to which bacterial toxins may actually cross the dialysis membrane.

The preparation of dialysate is greatly simplified for the home dialysis patient by the use of one of the proportioning systems manufactured for the purpose. These machines mix treated or untreated tap water in appropriate proportions with a concentrated solution of dialysate, heat the resulting solution to the correct temperature, de-gas the heated solution and supply it to the dialyser. It is convenient to have machines which incorporate a monitoring device necessary for safe unsupervised dialysis. These machines have become smaller and more compact for home use in recent years, even though it has not been possible to reduce the hydraulic components in size in the way in which it has been possible to miniaturize the electronics. The selection of machines is a matter of individual choice based upon the requirements outlined at the beginning of this section. Apart from the general layout, electrical safety and reliability of the machine, points to consider are whether the machine has any special electrical or drainage requirements which will be difficult for the individual patient's home, whether the water pressure in the patient's taps is likely to be adequate for the particular brand of proportioning system and whether the de-gassing system is adequate. Some types of proportioning system rely upon a pump which is driven by the water pressure from the tap. This can put a limitation upon the adaptability of some patients' homes. Such a system is usually less flexible in the ability to vary the dialysate concentration. On the other hand it should not be possible for a patient to vary the proportioning outside very narrow safe limits. Warming a solution prepared from tap water results in the release of dissolved air. This may appear as bubbles, particularly likely to appear when a negative pressure is exerted on the dialysate outflow by a pump, and the bubbles can effectively reduce the surface area of the dialyser membrane. Alternatively, some of the gas diffuses across the membrane. In consequence of a fall in pressure from the dialyser inflow to the venous return, the gas comes out of solution in the blood and causes foaming in the lines, sometimes severe enough to cause air embolism. In our experience this problem has been much more troublesome in home dialysis than in the hospital centre, probably because of the differences in the route of the water supply. Winter has been a particularly troublesome time because the colder water holds more gas in solution. The early approach to this problem was to pass warm dialysate through some sort of trap, either a mesh or pieces of ceramic which will encourage the formation of bubbles. Such systems usually prove inadequate and it is necessary to add an additional system, such as warming the dialysate above the required temperature followed by cooling or allowing the dialysate to pass into an expansion chamber which will encourage the release of dissolved air before it actually passes into the dialyser itself.

Although the dialysate does not need to be actually sterile, the equipment does need to be cleaned after dialysis to prevent a build up of bacterial growth, which cannot only cause serious contamination of dialysate but may actually lead to a build up of bacterial material in the tubing and connections of the machine, narrowing the lumen and interfering with function. The three approaches used in a proportioning system have been chemical sterilization, usually with formalin, sterilization by circulation of hot water, or sterilization with hot water under pressure – in effect autoclaving. Chemical sterilization is the cheapest approach, but formalin is unpleasant to use at home and the time taken up in preparation may be increased, although machines with semi-automatic chemical sterilizing systems are now available. One of the commonest arrangements for cleaning dialysate proportioning systems is the facility for recirculating water at about 90 °C through the system for 30 minutes or longer. This effectively destroys most bacteria but would be less effective in the presence of heavy contamination and ineffective against spore-forming bacteria. Although the use of hot water systems has been criticized as being little more than 'pasteurization' they have proved simple and effective as long as the equipment is kept clean and properly looked after. Machines with autoclaving systems tend to be more complex, more expensive and heavier, and, in our opinion, are something of a luxury.

The systems using continuous regeneration of dialysate by passage through charcoal columns allow a great reduction in the volume of dialysis equipment and in many ways meet some of the ideals for home dialysis. The machinery is light and compact, easily fitting into the luggage compartment of a patient's car so that he can take it away on holiday or to visit his friends. Little or no adaptation of the home is required as this equipment does not even need a running water supply, using only 5 litres of water at the start of treatment. In this equipment, urea is removed by treatment with urease and subsequent absorption of the ammonia thus produced by sodium zirconium phosphate. Unfortunately this system still has certain drawbacks. Firstly, the adsorbent cartridges are expensive and the cost of dialysis is nearly doubled. Secondly, because of the ion exchange for ammonia the sodium concentration tends to rise during dialysis and control of acidosis is more difficult because of the adsorption of bicarbonate or acetate. Nevertheless this type of equipment has been used for long periods for home dialysis and has a particular relevance for patients whose homes would require elaborate adaptation, who have limited space or who are likely to be transplanted within a relatively short space of time. Portability and simplicity of this equipment makes it popular for home dialysis patients and their families when it comes to taking holidays.

Water preparation

It would be inappropriate to talk about the supply of dialysate in the home without a brief discussion of the subject of water preparation. Whereas some domestic water supplies can be used virtually untreated to prepare dialysate, in hard water areas the removal of calcium and magnesium is mandatory. This is most conveniently done by the use of cation exchange water softeners of the type used domestically for many other purposes. The patients need to be trained not only to use the equipment but to check the need for regeneration. Failure to regenerate the softener may result in the 'hard water' syndrome[13]. With water softener failure and a rising dialysate calcium the patient develops over a few days or weeks nausea, vomiting and constipation, with a rise in blood pressure and sometimes muscle weakness. The syndrome is usually rapidly reversed by correcting dialysate composition, but if the patient's serum potassium has been unduly lowered by dialysis against low or zero potassium dialysate, cardiac arrest may occur. Ectopic calcification is another hazard of the induced hypercalcaemia.

Concern about the significance of other contaminants or ions in tap water has led to concern about the need for more adequate water treatment. Copper piping in water supply systems can lead to copper intoxication in chronic dialysis patients and in recent years the evidence that aluminium in dialysate may produce dialysis dementia and a type of dialysis bone disease has become very strong indeed[14,15]. Fluoride is added to many domestic water supplies and is undoubtedly taken up by the bones of patients on regular dialysis treatment, although it is not yet clear how important this is in bone pathology. Concern about these and other ions present in tap water has prompted the use of deionization systems or reverse osmosis for water preparation. These put up the cost and complexity of home dialysis equipment and preparation but may prove to be wise precautions, particularly where there are potentially hazardous impurities in the water. Finally, in addition to the chemical constituents, we have had problems with domestic water supplies in terms of particulate matter which has tended to clog the fine filters in most proportioning systems. To counter this we have often found it necessary to install some type of coarse filter in the water supply line. In most cities, and even in country areas, where dialysis is practised, bacterial contamination of the water supply is not a serious problem, although it should not be neglected. More serious has been the gradual growth of water-loving organisms such as *Pseudomonas* and *Serratia* in water softeners. Thorough cleaning and regular flushing of equipment is recommended, but once these organisms have contaminated the resin bed they may be very difficult to eliminate.

Monitoring dialysis at home

Monitoring of dialysis aims at ensuring that dialysis is proceeding under optimal conditions and at warning the patient or his supervisors of a possible hazard. It was the fact that dialysis could be fairly simply and safely monitored that made unsupervised home dialysis possible. Grimsrud et al.[16] have discussed the desirable features of dialysis monitors. The monitors for home dialysis should give clear and easily understood warning of malfunctions and should be designed to fail in an alarm condition should they go wrong.

Table 3 summarizes those aspects of haemodialysis which can be usefully monitored at home. There is, of course, a variation in the requirement between an unattended home dialysis and a supervised dialysis, and between short dialysis taking place during waking hours compared with overnight dialysis, while, it is hoped, the patient and relatives are asleep. The two functions which it is most essential to monitor at home are the temperature of the dialysate being delivered to the dialyser and the pressure in the line returning blood to the patient from the dialyser, usually monitored at the bubble trap. Variation in the pressure at the latter site will follow obstruction in the blood pathway due to kinking of the tubing by movement or to clotting and will pick up major leaks through the dialyser, or accumulations of air in the line. If the dialyser is being perfused from an arterial cannula without the use of a blood pump the venous pressure monitor will also detect falls in arterial pressure with disconnections in the inflow line to the dialyser. When a peristaltic pump is used to propel blood into the dialyser, as is inevitable with an arteriovenous fistula, variations off low proximal to the pump will only slowly be picked up by the venous pressure monitor. Some form of monitor on this part of the system is desirable, because if the flow of blood from the patient is inadequate to prevent the development of a negative pressure as a result of pump action, air could be drawn into the circuit and then pushed through the dialyser under pressure. It is therefore usual to have an additional monitor on the inflow side of the dialyser. The simplest device is the use of an expanded segment in the line which can be inserted into a microswitch alarm and which has sufficiently thin walls to collapse when the pressure in the line becomes negative. This type of monitor, affectionately known in dialysis centres as the 'mousetrap', suffers from a defect in that it is easily left out of the circuit by the patient when he is being troubled by excessive alarms due to poor blood flow. An alternative device is an arterial pressure monitor connection to a bubble trap, similar to that in the return line. This increases the complexity of setting up dialysis, but some centres prefer to monitor the blood line pressure at this point rather than at the venous return bubble trap, although we believe this has disadvantages.

Table 3 Desirable monitors for home dialysis

Essential
Pressure in venous return line
Dialysate temperature
Dialysate composition (conductivity)
Transmembrane pressure (or venous line + dialysate negative pressure)
Electricity and water supply failure

Desirable
Fall in arterial flow to pump
Blood-to-dialysate leak
Air in venous bubble trap

When dialysate is prepared continuously during dialysis, preferably even if it is being premixed, it is necessary to ensure that dialysate composition is within safe limits, which is best checked by measuring electrical conductivity, since sodium chloride is the major component.

If the patient is to understand and control ultrafiltration he needs some assessment of transmembrane pressure. This can either be provided by a monitor which gives a direct assessment of transmembrane pressure or by explaining to the patient the significance of the venous bubble trap pressure and the negative pressure produced by the dialysate circuit pump on the outflow system. The monitoring arrangement depends to some extent on the type of dialyser used, since with a coil dialyser, for example, a dialysate negative pressure is only meaningful with a closed system. Some types of machine do have an ultrafiltration measure by which the patient can get a direct assessment of the rate of fluid loss. A simple method of assessing ultrafiltration is, of course, to provide the patient with bedside scales which he can step on to during dialysis, or a luxury alternative would be some form of weighbed which we no longer regard as essential for home dialysis, except perhaps for children.

The risk of air embolism exists despite one's precautions and one example we mentioned earlier was from the diffusion of gas across the membrane when dialysate de-gassing has been inadequate. Patients can certainly be very worried about this risk, particularly when they are trying to sleep during dialysis. There are now relatively reliable monitors of the blood level in the venous bubble trap which will distinguish between blood and froth, and these will ensure additional safety at a price. Most patients feel happier if they have some form of blood-to-dialysate leak monitor. These are photo-electric devices and are liable to give false alarms, particularly from air bubbles, so that some type of time delay device is desirable.

For those types of monitor equipped with a high or low level of alarm setting, such as the blood line pressure or dialysate negative pressure, it is desirable that the patient cannot set these outside the safe limits or widen the difference between the two values beyond safe limits. In our early years of home dialysis at least one of our patients was liable to set his venous pressure alarm limits very wide apart so that he would not be woken if he turned over in his sleep and caused a change in pressure in the venous return line. Despite our warnings about the risks involved he did not mend his ways until a disconnection of the line nearly led to his exsanguination before the alarm sounded, but fortunately his wife came to check on him just in time. Likewise, although it is desirable to have an alarm silence to allow the patient to survey and correct the situation without being too flustered, it is necessary for the alarm to sound again if the fault is not corrected, otherwise the patient may ignore a fault and fail to correct it. Finally, alarms should be provided to give warning of failure of electricity or water supplies.

Pumps and lines

Several types of peristaltic pump are available for use in haemodialysis. Although there are many variations in the extent to which these cause damage to blood components it is doubtful whether the mild haemolysis thus caused is significant. The important consideration for home dialysis is that the pump is easily set up, that the patients and relatives are not likely to trap their fingers in the mechanism and that it is electrically safe and that occlusion of the line is adequate but not excessive. A quiet and reliable pump is obviously desirable. That the choice of blood lines is as much a subject of emotion as of common sense is shown by the extremely wide variation manufactured by the same as well as by different companies. For home dialysis simple lines with few or no inserts are preferable. We believe it is easier if priming and wash-back can be performed through the proximal end of the tube rather than through a separate insert. One does not usually undertake blood transfusion at home so no special infusion insert is necessary. Heparin can either be metered into the venous bubble trap or we believe it to be simpler to have a narrow bore side arm for this purpose. Dialyser inflow or arterial lines for use in home dialysis with a blood pump should not have any insert between the blood vessel and the blood pump. If this precaution is neglected it is always possible that the action of the pump could draw air in through the side arm, should any leak or disconnection occur.

Heparin is most conveniently given in home dialysis by the use of a syringe pump. The desirable dose of heparin for the patient should be estimated before the patient is established on home dialysis and he should be trained so that he automatically switches on his heparin pump at the start of dialysis rather than when the dialyser has clotted 1 hour later, and routinely checks the setting up and operation of the pump.

The choice of dialysate proportioning pump and of pumps used to draw dialysate through the dialyser depends upon the equipment to be chosen. These pumps should be electrically safe, should not be prone to leaks, should have a long life and be easily serviced, although not easily adjusted by patients who might thereby endanger themselves.

Adaptation of the home

The alteration of the patient's home for dialysis is obviously dependent upon facilities available and the type of equipment which is to be used, as well as the finance available for the purpose. We have recommended a minimum floor area of 8–9 m². With dialysate regeneration and the use of a small dialyser even this space could be reduced. It is desirable that the patient does not have to live with his equipment when he is not on dialysis, so the dialysis room should either be in a spare bedroom or should at least be screened off when not in use. The reasons for this isolation are as much psychological as hygienic.

Most home adaptations require some electrical rewiring to provide an adequate and reliable supply and outlet, usually of the type provided for electric cookers. Most dialysate proportioning machines require a minimum working head of water pressure of 5 lb per square inch or more. If other demands are made upon the water supply during the operation of the equipment it may cause undesirable fluctuations and we have suggested a head of water pressure close to 20 lb per square inch. Static water tanks should either be avoided or carefully covered because of the risk of contamination. The need for filtration of the water and water preparation has been dealt with in an earlier section. Drainage must be adequate to take the flow rate from single pass equipment. The type of drainage and its positioning is dependent upon the presence and type of a dialysate effluent pump. Plumbing of home dialysis installations must be of a high quality. We have had several disastrous floods which have been both costly and psychologically traumatic to the family. Leakages of brine from water softeners or dialysate are particularly damaging. We have made it our practice to provide water-proof floor covering. The floors must be strong enough to take the weight of the equipment which may exceed 200 kg. If not already present a telephone is installed so that the patient can contact the centre or his medical adviser in the event of dialysis mishaps.

It has sometimes proved easier to install the home dialysis unit outside the house in a small prefabricated building. In theory this might seem a good idea for a patient who is anticipating a renal transplant because the building could be removed and re-assembled elsewhere. In practice we have found that the provision of services for installation of such a cabin is as costly as most alterations inside the home.

Many of the problems of adaptation for the home are of an economic, social or psychological nature. Even if the patient is happy to accept alterations to his home for life-saving treatment – which is not always the case – it may cause a good deal of stress to the rest of the family, particularly if they are houseproud. Home adaptations can be expensive and problems may arise as to where the finance is to be found. In the United Kingdom the home adaptation is now financed from the National Health Service so that the patient is relieved of this burden, but, unfortunately, bureaucratic delays are by no means uncommon, particularly in areas where few home dialysis patients have been installed before. It is in looking at adaptation of the home and at the increasing cost of these modifications that one realizes how important it is that we should design compact portable equipment which can be used with little or no building or service alterations.

SELECTION OF PATIENTS FOR HOME DIALYSIS

If the goal is to achieve for our patients independence of the hospital centre, the design of equipment and the training of patients should be adaptable for use by all but the most disabled, or intellectually or emotionally disadvantaged patients. To have to select only those patients considered 'suitable' is an admission of our failure to design anything like ideal haemodialysis equipment. In practice there must be few if any centres running home dialysis programmes which do not practise some form of patient selection. This selection is made along a variety of lines and is influenced by the availability of alternative treatment. Thus the presence of nearby centre dialysis facilities or self-care hospital facilities would make home dialysis less attractive for the patient than for one who lived many miles from any dialysis facility. For the patient expecting or hoping for an early renal transplant, the time and expense of home dialysis training and installation would scarcely be worthwhile and psychologically we have found such patients less amenable to home training. Other considerations in patient selection are relative and as much influenced by the practice of the centre, the type of equipment and the attitude of the patient, family and physician as by medical reasons. If home dialysis is to be successful frequent return to the dialysis centre or home visits by medical, nursing or technical staff are to be avoided. Selection will therefore tend to favour patients who are or who expect to be stable on dialysis and unlikely to experience major medical complications. Whilst we have successfully maintained patients at home with past histories of depressive illnesses or episodes of anxiety or obsessional behaviour, severe psychotic disorders are a clear barrier to home treatment. The intelligence and educational level of the patient probably influenced selection more in the early days of home dialysis than now. Although an independent survey of our patients' intelligent quotients showed good correlation with the renal unit staff's assessment of how well they had coped with home dialysis, personality traits are probably a more important influence. If the patient can cope or seems likely to be able to cope with ordinary daily mechanical tasks, such as driving a car or using a washing machine, he or she should be able to manage home dialysis. Familiarity with the machines of modern life makes acceptance of the training for home dialysis easier, but education has only a minor influence and illiterate, deaf and dumb, as well as blind patients, have coped with home dialysis, albeit the latter requiring some assistance.

Severe degrees of anxiety, over-dependence and excessive independence are traits which may make home dialysis very difficult, whereas mild obsessional tendencies are probably an advantage. Social circumstances and family background are important influences. It is obvious that home dialysis is not possible if the patient does not have a home and it is always desirable, though not always possible, that there is sufficient space for the patient to be able to arrange that the equipment does not intrude upon his life between dialyses. Patients can be trained to run the dialyses even though they live alone, although with most types of equipment we do not consider solitary dialysis desirable because of the slight risk of a mishap, such as a fit or faint, which may incapacitate the patient during the course of a dialysis. On the other hand, whilst it is desirable that a relative or friend is present in the home during dialysis, and they usually help at least with starting dialysis, a sense of dependence on this relative may bring a host of problems and we prefer to train the patient to run his own dialysis either unaided or with a relative or friend acting as relatively unskilled assistance. An exception to this may be the need for the assistant to puncture an arteriovenous fistula, and for all except the older children one would expect the parents to set up and supervise the dialysis. Children have in fact adapted very well to home dialysis and it is likely to produce less disruption to their lives and to schooling than regular trips to the hospital.

TRAINING FOR HOME DIALYSIS

A well-planned training programme is the essence of a successful home dialysis. Whatever equipment is selected, the patient needs to have a simple but clear and adequate understanding of the nature and aims of regular dialysis treatment, including fluid balance, familiarity with the operation of his equipment, simple fault finding and correction and a knowledge of the potential hazards to be avoided or coped with. Training may either be undertaken in the main hospital centre, in a separate training area in that centre or in a training area out of the hospital environment altogether or even at home. Each of these sites has advantages. The best and quickest results are probably achieved when the patients start their training in the hospital centre from their first dialysis and when they can join together in groups so that the atmosphere of mutual help as well as of competition for success can be developed.

Attitude to training

The attitude of the patient to training is a very important determinant of success – more so than the intelligence level. For this reason the psychological approach to the patient and the relationship between patient and staff is important. The overdependent patient or the one who reacts to his illness with aggression or denial is difficult to train and tends to engender hostile reactions in the staff. Apart from these psychological traits the problem of retention and recall often arises in training uraemic patients. Loss of the powers of mental concentration is a feature of chronic uraemia and we have found it particularly a problem in patients who have had long periods of symptomatic uraemia and protein restriction before coming on to dialysis. These patients can be taught the same simple task over and over again and still make errors of recall which seem incompatible with their premorbid attainments. These patients require a great deal of patience on the part of the training staff, but this disability is not usually permanent unless compounded by co-existing cerebral vascular disease, as in the more elderly patients or those with a long history of hypertension. This difficulty provides one more argument for starting training and regular dialysis earlier rather than later in the course of the uraemic illness.

The attitudes of the staff to training are also very important. Training staff need to be fully conversant with the reactions of patients to the illness and need to be able to cope without either hostility or disproportionate sympathy. Some staff have a flair for training patients, some are never able to explain ideas or techniques to patients without muddling them, however hard they try. Most staff can train patients for home dialysis but first need training themselves. The trainers need to be able to hold back and let the patients set up and run equipment, even if they make mistakes, as long as they are not dangerous ones. Holding back and letting the sick patient try to cope with his problems does not come naturally to many nurses and they need to be appropriately indoctrinated and be able to give gentle but firm encouragement, interfering only when necessary.

Programme of training

Practical training should begin with the patient's very first dialysis, but many patients may have been able to start a training programme before they need to start haemodialysis. In this introductory stage they should meet and establish good relationships with the staff and have an opportunity to discuss home dialysis with patients and relatives already familiar with it. The patient should be given a simple introduction and background to the problems of renal failure and its treatment, including diet. This part of the training can be undertaken in small groups, given in the form of programmed learning or by a slide demonstration. Practical training should begin with the mastery of the simpler aspects, such as the interpretation of monitors and the setting up and the priming of the dialyser.

As the patient progresses it is wise to have a check-list to ensure that he has been taught and become proficient at the various procedures, including as many alarm situations as occur or can safely be simulated.

The time taken to train a patient for home haemodialysis depends upon the health and aptitude of the patient, his motivation and type of equipment. Our personal record is just over 2 weeks. An average time is 6 to 8 weeks, although training to needle the fistula may take much longer.

ORGANIZATION OF HOME DIALYSIS

As with any of the more complex forms of medical treatment, the success of home dialysis is directly related to the enthusiasm and the attention to detail with which it is applied. These are more important than the actual way the programme is organized, which must depend upon local, regional and national circumstances and the availability of alternative therapies. Home dialysis can proceed successfully remote from the training centre – even in another continent. The remote patient must receive a thorough training, equipment must be chosen to suit his home circumstances and a local physician and technician enlisted to deal with any problems once the patient is home. These latter individuals may be able to attend the dialysis centre for indoctrination, but it is more likely that they will have to receive their indoctrination in the form of a manual prepared by the training centre. Such a manual for the patient's regular medical attendant is a desirable part of programme organization, even for patients near the centre, although in the latter situation technicians are likely to be part of the renal unit staff, or working regularly for the unit. Even more important is the provision for the patient of a manual to reinforce training and to act as an aide memoire to dialysis, diet, drug therapy, etc.

Table 4 Personnel in a home dialysis programme

Staff	Role
In centre	
Centre medical staff	Overall responsibility Selection and background training Medical supervision and follow-up
Centre nurse	Training and supervision of dialysis
Dietician	Advises patient and family; follow-up advice on diet
Social worker	Identifies and anticipates problems and needs
Administrator	Organizes home adaptation and finance Later organizes supplies to home
Plus supporting staff (laboratory, clerical, diet kitchens, etc.)	
At home	
Family physician	Available if needed Routine follow-up (e.g. blood pressure checks, biochemistry)
Home dialysis nurse	May supervise first dialysis Visits for support, supervision and advice
Technician	Services machine, repairs and preventive maintenance
Social worker	As above

Very remote home dialysis is most often applied to patients in developing countries, where local resources are few or non-existent, or to patients in very remote, sparsely populated areas. These patients are either very privileged or very independent or both. For most home dialysis programmes the distances may be considerable, but contact with and travel to the parent centre is relatively easy. In the United Kingdom, where home dialysis is a popular approach to the treatment of end-stage renal failure, most programmes are now based on a regional centre dealing with patients within a radius of 200 miles or less. Such a programme can be integrated with the centre dialysis and renal transplant service and the most appropriate therapy selected for each patient[17]. With a regionally-based programme it is possible for the main centre to give the patients more support with social and medical problems, including vascular access problems and longterm complications such as bone disease. The home adaptation can be supervised by the centre to conform more closely with the standards and layout known to give the best results, and a nurse or technician based on the hospital centre can be present for the initial dialysis to ensure that the equipment is functioning and the patient can cope in the home setting. Such initial visits are not essential but have been valuable in giving the patient confidence and forestalling later problems. Later, the home dialysis nurse can visit the patients at home to reinforce training, to ensure that safe standards are being maintained and often to anticipate social, domestic or psychological problems before they become severe.

Involvement of the patients' family physician can reduce the demands on the hospital centre, but periodic follow-up visits by the patient to the centre are desirable to check the patient's progress and anticipate or deal with any special problems, such as osteodystrophy. Such visits, which usually need not be more often than once every 2 or 3 months, or longer, should aim to give the patient the feeling that he is not alone with his problems, yet help rather than hinder his relative independence of hospital support.

The potential staff and their respective roles in a large home dialysis programme are summarized in Table 4. A team of this size, involving also the primary care health workers and welfare organizations when necessary, can maintain a programme of more than 100 patients on home dialysis.

One of the drawbacks of home dialysis is the restriction on the patient and family for travel and vacation. Patients can often dialyse in other centres by special arrangement or in special dialysis vacation centres which have opened in recent years. The risk of contracting hepatitis by such contacts has tended to restrict this practice, although the availability of sensitive hepatitis antigen tests has allowed a little more freedom. Nevertheless, it has been UK policy to restrict 'itinerant' dialysis for this reason. Several large centres have arranged vacation facilities for their home dialysis patients, who can travel to a vacation area and use the same type of equipment as they do at home. The development of adsorbent regeneration of dialysate (see above) or the use of 'suitcase equipment' for short dialyses has given the patient the opportunity to travel more freely with this portable equipment, if he can find hotels, camping sites or friends who will allow him to visit and dialyse.

Relatives may be able to take a vacation if the patient temporarily returns to the centre. The need for periodical returns to hospital for this reason or for medical complications, particularly access site problems or occasional blood transfusions, requires available 'back-up' hospital beds to support the home programme. How many beds are required depends upon facilities elsewhere and the type of patient treated at home. Our experience with a regional service training relatively unselected patients to go home suggests that one may need one bed available for every ten patients at home. Very often these beds will not be used at all, but problems have a nasty habit of coming all at the same time so one may find several patients requiring access site surgery, treatment for pneumonia or septicaemia and for unrelated medical problems requiring admission in the same week.

THE RESULTS OF HOME DIALYSIS

Haemodialysis is a potentially hazardous procedure, but any doubts about the wisdom of home dialysis have been dispelled by its outstanding success. The survival rate of patients on home haemodialysis exceeds that of all other methods of treating end-stage renal failure. The European Dialysis and Transplant Registry statistics[18] show a survival rate of 74% at 5 years. Only live related donor transplants give comparable figures and survival rates after more than 5 years for this latter group do actually appear to be better than for dialysis. Survival of home dialysis patients is, not unexpectedly, better for the younger age groups than for patients over 55. These figures are influenced by selection, but it is doubtful whether this is the whole explanation.

Rehabilitation figures are also very impressive for home dialysis patients[18], although successful transplantation has an undoubted advantage in terms of patient well-being and rehabilitation. This is at least in part explained by the anaemia of dialysis patients and the lethargy which may follow dialysis.

Major disasters on home dialysis are fortunately rare. In over 50 000 home dialyses on our programme major mishaps have been very rare. A physician has only been called to give assistance on four occasions. One of these was due to bleeding from a duodenal ulcer as a result of heparinization. One patient had a fatal cardiac arrest on dialysis which remained unexplained, although he had extensive occlusive coronary atheroma. Other problems have occurred in this group of patients on or off dialysis but have usually been dealt with over the telephone or by the patient visiting his physician or the hospital centre straight away or after an interval, as appropriate. Emergency calls because of technical problems are more frequent. Some of these are false alarms, particularly in the first few weeks of home dialysis if the patient lacks confidence. Some patients telephone with imagined problems several times daily at first, yet after a few weeks one ceases to hear from them for months on end. It is important to give the patient support through this stage and either a visit by the home dialysis nurse or recall to the training centre may be necessary. More remote patients tend to be much more independent and self-reliant.

The frequency of genuine technical problems depends upon the type of equipment and the adequacy of back-up servicing rather than upon mistakes by the patient. In a regional programme about 50% of these problems can be solved by discussion over the telephone with the technical staff during dialysis. For most of the remainder the dialysis has to be discontinued and a visit made by the technician the next day. Only rarely is it necessary to return the patient to hospital for dialysis pending a major overhaul of the installation. Problems with dialyser membrane rupture and with conductivity metering are now rare, and pump or electrical faults are the main problems. With the use of well-tried and well-designed equipment these problems diminish.

The number of patients who have to return permanently to hospital centre dialysis are few, but this depends upon the selection of patients. We have had five patients out of 150 who have to be assimilated back into the hospital unit. Two of these were for cerebral vascular disease, in one a complete hemiplegia. One patient had continual access site problems. In only two has readmission to hospital been necessary for social and psychological reasons. In a much larger series[19] the reasons were domestic in 65 out of 140 and medical in 32, of which problems with vascular access were responsible in 13.

Most of the medical complications to which the regular dialysis patient is prone occur also in the home dialysis patient. Thus renal osteodystrophy and occlusive vascular disease occur in both groups. Infective complications are fewer in the well-trained home patient probably because of the reduced cross-infection risk.

The well-trained, well-motivated patient seems to have fewer problems and complications than the hospital patient, and those who have carefully adhered to the dialysis regime and dieting and fluid restrictions look impressively fitter after several years of RDT. But even carefully selected dialysis patients do not always behave as one would wish and may come to resent or ignore dietary and fluid restrictions, wash-back or re-use instructions, or not uncommonly 'cheat' on dialysis times. Patients may become impatient or uncomfortable after several hours and begin to curtail their dialyses. Not uncommonly they deny, even to themselves, that they are doing this. The underdialysis syndrome, with severe anaemia, pericarditis, chronic fluid overload, or even neuropathy, may then supervene. Another cause of this syndrome in home dialysis patients is an inadequate shunt or fistula. This may result in poor blood flow rates unrecognized by the patient and thus poor clearances by the dialyser.

A particular problem of home dialysis is the disruption caused by performing dialysis in the domestic environment. Our early enthusiasm about the success of home dialysis led us to focus upon the well-adjusted patients to whom home dialysis was 'little more trouble than turning on the television' (to paraphrase one of our patients – a successful farmer). The family gathered round these patients and relationships sometimes actually become closer, especially in families with dependent children. But this ignores that sizeable minority of patients to whom the chore of regular preparation for dialysis and the hours spent 'on the machine' become a nightmare. The stresses then spread to involve and disrupt the family. Marriages, already insecure, may break up or be held together only by guilty feelings about deserting the sick partner. Resentments develop, even in close relationships, with resulting ambivalence in attitude to the patient.

To avoid these problems it has usually been recommended that one trains the patient to be responsible for his own dialysis. We were interested to find from an independent survey of the pattern, once our married patients were established at home, that the dialysis was managed by the previously dominant partner, whether this was the patient or the spouse. The involvement of the family was shown in a survey on sleep patterns in overnight dialysis. On dialysis nights the patient usually achieved more sleep than relatives in the same house, even if these relatives were not in the dialysis room.

THE PRESENT AND FUTURE OF HOME HAEMODIALYSIS

Home haemodialysis was introduced as a means of lowering the cost and increasing the availability of dialysis. It is difficult to cost medical treatment accurately, and in these inflationary times actual cost figures would not remain meaningful. Home haemodialysis is probably three-fifths the cost of hospital dialysis per annum and twice the cost of a successful transplant. Transplant failures, however, are very expensive. Home peritoneal dialysis is discussed elsewhere (see Chapter 3). The problems and costs are similar in many ways. The introduction of chronic ambulatory peritoneal dialysis, however, may alter our approach to home dialysis. This technique is quickly learnt and does not require elaborate preparations nor costly equipment and adaptations. If the main problems, particularly peritonitis, are solved, we may have to reconsider our enthusiasm for home haemodialysis for any patient with an intact peritoneal cavity.

Enthusiasm for home dialysis has varied. In the UK it has been popular because centre dialysis facilities have been limited – indeed the very success of home dialysis may have been a factor in this limitation by reducing demand. The nature of housing in the UK and the availability of state and welfare support has favoured this development. In other countries housing patterns or financial disincentives or disadvantages to home as opposed to centre dialysis have been a factor in discouraging this development. An alternative approach has been the self-care or satellite centre. The latter is near the patient's home, and after initial training in the patient centre or in a separate part of the unit, the patient conducts his own dialysis as though he were at home, with minimum supervision. These units differ in the extent to which preparation and cleaning up is left to the patient, but there is no doubt that for many individuals this approach is a very satisfactory compromise.

Because of the excellent results of home dialysis and the 'capital investment', physicians have often been reluctant to recommend these patients for transplantation. At one time we found unsuccessful transplantation to be the largest single cause of death in our home dialysis programme[20] even though the transplant unit was obtaining average or better than average survival results. However, all but a few home dialysis patients look forward to the day when they will have a functioning graft. With the more cautious immunosuppressive regimes adopted in the last few years, preliminary blood transfusions and tissue matching, there is no doubt that the best results can be achieved by an integrated home dialysis and transplant programme[17]. The patient is in good health before his transplant and can await a suitable cadaver graft from a national matching programme. Subsequently, if the graft is rejecting he can readily return to dialysis and there is less temptation to use excessive or prolonged immunosuppression in the faint hope of preserving a failing graft.

The future of home haemodialysis must depend upon the relative success of transplantation and continuous ambulatory peritoneal dialysis. The design of satisfactory portable or wearable equipment with reduced preparation time will continue to make home dialysis a satisfactory approach to end-stage renal disease, and, for those with immunological or anatomical barriers to transplantation, the definitive treatment.

References

1 Merrill, J. P., Schupak, E., Cameron, E. and Hampers, C. L. (1964). Hemodialysis in the home. *J. Am. Med. Assoc.*, **190**, 468–470

2 Baillod, R. A., Comty, C., Ilahi, M., Konotey-Ahulu, F. I. D., Seviett, L. and Shaldon, S. (1966). Overnight haemodialysis in the home. *Proc. Eur. Dial. Transplant Assoc.*, **2**, 99–104

3 Eschbach, J. W., Barrett, B. M. S., Daly, S., Cole, J. J. and Scribner, B. H. (1967). Hemodialysis in the home. *Ann. Intern. Med.*, **67**, 1149–1162

4 Quinton, W. E., Dillard, D. H., Cole, J. J. and Scribner, B. H. (1962). Eight months' experience with Silastic–Teflon bypass cannulas. *Trans. Ann. Soc. Artif. Intern. Organs*, **8**, 236–242

5 Brescia, M. J., Cimino, J. E., Appel, K. and Hurwich, B. J. (1966). Chronic haemodialysis using venepuncture and surgically created arteriovenous fistula. *N. Engl. J. Med.*, **275**, 1089–1092

6 Robinson, B. H. B. (1971). Intermittent haemodialysis in the home. *Br. Med. Bull.*, **27**, 173–180

7 Rowley, R. T., Sterioff, S. and Williams, G. M. (1976). Arteriovenous fistulas for dialysis using modified bovine arteries. *Surg. Gynecol. Obstet.*, **152**, 700–703

8 Baker Jr, L. D., Johnson, J. M. and Goldfarb, D. (1976). Expanded polytetrafluoroethylene (PTFE) subcutaneous arteriovenous conduit: an improved vascular access for chronic hemodialysis. *Trans. Am. Soc. Artif. Intern. Organs*, **22**, 382–387

9 Kopp, K. F., Gutch, C. F. and Kolff, W. J. (1972). Single needle dialysis. *Trans. Am. Soc. Artif. Intern. Organs*, **18**, 75–78

10 Whelpton, D. (1978). National and international electrical safety requirements in dialysis. In Frost, J. (ed.) *Technical Aspects of Renal Dialysis*, pp. 235–241. (Tunbridge Wells: Pitman Medical)

11 Dobbie, A. K. (1973). Patient monitoring equipment: problems of interference and electrical safety. *Proc. R. Soc. Med.*, **66**, 981–982.

12 Wing, A. J., Brunner, F. P., Brynger, H., Chantler, C., Donckerwolcke, R. A., Gurland, H. J., Jacobs, C. and Selwood, N. H. (1978). Mortality and morbidity of re-using dialysers. *Br. Med. J.*, **2**, 1853–1855

13 Freeman, R. M., Lawton, R. L. and Chamberlain, M. A. (1967). Hard-water syndrome. *N. Engl. J. Med.*, **276**, 1113–1118

14 Allfrey, A. C., LeGendre, G. R. and Kaehny, W. D. (1976). The dialysis encephalopathy syndrome: possible aluminium intoxication. *N. Engl. J. Med.*, **294**, 184–188

15 Flendrig, J. A., Kruis, H. and Das, H. A. (1976). Aluminium intoxication: the cause of dialysis dementia? *Proc. Eur. Dial. Transplant. Assoc.*, **13**, 355–361

16 Grimsrud, L., Cole, J. J., Eschbach, J. W., Babb, A. L. and Scribner, B. H. (1967). Safety aspects of hemodialysis. *Trans. Am. Soc. Artif. Intern. Organs*, **13**, 1–4

17 Oliver, D. O. and Morris, P. J. (1978). The organisation of results of an integrated home dialysis and transplant service. In Davidson (ed.), *Dialysis Review*, pp. 32–39. (Tunbridge Wells: Pitman Medical)

18 Brynger, H., Brunner, F. P., Chantler, C., Donckerwolcke, R. A., Jacobs, C., Kramer, P., Selwood, N. H. and Wing, A. J. (1980). Combined report on regular dialysis and transplantation in Europe. X. 1979. *Proc. Eur. Dial. Transplant. Assoc.*, **17**, 4–84

19 Wing, A. J., Brunner, F. P., Brynger, H., Chantler, C., Donckerwolcke, R. A., Gurland, H. J., Hathway, R. A., Jacobs, C. and Selwood, N. H. (1978). Combined report on regular dialysis and transplantation in Europe. VIII. 1977. *Proc. Eur. Dial. Transplant. Assoc.*, **15**, 4–76

20 Naik, R. B., Barnes, A. D., Hawkins, J. B., Little, G., Mahood, C. B. and Robinson, B. H. B. (1976). The effect of renal transplantation on a home dialysis programme. *Proc. Eur. Dial. Transplant. Assoc.*, **13**, 143–150

7

Immunogenetics of tissue grafting

F. H. Bach

One of the major factors, which is clearly important in determining the fate of an allograft, is the degree of compatibility between donor and recipient at the major histocompatibility complex (MHC). In man, the MHC is referred to as HLA. It has been known for more than a decade that siblings who inherit the same HLA haplotypes from their parents, and are thus genotypically identical for HLA, are close to ideal in the very great majority of cases for donating or receiving a kidney from each other. Long-term graft survival in such instances is approximately 90%. Any degree of disparity for HLA, such as that found in siblings sharing one HLA haplotype but differing by the second, is associated with significantly decreased graft survival. The overwhelming import of matching donor and recipient for HLA is thus clearly established.

The biological basis which accounts for the importance of HLA matching is presumably that HLA genes code for cell surface antigens that are recognized as histocompatibility (H) antigens and which in turn incite a rejection response in the recipient. It is the genes of the MHC which are thought to code for the strongest H antigens; the biological basis of this great 'strength' will be discussed later. Although it is clear that matching for the entire genetic segment that constitutes the MHC is of great importance, it is still not clear which of the antigens encoded by MHC genes are most important in terms of matching. Indeed, it is still not known whether the antigens of greatest importance have yet been defined.

The major approaches used for detection of MHC-encoded antigens involve serological methods. There are some serologically detected determinants that are recognized on essentially all cells of the body and others that have an apparently more restricted tissue distribution[1-3]. In addition, there are cellular methods, studying activation of T lymphocytes in mixed leukocyte culture (MLC), that can be used to define MHC encoded determinants. Here, also, determinants can be divided into two categories, including those that activate much of the proliferative response in a primary MLC in which the donors of the responding and stimulating cells differ by an entire MHC, and those that are recognized by cytotoxic T lymphocytes[4].

There is substantial evidence to suggest that determinants recognized serologically and those recognized by T lymphocytes are not identical. Conceptually, therefore, we must deal with two methods of detection, serological and cellular, with two different 'types' of antigens recognized by

Table 1   HLA – detection of antigens

Method	Region(s)	
	ABC	D
Serological	SD	DR (Ia-like)
Cellular	CD	LD

each of the methods. In order to have a uniform nomenclature that allows us to refer to these various types of determinants in any species, the designations given in Table 1 have been used. These differentiate between the serologically defined antigens found ubiquitously on essentially all cell surfaces, referred to as the S determinant (SD) antigens, and the serologically detected antigens with a much more limited tissue distribution, encoded by HLA-D related (DR) genes. The antigens detected by T lymphocyte reactivities are referred to as L determinants (LD) and C determinants (CD) as listed.

HLA – THE MAJOR HISTOCOMPATIBILITY COMPLEX IN MAN

Presented in Figure 1 is a schematic representation of the HLA complex. In man, as in mouse, serological and cellular methods have been used for the definition of the various antigens and molecules encoded by HLA genes. The HLA-A, -B and -C loci code for antigens that are present on essentially all cells of the body and that show sequence homology with the H-2K/D antigens. The HLA-D locus was first defined using cellular techniques, i.e. proliferation in a primary MLC; thus, the antigens associated with HLA-D that can be detected by serological methods have been referred to as the DR (D-related) antigens. The DR antigens are thought to be homologues of Ia antigens in the mouse.

Presented in Table 2 are the currently recognized antigens of HLA, as detected both by serological methods and by the primary mixed leukocyte culture response to homozygous typing cells (HTCs)[3]. As noted, the HLA-A and -B loci are very markedly polymorphic with a continuing finer definition of determinants that can be recognized by different sera. The HLA-C locus does not appear to be as polymorphic as HLA-A and -B.

HLA

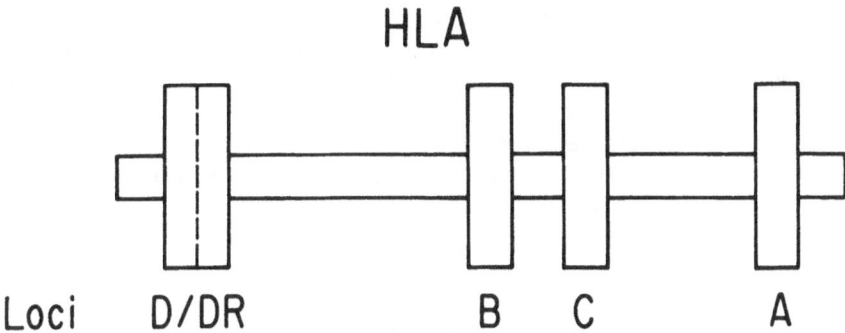

Figure 1 A schematic representation of the HLA complex. See text for discussion

The HLA-D locus is formally defined by response in a primary mixed leukocyte culture to HTCs. The HTC technique[5] involves the use of stimulating cells that are homozygous for HLA-D antigen(s). The rationale behind HTC testing is that, if one given individual does not carry the antigen(s) present on the HTC, there should be a strong response by the cells of that individual to that particular HTC. If, on the other hand, a

Table 2 Recognized HLA-A, -B, -C, -D and -DR specificities

HLA-A		HLA-B	HLA-C	HLA-D	HLA-DR
HLA-A1	HLA-B5	HLA-Bw46	HLA-Cw1	HLA-Dw1	HLA-DR1
HLA-A2	HLA-B7	HLA-Bw47	HLA-Cw2	HLA-Dw2	HLA-DR2
HLA-A3	HLA-B8	HLA-Bw48	HLA-Cw3	HLA-Dw3	HLA-DR3
HLA-A9	HLA-B12	HLA-Bw49(w21)	HLA-Cw4	HLA-Dw4	HLA-DR4
HLA-A10	HLA-B13	HLA-Bw50(w21)	HLA-Cw5	HLA-Dw5	HLA-DR5
HLA-A11	HLA-B14	HLA-Bw51(5)	HLA-Cw6	HLA-Dw6	HLA-DRw6
HLA-Aw19	HLA-B15	HLA-Bw52(5)	HLA-Cw7	HLA-Dw7	HLA-DR7
HLA-Aw23(9)	HLA-Bw16	HLA-Bw53	HLA-Cw8	HLA-Dw8	HLA-DRw8
HLA-Aw24(9)	HLA-B17	HLA-Bw54(w22)		HLA-Dw9	HLA-DRw9
HLA-A25(10)	HLA-B18	HLA-Bw55(w22)		HLA-Dw10	HLA-DRw10
HLA-A26(10)	HLA-Bw21	HLA-Bw56(w22)		HLA-Dw11	
HLA-A28	HLA-Bw22	HLA-Bw57(17)		HLA-Dw12	
HLA-A29	HLA-B27	HLA-Bw58(17)			
HLA-Aw30	HLA-Bw35	HLA-Bw59			
HLA-Aw31	HLA-B37	HLA-Bw60(40)			
HLA-Aw32	HLA-Bw39(w16)	HLA-Bw61(40)			
HLA-Aw33	HLA-Bw39(w16)	HLA-Bw62(15)			
HLA Aw34	HLA B40	HLA-Bw63(15)			
HLA-Aw36	HLA-Bw41				
HLA-Aw43	HLA-Bw42	HLA-Bw4[a]			
	HLA-Bw44(12)	HLA-Bw6			
	HLA-Bw45(12)				

second individual does carry the antigen(s) present on that HTC, there should be a relatively weak, or absent, response by the cells of that second individual to the same HTC.

Although the results obtained with most HTCs which are either genotypically or simply phenotypically homozygous for HLA-D are not as 'clean' as suggested by the prototype results given above, it is possible to obtain useful information, and a number of different HLA-D antigens (or antigenic clusters) have been defined by utilizing HTCs. These are listed as HLA-Dw1 to Dw12 in Table 2.

Seven different antigens have been serologically recognized which are associated with the HLA-D locus and are referred to as HLA-DRw1 to HLA-DRw7, with some still carrying the workshop (w) designation. Very recently, a second series of HLA-DR antigens has been proposed. The evidence for the existence of this second series (MB) was further analysed at the Eighth International Histocompatibility Workshop in 1980[18].

The relationship of HLA-D to HLA-DR antigens is not well elucidated. Whereas a given HLA-D antigen is most frequently found in a given population with a given HLA-DR antigen (for the sake of convenience, one refers in most instances, to an individual having HLA-Dw1 as also having HLA-DRw1), there is evidence to suggest that the determinants recognized by cellular response and serological response are different. This evidence is based on both a very few putative recombinants within the HLA-D region[6,7], as well as the existence, within Caucasians and other populations, of associations between HLA-DR and HLA-D other than those most commonly found in the Caucasian population. For instance, in the Oriental population, the antigen HLA-DRw2 is frequently found with the D specificity referred to as Dw12. Whereas this association is also found in the Caucasian population, the most common association in Caucasians with DRw2 is, again by convention, the Dw2 specificity.

An additional method that has provided information about the HLA-D region has been primed LD typing (PLT)[8,9]. This method uses 'sensitization' of lymphocytes *in vitro* in a primary mixed leukocyte culture in which donors of responding and stimulating cells differ by only a single HLA haplotype. The cells resulting 10 days after the initiation of the primary MLC are thought to represent 'secondary-type' responding cells. These will give a rapid, measurable by 24 or 48 hours, proliferative response to those antigens initially recognized by the responding cells or the stimulating cells during the sensitization phase. Although PLT reagents can respond to antigens other than those encoded by the HLA-D region, most of the responses are associated with HLA-D region-encoded determinants.

PLT reagents can be prepared, each against a different HLA-D haplotype, and used to 'define' PL antigens associated with HLA-D. A number of different PL antigens have been defined in this manner[9], most of which are highly associated with a given HLA-D antigenic cluster.

The PLT test can be used to detect both antigens associated with HLA-D and those associated with HLA-DR. This can be demonstrated by studying the situation mentioned immediately above in which DRW2 is associated with Dw12 in Orientals but primarily with Dw2 in Caucasians. PLT reagents can be prepared against either the DRw2–Dw2 or the DRw2–Dw12 complex and then tested for their responsiveness to each of these two types of stimulating cells. Under these conditions, there appears to be a clear response associated with DRw2. However, the magnitude of the response is also affected by the presence of the priming D specificity on the restimulating cells. Further information regarding reactivity with D, or a factor associated with D, is obtained if priming is done against only Dw2 or Dw12, with respect to these determinants. Under these conditions, the resulting PLT reagents react only with Dw2 and not with Dw12 if primed to Dw2 and vice versa[10].

A finer analysis of D-associated antigens is promised by the recent advent of cloning of PLT cells. Day 4 blasts are isolated from a regular MLC during the sensitization phase and then cloned in the presence of T cell growth factor (TCGF)[11]. Under these conditions, presumed single precursor cells can be grown to very large numbers. In many cases, the resulting 'monoclonal' PLT reagents give highly significant PLT-type responses providing a dissection of the D region hitherto unavailable with cellular reagents[12]

Table 3 Proliferative response of non-cloned PLT vs limiting dilution 'cloned' alloactivated cells

Responding cells	Restimulating cells			
	A_x	B_x	C_x	D_x
Original PLT	173	5152	831	207
'Clones'				
40-10E	543	6000	536	375
40-7E	641	44681	906	489
40-8E	576	3842	2313	710
40-4E	814	4634	2475	683
40-9D	881	999	993	742

'Clones' were obtained from limiting dilution of day 4 MLC blast cells and were grown in Terasaki microtitre wells in the presence of feeder layers and TCGF. The cells were derived from wells which received on average 40 cells per well at the time of dilution into Terasaki plates. 40-9D is an example of a clone giving no proliferative response

(Table 3). In Table 3, the original PLT cell, in which cells of Individual A were sensitized to cells of Individual B, gives a strong response when restimulated with cells of Individual B, as compared with restimulation with autologous cells of Individual A, but also gives a weak, albeit significant, response to cells of third-party Individual C. Cells of Individual D do not stimulate a proliferative response significantly different from that found in the control restimulation with cells from Individual A.

Such intermediate values of restimulation, e.g. as found with Individual C, have been difficult to interpret. The results of PLT tests using various clones suggest strongly that the low-level restimulation with cells of Individual C, as compared with the reference restimulation with the initial sensitizing cells, B, represent either sharing or cross-reactivity of antigens between B and C as recognized by A. Some clones, such as 40-10E and 40-7E, recognize only antigens on cells of Individual B; restimulating cells of

PRIMARY RESPONSE

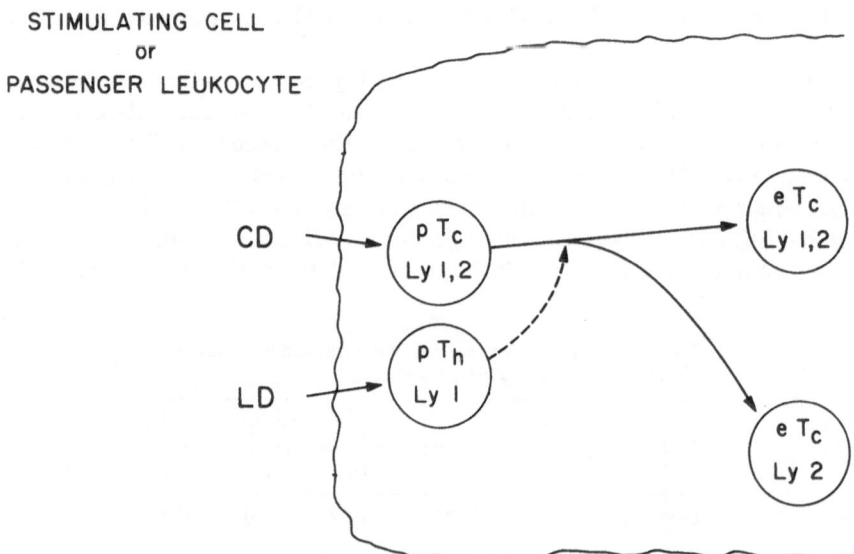

Figure 2　Schematic representation of the cells involved in the generation of a cytotoxic response. Precursor cytotoxic cells (which in mouse are Lyl^+2^+, i.e. marked by the presence of the differentiation antigens referred to as Lyl and Ly2) respond to CD antigenic determinants; precursor helper T lymphocytes (Lyl^+, 2^- in mouse) respond primarily to LD. Collaboration between the two types of cells, as discussed in the text, leads to the generation of effector cytotoxic T lymphocytes

Individuals C and D do not restimulate significantly. Other clones, such as 40-8E and 40-4E, are restimulated significantly by cells of both B and C. These two clones presumably represent ones which recognize the shared or cross-reactive antigen. It should be noted that in other experiments such clones respond equally well to the reference cell[13] and to the third-party cell. The use of cloned PLT reagents must be considered at its inception and thus much further analysis is needed to evaluate its practical usefulness.

Cellular response to MHC encoded antigens

Much of the interest relating to different 'types' of antigens that are encoded by MHC genes is based on the differential response of helper T lymphocytes (T_h) and cytotoxic T lymphocytes (T_c) to antigens associated with different subregions of the MHC. The findings can be summarized[4] as follows.

(1) HLA-D region-encoded LD antigens are primarily responsible for activating the vast majority of the proliferating cells in a primary MLC where the donors of the responding and stimulating cells differ by the entire MHC.

(2) The strongest cytotoxic responses are aimed at ABC region encoded CD antigens.

(3) The combined presence of ABC region differences plus D region-encoded difference on the stimulating cells results in the generation of a much stronger cytotoxic response than does the presence of ABC region-encoded antigens alone[4,13]. This phenomenon was referred to as LD–CD collaboration. The cellular counterpart of LD–CD collaboration is seen in the interaction of LD-responsive T_h and CD-responsive T_c. It is the combined response of T_h and T_c that leads to the strongest cytotoxic activity (see Figure 2). ABC region differences alone lead to cytotoxic responses only in some cases[14].

THE RELEVANCE OF HLA MATCHING TO GRAFT SURVIVAL

An enormous number of studies have been performed attempting to relate degrees of matching for the HLA-A and -B antigens, as detected serologically, to the success of allograft survival. It would have to be concluded in a summary of all those studies that most centres, in the United States at least, have failed to show a significant association between matching for the HLA-A and -B antigens and kidney allograft survival, with a few notable exceptions, such as the studies published from Minneapolis[19]. Such differences can be explained by many factors, including the degree of genetic heterogeneity in the population under study. In Europe, many more centres, including the very large Eurotransplant Programme, have found significant associations, i.e. that a graft survives longer given a four antigen match (often referred to as a full-house match for HLA-A and -B) than with lesser degrees of matching. In sequence, a match for three or two antigens is better than a match for one or none.

During the last few years, attempts have been made to match for the HLA-D region to investigate whether minimizing disparity for D region-encoded antigens may correlate with graft survival[15]. Two lines of approach have been taken. First, matching in primary MLC in living related donor–recipient combinations, and second, matching of the HLA-DR antigens for cadaver transplantation. Results obtained by our own group in Madison[16] compared graft surival in one haplotype disparate, intrafamilial, donor–recipient combinations. The degree of MLC stimulation between the recipient and the donor was related to the average MLC response the recipient demonstrated against a series of unrelated cells. This ratio, expressed as an incompatibility index, was classified as low, medium or high, based on being less than 0.4, between 0.41 and 0.8, or greater than 0.8. A significant correlation was found between a low incompatibility index and improved graft survival. Of very great importance from the clinical transplantation point of view was the observation that graft survival was not significantly different in HLA identical siblings and donor–recipient pairs falling into the low incompatibility index group. This demonstrated that low degrees of incompatibility were consistent with excellent graft survival. A large number of different studies have demonstrated similar findings.

An alternative method of matching for the HLA-D region has been to type donor–recipient for the HLA-DR antigens and compare graft survival in donor–recipient combinations sharing two DR antigens, one DR antigen or no DR antigens. The results of these particular studies must be considered preliminary; in Europe, several centres have suggested that a two-DR antigen match (i.e. a zero DR antigen mismatch) correlates with better graft survival than either other group, and a one-DR antigen match is better than a zero-antigen match.

Although these two types of approaches, the cellular and serological, may not measure exactly the same determinants, certainly serological typing for the HLA-DR antigens provides a very convenient guide to other determinants usually found in association with the given DR antigen on the HLA-D haplotype. Some results of both types of study suggest that matching for the HLA-D region may have a highly significant effect on the outcome of graft survival when the data from individual centres are considered. The lack of such a finding in the international co-operative trial will need further investigation. It would be worthwhile to reserve final judgement in this regard until the results of a carefully planned, preferably prospective, trial are evaluated. This should certainly be performed with regard to kidney transplantation in both Europe and the United States.

One major difficulty in interpreting the data from primary MLC tests and comparing it with matching for DR antigens, for instance, concerns the question of 'strength' of the H antigens. First, it may well be that if LD–CD collaboration, as discussed above, obtains *in vivo* in terms of leading to graft rejection, the strength of the overall rejection response is a measure of the interactive events taking place in LD–CD collaboration. From *in vitro* studies, it would appear that the strength of the LD stimulus, i.e. the stimulation of the helper T lymphocytes, is a limiting factor in the overall response[17]. Whether this can be extrapolated to the *in vivo* situation, such that matching for HLA-D is most important in terms of limiting the overall rejection response, must be considered highly speculative at the present time. Second, there is the more fundamental question concerning the differential strength of either LD (HLA-D region encoded) or CD (HLA-ABC region encoded) antigens. In any type of enumeration where the number of antigens mismatched between donor and recipient is used as the measure of compatibility, such considerations of differential strength of CD or LD antigens is not considered. On the other hand, matching with a primary mixed lymphocyte culture test does appear to provide, at least by some standard, a biologically meaningful measure of disparity. It may be that we shall need to evaluate the relative strength of the various antigens that we measure by such biological tests and the possible variation of antigenic strength depending on the phenotype of the responder.

SUMMARY

A variety of markers are associated with HLA genes which have allowed construction of the genetic map presented in Figure 1. Primarily it has been the use of antisera that has allowed this dissection. In the process of performing such investigations, it has become apparent that there are two types of antigens, differentiated initially on the basis of their tissue distribution. In addition, two 'types' of antigens are differentially active in stimulating proliferating and cytotoxic cells. The role of these antigens in stimulating T cells *in vitro* and in matching donor and recipient for transplantation are discussed.

Acknowledgements

This work was supported by NIH grants AI 08439, CA 09106, CA 16836 and AI 15588. This is paper No. 228 from the Immunobiology Research Center, University of Minnesota, Minneapolis, MN 55455.

References

1 Terasaki, P. I. (ed.) (1970). *Histocompatibility Testing 1970*. (Copenhagen: Munksgaard)
2 Kissmeyer-Nielsen, F. (ed.) (1975). *Histocompatibility Testing 1975*. (Copenhagen: Munksgaard)
3 Bach, F. H. and van Rood, J. J. (1976). The major histocompatibility complex—Genetics and biology. *N. Engl. J. Med.*, **295**, 806, 872, 927
4 Bach, F. H., Bach, M. L. and Sondel, P. M. (1976). Differential function of major histocompatibility complex antigens in T-lymphocyte activation. *Nature (London)*, **259**, 273

5 Mempel, W., Grosse-Wilde, H., Baumann, P., Netzel, B. and Steinbauer-Rosenthal, I. (1973). Population genetics of the MLC response: typing for MLC determinants using homozygous and heterozygous reference cells. *Transplant. Proc.*, 5, 1529

6 Reinsmoen, N., Noreen, H., Friend, P., Giblett, E., Greenberg, L. and Kersey, J. (1979). Anomalous mixed lymphocyte culture reactivity between HLA-A, B, C, DR identical siblings. *Tissue Antigens*, 13, 19

7 Festenstein, H. (1978). *Histocompatibility Testing 1977*, p. 360. (Copenhagen: Munksgaard)

8 Sheehy, M. H., Sondel, P. M., Bach, M. L., Wank, R. and Bach, F. H. (1975). LD (lymphocyte defined) typing: a rapid assay with primed lymphocytes. *Science*, 188, 1308

9 Bach, F. H., Jarrett-Toth, E. K., Benike, C. J., Shih, C. Y. and Valentine, E. A. (1977). Primed LD typing: reagent preparation and definition of the HLA-D region antigens. *Scand. J. Immunol.*, 6, 469

10 Reinsmoen, N. L., Noreen, H. J., Sasazuki, T., Segall, M. and Bach, F. H. (1979). Roles of HLA-DR and HLA-D antigens in haplotype-primed LD typing reagents. In Gordin Kaplan, J. (ed.) *The Molecular Basis of Immune Cell Function, Proceedings of the 13th International Leucocyte Culture Conference*, p. 529. (Amsterdam: Elsevier/North-Holland Biomedical Press)

11 Morgan, D. A., Ruscetti, F. W. and Gallo, R. C. (1976). Selective *in vitro* growth of T lymphocytes from normal human bone marrows. *Science*, 193, 1007

12 Bach, F. H., Inouye, H., Hank, J. A. and Alter, B. A. (1979). Human T lymphocyte clones reactive in primed lymphocyte typing and cytotoxicity. *Nature (London)*, 281, 307

13 Eijsvoogel, V. P., du Bois, R., Melief, C. J. M., Zeylemaker, W. P. and Raat-Koning, L. (1973). Lymphocyte activation and destruction *in vitro* in relation to MLC and HL-A. *Transplant. Proc.*, 5, 1301

14 Long, M. A., Handwerger, B. S., Amos, D. B. and Yunis, E. J. (1976). The genetics of cell mediated lympholysis. *J. Immunol.*, 117, 2092

15 *Transplant. Proc.*, vol. 11, No. 1, March 1979.

16 Segall, M., Bach, F. H., Bach, M. L., Hussey, J. L. and Uehling, D. T. (1975). Correlation of MLC stimulation and clinical course in kidney transplants. *Transplant. Proc.*, 7, 41

17 Bach, F. H., Gose, J. E., Alter, B. J., Sondel, P. M. and Bach, M. L. (1979). Past, present and future aspects of histocompatibility. *Transplant. Proc.*, 11, 1207

18 Terasaki, P. I. (ed.) (1980). *Histocompatibility Testing 1980*. (UCLA)

19 Ascher, N. (1979). Effects of HLA-A and B matching on success of cadaver grafts at a single center. *Transplantation*, 28, 172

8

Renal transplantation

J. E. Castro

HISTORICAL

The concept of replacing diseased and worn-out organs is a problem that has fascinated the minds of clinicians, scientists and philosophers for many years. It is exemplified by the chimera of Greek mythology; a monster with a goat's body, lion's head and serpent's tail, which roamed the streets of Lycra. Similarly, the second-century BC reports of cardiac transplantation by Pien Ch'iao and Hua T'o must be regarded as examples of medical mythology; so too the exploits of Cosmos and Damien, who replaced the leg of a devout person with the leg of a Moor, recently dead. These twin Arab brothers were converted to Christianity and subsequently martyred in AD 303. In the tenth century they were canonized by Pope John XVI and later became the patron saints of the barber surgeons.

Experimental kidney grafting started in dogs in 1902 when Ullmann used Payr's canulae to join transplanted kidneys to the main vessels in the neck. The same year Carrel described his methods of vascular anastomosis in *Lyon Medicale* and subsequently the techniques were successfully used by Floresco, who anastomosed the renal vessels to the femoral blood vessels, bringing out the ureters of the transplanted kidney as a cutaneous ureter-ostomy. Subsequent experiments in renal transplantation were designed to define the optimal techniques by which permanent graft survival could be achieved. Workers like Carrel and Guthrie in 1905, Stich in 1907, Borst and Enderlen in 1909, Unger in 1910 and Neuhof in 1923 were active in this respect.

It was another 50 years before these techniques were applied to man, but in 1955 details of nine renal transplants were reported[1]. All the grafts were from cadavers; there was no immunosuppression and the only tissue match-ing was of ABO blood grouping. However, five of the grafts survived for periods of 30–120 days. This report showed the operative techniques to be satisfactory but still organ grafting was dogged by tissue rejection.

In 1901 Lansteiner discovered the human blood groups. As early in 1903 Jenssen suggested that immunological mechanisms may be involved in rejection. By 1927 Gorer identified the first histocompatibility antigen and observed that genetically determined factors present in the graft, but not in the host, were capable of eliciting a response which resulted in the destruction of the graft. In 1945 some 40 years of experimental and clinical work was summarized by Leo Loeb, who attempted to define 'organismal differentials' which he thought constituted the somatic basis of individuality within strains and species. Modern transplantation immunology resulted mainly from the pioneering work on skin graft rejection by Medawar and his colleagues in the 1940s and 1950s. Comparisons of these changes with those dominant in kidney graft rejection were carried out by Dempster in 1953 in dogs[2].

Another line of investigation was the attempts made to suppress immunological rejection. In 1959 Hamburger[3] used whole-body irradiation of the recipient to achieve prolonged survival of a kidney graft. Subsequently cortisone and azathioprine have become the standard forms of immunosuppression.

TRANSPLANT RECIPIENTS

The incidence of end-stage renal failure is difficult to estimate. In the United States, estimates for the annual death rate from kidney-related illnesses vary from 50 000 to 100 000[4,5]. The number suitable for transplantation is probably between 7000 and 10 000 per year, dependent upon the criteria of acceptability. In the UK, and similar figures probably apply to Europe, it has been estimated that 40 per million population under the age of 60 develop renal failure each year. In 1978 in the UK 1257 recipients were on file awaiting transplantation and 788 transplants were carried out. In every country the number of patients suitable for transplantation still exceeds, by far, the number who undergo transplantation. This is due to the shortage of organs, financial constraints, and unawareness of the current status and benefits of transplantation by the medical profession and public.

From 1963 to 1977, 25 108 kidney transplants were registered with the American College of Surgeons/National Institutes of Health Registry, from centres worldwide. The longest survivors now approximate to 20 years. Of transplants carried out in the UK and Europe, 10% are from living related donors. In the United States, this figure approaches 40–50% although the introduction of health-care programmes has decreased this proportion, but in Australia the surfeit of cadaver donors means that only 2% of transplants are from living related donors. Most recipients are between 20 and 60 years of age, but in the recent past increasing numbers of transplants have been undertaken in children. There is also a trend to transplant older patients, but in Europe 70% of centres still reserve kidneys for patients under 55 years. Scandinavian countries and Switzerland are more prepared to transplant older patients and this is reflected in the average age of recipients, which exceeds 40 years in these countries.

Patients with renal disease secondary to almost every type of systemic disease have undergone successful transplantation although the success rate is higher with certain disorders. The commonest cause of end-stage renal failure treated by transplantation is glomerulonephritis, followed by pyelonephritis/interstitial nephritis, but significant numbers of transplants are performed for drug-induced nephropathy, cystic renal disease, hereditofamilial nephropathies including Alport's syndrome, inborn errors of metabolism, such as cystinosis and oxalosis, renal vascular disease and a range of others.

In recent years a more liberal policy has been adopted regarding the transplantation of patients with systemic disease. Of European centres, 25% excluded all diabetics from transplantation, and 25% also excluded all patients with other multisystem diseases. Even centres with an active transplant programme are selective regarding patients with diabetes or other multisystem diseases who are offered transplantation. In 'diabetes, data from Minneapolis[6] show that the results of transplantation are superior to those of haemodialysis, but both patient survival and graft survival are inferior to non-diabetics. A recent study[7] showed patient survival of transplanted diabetics at 1 year was 60% and at 2 years 50%. One-year survival with living donor transplants was 84%. Survival was significantly reduced in diabetic patients with heart disease, impaired vision and a long history of diabetes. Survival was not influenced by sex, age, neuropathy or pretransplantation dialysis. Diabetic retinopathy progressed slowly after successful transplantation and more than 90% had stable vision 1–2 years after transplantation. Progression of peripheral circulatory insufficiency was common.

In patients with amyloidosis, renal failure, or its complications, is the usual cause of death. Triger and Joekes[8] found the mean duration of survival with amyloidosis was 44 months after the first clinical features of the disease. In 1977 Kennedy and Castro[9] were able to trace the outcome of 24 transplants undertaken for this condition and concluded that survival after transplants in patients with amyloidosis was less than for patients with renal failure from other causes. However, the results were sufficiently encouraging to recommend its continuation, but myocardial amyloidosis in older patients was associated with a poor prognosis.

Renal transplantation has been carried out in a few patients with scleroderma[10] and the progress of the disease slowed after successful operation. Whether the disease recurs in the transplant is unknown. A few transplants have been done in patients with enzyme deficiency diseases, not because of renal failure, but as a possible means of enzyme production.

The only absolute contraindication to renal transplantation is the presence of uncontrolled infection or of malignancy. In these situations, transplantation can be considered if the patient has been free of infection for some months or there has been no tumour recurrence for several years. Penn[11] advocates a 1-year delay following the treatment of malignancy before transplantation, and exploratory laparotomy before grafting may be indicated. There have been several reports of transplantation for renal tumours alone[12] and in association with Lindau von Hippel disease[13].

Recurrent glomerulonephritis

In selecting patients with glomerulonephritis for transplantation, it is important to consider the incidence of recurrent glomerulonephritis recurring in the transplanted kidney. In the majority of patients, the original disease probably started many years before transplantation and the patient presents with small contracted kidneys, without active disease. In these patients, the incidence of recurrence is low. In those with evidence of recent activity such as Goodpasture's syndrome, anti-glomerular basement membrane nephritis, anti-tubular basement membrane nephritis, SLE, IgA nephropathy and membranoproliferative glomerulonephritis, there may be a substantial risk of histological recurrence and even graft failure due to disease recurrence[14,15]. In these diseases kidney transplantation is not absolutely contradicted, but it would seem sensible to wait until the disease is relatively quiescent. There is no definite evidence that bilateral nephrectomy of the diseased kidneys influences the incidence of recurrent glomerulonephritis in the diseases mentioned.

Transplantation and HBsAg antigenaemia

As 10–90% of dialysis patients may develop HBsAg antigenaemia, it is likely that some of the transplant recipients will be HBsAg-positive and this will persist during immunosuppressive therapy during the postoperative period[16]. In other patients HBsAg develops after transplantation. An increased virulence of some viruses in immunosuppressed renal allograft recipients and the known hepatotoxicity of azathioprine have been the reasons for concern about the outcome of hepatitis and the advisability of transplantation in these patients. However, most authors report a benign course for the hepatitis and few have noticed a high incidence of death. In the majority of instances, the symptoms are absent or mild and there are no deaths directly attributed to liver failure. No serious hepatic functional abnormality was noted in the group that was positive before transplantation or in the group in which persistent antigenaemia developed following transplantation. However, precautions to protect other patients and staff must be observed.

Transplantation into an ileal conduit

Urinary diversion is rarely used in kidney transplant patients but occasionally transplants into an ileal conduit are necessary in patients with urinary outflow tract abnormalities and in those that develop urological complications after transplantation. Our own experience[17] was with eight transplants in seven patients. The technique used is shown in Figure 1. In six instances the diversion was required either because the bladder had previously been removed or there was gross abnormality of the outflow tract: in

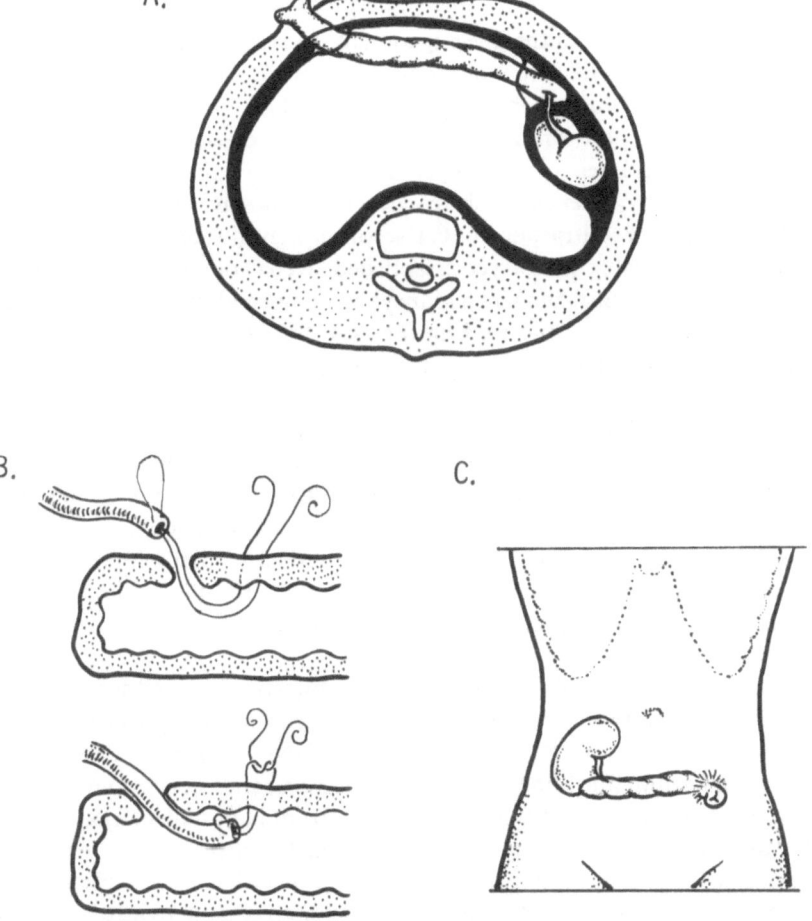

Figure 1 The technique of ureteroileostomy in kidney transplantation. The proximal end of the ileal loop is brought through the peritoneum so that the site of the ureteric implantation is extraperitoneal (A). The ureter is implanted into the loop through a 5 mm stab incision and is anchored by a mattress suture (B). The ileal stoma is in the left iliac fossa when the kidney is transplanted to the right side (C).

two it was successfully employed to deal with difficult post-transplantation urinary fistulae. Four patients died: three within 2 months and one at 9 months after the operation. Infection with organisms indistinguishable from those cultured from the ileal loop was a common complication and, although there were other significant factors which contributed to the mortality, retrospective consideration suggests that energetic prophylactic antibacterial therapy should be instituted when kidney transplantation with ileal urinary diversion is undertaken.

Assessment of the recipient

The extent and scope of the investigation of the recipient depends upon the disorder present. The essential factor is to exclude any reversible factors leading to renal failure. Renal evaluation should include determinations of serum creatinine, creatinine clearance, urinary excretion of total proteins and urine electrolytes, urine analysis and culture. High-dose pyelography with tomography, to exclude obstruction or calculi and also to judge renal size, is mandatory. Ultrasound or CT scanning may give useful information, although their value is not yet established. Renal biopsy is a matter for debate but should be taken when kidneys are of normal size. Immunological studies may include anti-AGM antibodies, ASO titres, complement and antinuclear antibodies as well as tests for lupus erythematosus and rheumatoid factor.

Urological evaluation depends upon the underlying disease; voiding cystography may be useful in patients with recurrent infections and occasionally cystoscopy and urodynamics may be indicated if there are radiological abnormalities of the bladder. Because of the high incidence of hyperparathyroidism, X-rays of the hands and acromioclavicular joints, as well as serum calcium, phosphate and plasma proteins should be undertaken. An extensive search should be made for evidence of infection, including tuberculosis.

The high incidence of gastrointestinal complications has led some centres to investigate gastric acid secretion in depth. Our own experience suggests predictive tests are of little value[18]. We investigated a history of dyspepsia, abnormal barium meal findings or gastric hypersecretion and found that it was not possible to identify patients at risk from peptic ulceration or life-threatening alimentary complications after renal transplantation. Thus, the routine screening of these patients for peptic ulcer has no practical value, and the incidence of fatal complications is not high enough to justify routine prophylactic anti-ulcer surgery aimed at reducing acid secretions before renal transplantation.

If peptic ulceration is diagnosed during the period of dialysis, then treatment is required before transplantation. A reasonable approach would be to give a full therapeutic dose of the H2 antagonist, cimetidine, for 6 weeks followed by repeated endoscopy. Cimetidine is excreted by the kidney and the recommended dose would be 200 mg twice daily, with the maintenance dose being 200 mg at night. If healing occurs after 6 weeks therapy maintenance should be continued for 6 months, using endoscopy as the criterion of success. Failure to heal, or recurrence, are indications for surgery.

Prophylactic cimetidine after transplantation is now frequently used.

Recipient nephrectomy

Removal of the patient's own kidney may be necessary if there is persistent infection or vesicoureteric reflux associated with recurrent infections. Occasionally in polycystic renal disease nephrectomy is required to make room for the graft. In some cases of hypertension removal of the diseased kidneys is necessary. Hypertension is found in 80% of patients presenting for maintenance haemodialysis. In approximately 80–90% of these, hypertension can be well controlled with salt and water depletion and small doses of antihypertensives. The remaining cases may present problems. Bilateral nephrectomy is indicated if blood pressure is inadequately controlled and if control is associated with intractable thirst, unexplained progressive weight change or severe hypertension during dialysis. The value of plasma renin measurements for predicting the response to nephrectomy is still a matter for debate[19,20]. Whilst it correlates with a renovascular cause of hypertension in most cases, this is not true for all[21]. Occasionally, patients become hypotensive postoperatively and require large volumes of fluid.

For bilateral nephrectomy of small kidneys we usually employ a lumbar approach removing both kidneys at the same time. If total nephroureterectomy is required, I usually remove the left kidney and ureter through an extended loin incision as a primary operation, and remove the right kidney and ureter at the time of transplantation. Should the kidneys be a source of infection, this scheme requires modification. A polycystic kidney can be removed at the same time as transplantation by an extraperitoneal extended hockey-stick incision. Some clinicians advocate bilateral nephrectomy only after the establishment of a functioning transplant[22].

Splenectomy and appendicectomy are routinely carried out in some units, but evidence of benefit is lacking. It is claimed that splenectomy reduces the incidence of leukopenia and thrombocytopenia.

Mendez et al.[23] have shown a very high mortality rate in patients with end-stage renal failure due to polycystic kidney disease who do not undergo nephrectomy. These workers now advocate routine bilateral nephrectomy in all of these cases. Our own experience[24] showed that transplant function was better at all times in patients with end-stage renal failure from adult polycystic disease than a matched group with chronic renal failure from other causes. The only indications for removal of polycystic kidneys in graft recipients were persistent or recurrent infection, erythremia that failed to respond to conservative treatment and to make room for the transplant.

CADAVER DONORS

Kidneys from cadavers must be removed as soon as possible after death whilst adequate circulation persists so that tubular damage is avoided and the kidneys excrete urine soon after transplantation. An age limit for donors varies – some suggest a maximum of 60 years[25] but, because of the shortage of kidneys, our policy is to remove kidneys from cadavers of all ages and examine them after removal for obvious defects. Criteria for excluding potential donors are those with a history of malignancy (except for tumours of the CNS) and those with a history of renal disease or insulin-dependent diabetes. Hypertension requiring drug therapy makes a donor unsuitable, but terminal hypertension accompanying a head injury does not debar the kidneys from use. The presence of localized infection adequately treated with antibiotics does not exclude. Criteria vary with different units – for example, some will accept donors whose malignancy was more than 5 years ago. An additional criterion for exclusion is evidence of trauma to the kidneys. Intravenous urography may be helpful in this respect, although surgical exploration is the only absolute method for determining the satisfactory condition of the kidneys. Macroscopical or microscopical haematuria does not rule out the possibility of kidney donation because injury to the bladder or lower urinary tract may be responsible.

Despite the continuing shortage of suitable cadaver kidneys for transplantation, there is still widespread reluctance to transplant kidneys from donors in the paediatric group into adults. Boczko et al.[26] transplanted 31 single kidneys from donors between the ages of $1\frac{1}{2}$ and 9 years. Kidneys from donors 3 years of age and younger developed a creatinine clearance rate of 20 ml/min in 12 days or less when transplanted into adults. Maximum creatinine clearance rates for kidneys from donors of the paediatric age-group equalled those of adult donors. It appears that single kidneys from donors as young as 18 months of age can be transplanted without special difficulties and they can provide excellent renal function for adult recipients. However, some workers suggest that paediatric kidneys should be transplanted as a pair into the adult recipients. With increasing paediatric transplantation being undertaken it is probably correct that such kidneys should be reserved for child recipients. There is some evidence that the older the donor kidney the smaller the chance of successful kidney transplantation[27].

During the agonal phase it is important that the transplant clinician is not involved in the management of the prospective donor. Some indication of renal function is useful, especially with the patient adequately hydrated. Measurement of urine output (> 50 ml/h), urinary urea and serum creatinine are useful. Once the diagnosis of death has been made, supportive therapy can be directed at protection of the kidneys. Adequate hydration, maintenance of blood pressure and preservation of peripheral perfusion with phenoxybenzamine may be useful. A recent study by Filoso and Cho[28] showed that 75 kidneys discarded because of poor flow characteristics on pulsatile perfusion, 25 had been pretreated *in vivo* with phenoxybenzamine, methylprednisolone or phentolamine, whereas the remaining 50 had not. In the same study, of 356 kidneys transplanted 70% had received the treatment whereas 30% had not. There is also evidence that pretreatment of the donor with steroids and cytotoxic drugs may decrease the immunogenicity of the kidney and so decrease rejection after transplantation. There is no doubt that such treatment leads to extra work, which in some countries (e.g. Holland) is financially rewarded.

Brain death

The subject of brain death is contentious and emotive, and has been the subject of considerable publicity in the media in this country. The full potential of transplantation surgery is at present hampered in the United Kingdom by the lack of donor organs. Some 600 kidneys are transplanted each year in the UK. There are 1200 patients (the majority between 30 and 50 years of age) on file awaiting transplantation and it is estimated that 2500 patients could benefit from transplantation annually. Even the proportion of the annual 6000 fatal road traffic accidents, let alone the patients dying of cerebrovascular disease or cerebral tumours, would totally satisfy the transplantation needs of this country.

Because of the shortage of kidneys, there is no doubt that units use kidneys which in a more favourable situation might have been turned down. In the recent past it has been shown that 17% of kidneys transplanted in this country never function, many because of excessive warm ischaemia[29]. In the United States and some parts of Europe, primary transplant failure due to ischaemic heart damage is very rare, since the public has accepted the concept of brain death, and most kidneys come from patients with irreversible complete brain death but an intact circulation.

There has been much philosophical argument about the diagnosis of death and the situation has been well discussed by the Medawars[30]:

Being alive is a system property, i.e. a characteristic that can be attributed only to an organized system. This does not mean, however, that parts of such a system may not also enjoy the same property, for it is characteristic of living things that they are hierarchically organized; thus societies are made up of men and women, and individual human beings are made up of organs which have a certain wholeness and functional unity of their own. Organs and tissues in their turn are composed of cells which also have a high measure of autonomy. It is perfectly understandable that a society should die – that is, disintegrate – before any of its individual members and that a human being should die before one or other of its organs – e.g. kidney has lost its capacity to work in another human being as it did in its original owner. Transplant donation would be impossible but for this dispensation.

It is now agreed that permanent functional death of the brainstem constitutes brain death and, once this has occurred, further artificial support is fruitless and should be withdrawn. There have been several useful guides detailing the criteria for this diagnosis, but the exact details are still matters of debate. Brain death should particularly be suspected when the patient is deeply comatose, or when spontaneous respiration has become inadequate and assisted ventilation is required[31]. The diagnosis is based on the absence of all brainstem reflexes and it is customary to repeat the tests to ensure that there has been no observer error. It is well established that spinal cord function can persist despite irretrievable destruction of the brainstem. Indeed, spinal reflexes may persist or even return after an initial absence. Hypothermia is not common in these patients, but it is recommended that body temperature is not less than 35°C when testing for the diagnosis of brain death. Most neurologists believe that the electroencephalogram is not necessary for the diagnosis and there is now a clear consensus of medical opinion on the requirements for such a diagnosis. It is hoped that this will put an end to the confused thinking and inadequate expert advice that has punctuated public comment.

The diagnosis can usually be made by experienced clinicians, particularly in the intensive care unit and accident ward where most of these patients will be sustained. The decision to withdraw artificial support should be made either by the consultant in charge of the case and one other doctor, or, in the absence of the consultant, a deputy who should have been registered for at least 5 years[32]. A survey of public attitudes to renal transplantation showed that 80% of those questioned had no objection to it, yet only 4·4% carried a completed donor card agreeing to their kidneys being available for grafting after death. The main reason why people did not carry a card was the fear that organs might be taken before they were really dead[33]. Uncertainty in the minds of doctors about brain death may be the reason for this. Certainly the willingness of the community to co-operate has not fully developed anything remotely approaching its full potential. The law pertinent to removal of organs for transplantation varies in different countries and has been well summarized[34–36].

Donor pretreatment

It has been demonstrated experimentally that important immunogens reside in the interstitial compartment of the kidney. These are derived from the haemopoietic system and are known as passenger leukocytes. The pretreatment of brain-dead, mechanically ventilated donors with high doses of cytotoxic drugs has been carried out in an attempt to reduce allograft immunogenicity by altering passenger leukocytes. In two uncontrolled studies[37,38] it was shown that pretreatment was advantageous. In a small, prospective, controlled, multicentre trial it was initially found that pretreatment markedly improved graft survival. However, two subsequent small studies by the same group demonstrated no significant difference in survival[39]. A larger-scale multicentre study is planned to elucidate this problem.

At present the principal drugs used for pretreatment are cyclophosphamide at 50–70 mg/kg followed by methylprednisolone 50–70 mg/kg with a delay in the time of nephrectomy of 5 h. There is no evidence that these high doses are nephrotoxic when used in this situation.

Cadaver donor nephrectomy

Today kidneys are usually only removed from patients with assisted ventilation; dehydration should have been corrected. If the kidneys are to be removed from a 'heart-beating' cadaver, great haste is not necessary. Several techniques are used.

The kidneys are removed transabdominally. Either a long midline incision, bilateral subcostal incisions, or a combination of both to form a cruciate incision, may be used. The object is to remove both kidneys with the full length of the main renal artery and vein. Preferably the vessels should include cuffs of the aorta and vena cava to limit the possibilities of the damage to accessory vessels and to allow a choice in the technique of anastomosis.

When the abdomen is opened, laparotomy is performed to exclude sepsis or malignancy. The small bowel and mesentery are all retracted to the right and the posterior parietal peritoneum incised over the great vessels. The duodenum and pancreas are retracted superiorly and the proximal aorta freed to above the coeliac axis by clamping and dividing the superior mesenteric and coeliac arteries. The aorta and vena cava can then be isolated and clamped above the iliac birfurcation and around the proximal aorta. At this stage perfusion and cooling of the kidneys may be started. The kidneys are then mobilized. The ureters are freed as far down to the bladder as possible. A considerable amount of periureteric tissue should be included in the mobilization and care taken to avoid dissection in the renal hilum. When the kidneys and ureters are completely mobilized the aorta and vena cava are divided between ligatures. The block is displaced forwards to expose the lumbar vessels which are then divided. Detailed examination and dissection may then take place. Spleen and lymph node samples required for testing should be removed. When a child's kidney is removed, the technique is essentially the same, but vascular patches are essential because of the small size and possible disparity of the vessels.

Kidneys from adult donors may be transplanted into children as young as

2 years. Kidneys from paediatric donors less than 5 years can be used for adolescent and adult recipients. When donors are below the age of 3 years, they are sometimes transplanted *en bloc* into adult recipients.

Renal preservation

Techniques for renal preservation fall into two groups: (1) those using cold storage solutions, and (2) those using machine preservation.

Cold storage solutions are satisfactory for short-term preservation when warm ischaemic time has been minimal. In general, if kidneys can be obtained with short warm ischaemic times and they can be transplanted within 4–6 h after procurement, flushing with an extracellular electrolyte solution, such as Ringer lactate, is satisfactory. If cold ischaemic times are to be longer, then fluids with a intracellular electrolyte composition such as Collins' C3 solution[40] or the hyperosmolar polyelectrolyte solution of Sacks[41] is recommended and transplantation can then be carried out within 24–48 h.

Preservation by a pulsatile perfusion machine allows the observation of functional characteristics for 48 h or more after procurement. Machine preservation has the advantage that kidneys of doubtful viability can be observed and the perfusion characteristics may suggest which are suitable for use. It has not yet been established whether these characteristics should be the sole criterion of acceptability.

There is a shortage of good comparative studies on the merits of the different methods of preservation. In the retrospective analysis of 108 centres, kidney survival was better at 1 month in the group treated by a cold flush compared with machine preservation[42]. However, this study suffers from all the problems of retrospective data. In a controlled trial of preservation techniques from a single centre there was no significant difference between the preservation methods[43]. Whether the addition of PPF, allopurinol or other manipulations will improve machine preservation is yet to be decided. It is known that high doses of corticosteroids in the machine perfusate have adverse effects[44] and if the perfusate contains antibody against the donor there may be renal damage[45].

It is not yet clear what the risks of tissue damage are, and how long-term renal function is affected by the method of preservation or the period of cold ischaemia. It is likely that the selective use of machine-preserved kidneys by experienced teams together with cold flush solutions used for most cases will continue to be common practice.

LIVE DONORS

There is little doubt that the most successful transplants involve living related donors. It is important that the donor should volunteer, and subtle pressures from family, friends and clinicians must not be applied. Frank discussion on the hazards of donation, as well as a clear description of results of the transplantation, are mandatory. It is our policy not to accept donors under the legal age of consent. The decision of whether to accept relatives' offers to donate depends upon the motivation of the potential donors, the other forms of treatment available to the recipient, as well as the clinical and immunological criteria. We transplant from parents to children, sibs to sibs and occasionally from child to parent. The investigation of the potential donor is summarized in Table 1.

Table 1 Investigations for a potential live related kidney donor

---

1. Clinical history – renal disease, hypertension, malignancy, sepsis
2. Physical examination – blood pressure
3. ABO blood group, tissue typing, leukocyte cross-match, immunological assessment
4. Blood examinations – creatinine, urea, biochemical profile, Australia antigen, full blood count
5. Urine examination – analysis, culture and microscopy, 24 h protein excretion, creatinine clearance
6. Chest X-ray, intravenous urography
7. ECG
8. Aortography

Angiography is only undertaken if preliminary studies are satisfactory. It is our practice to perform abdominal aortography via a transfemoral catheter. The indications for angiography are to ensure the kidney left behind in the healthy donor is structurally sound and to assess the vascular supply to the kidney available for donation. Multiple renal vessels are found in 24% of renal angiograms[46]. If multiple vessels are unilateral it is generally better to choose the contralateral kidney with a single artery. Rapid serial films are taken following pressure injection of contrast medium into the aorta. Only if there is any doubt about renal abnormality or multiple vessels is a selective renal arteriogram done. The renal angiographic and operative findings in our first 88 live kidney donors were compared[47]. Fifty patients had normal arteriograms and uneventful nephrectomies. Abnormal renal parenchymal (solitary cysts) or main artery lesions were found in eight donors (9%). These included four renal artery stenoses, and the kidney distal to the lesion was used for transplanting. Thirty-one patients (35%) had multiple renal vessels – if these were limited to two vessels of approximately equal size we proceeded to nephrectomy; more vessels than this we consider a bar to donation.

Live donor nephrectomy

Preparation for operation is similar to that for any major elective surgery. Some centres administer immunosuppressive drugs to the donor for 1–2 days before nephrectomy; we do not. Shortly before operation, blood is taken for transfusion, cross-match and a final lymphocyte cross-matching with the recipient.

An extraperitoneal low approach, either through the bed of the 12th rib or the intercostal space above it, is used. The kidney is mobilized from the perinephric fat. The ureter is identified and freed, with adequate peri-ureteric tissues, as far as the pelvic brim. The renal vein or veins are identified and on the left side ligation and division of lumbar, adrenal and ovarian or testicular vessels will be necessary. Where two renal veins are present, the smaller one, or either one of two veins of equal size, may be safely ligated, because of ample intrarenal venous communications. The renal artery is mobilized to the aorta. Minute polar arteries supplying an area less than 1 cm in diameter may be ligated; larger vessels must be preserved. The mobilized ureter and vessels are only divided after the recipient is prepared. After careful clamping of the artery and the vein with modified vascular clamps, the vessels are ligated and divided with right-angle scissors. The kidney is surrounded by ice slush. The kidneys can then be used immediately or flushed with one of the solutions previously described. During transplant nephrectomy, it is important to maintain urinary flow at a rate of 2 ml/min, or more, by adequate hydration and diuretics. If vasospasm occurs, time should be allowed for this to recover. We do not heparinize the donor, although the use of subcutaneous heparin for prophylaxis against venous thrombosis is advocated by some clinicians.

Complications are few[48,49] and our experience has confirmed this. However, in this unique situation of a patient undergoing operation for the benefit of another, constant vigilance is essential. In the long term, we have found no significant problems, provided the patients are adequately screened. We have not accepted relatives from patients with end-stage renal failure due to polycystic disease until they are more than 40 years old, and have both normal ultrasound and arteriogram. In relatives with Alport's syndrome we have routinely undertaken audiometry. Edgren et al.[50] showed that compensatory renal hypertrophy took place in donors up to the age of 74 but the greatest changes were in donors under the age of 40. The total renal function decreased postoperatively to about 77% of the initial level but function remained normal in all cases.

TRANSPLANTATION

The operation of renal transplantation is now fairly standardized (Figure 2). If the operation is planned then the patient should be well dialysed. The serum electrolytes and lymphocyte cross-match should be checked in all cases and patients should be examined clinically and bacteriologically for infection. Blood for transfusion is required.

It is our practice to give immunosuppression with the premedication. When the vascular anastomoses are completed and haemostasis is certain we give 1 g methylprednisone i.v. and 150 mg azathioprine. The role of prophylactic antibiotics given with premedication is not yet established but our preliminary studies suggest that they are useful. Some clinicians take culture swabs from the kidney graft and subsequently give appropriate antibiotics.

We have not given anticoagulants to avoid vascular complications in the recipient and these have not been a problem in our experience. Some units use 5000 units of heparin s.c. 1 h before the operation and at 12 h intervals for the next 5–7 days. In addition some institute Warfarin after 3 days. At the beginning of the operation we insert a Foley catheter, connected to a

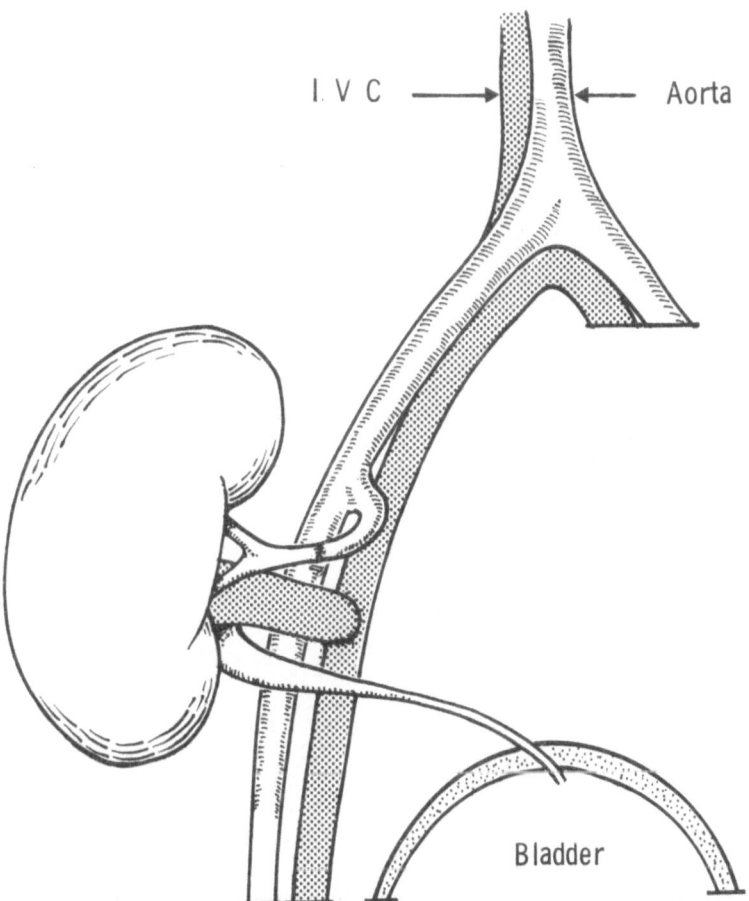

Figure 2 The most commonly employed technique of renal transplantation. The renal artery is anastomosed to the internal iliac artery and the renal vein to the external iliac vein. The ureter is implanted into the bladder

closed irrigating system so the bladder can be filled at the appropriate time for bladder dissection. Others merely irrigate the bladder, or fill it and withdraw or spigot the catheter.

In preference we use the right iliac fossa for the first transplant; the left for a second. The iliac vessels are exposed retroperitoneally through an oblique

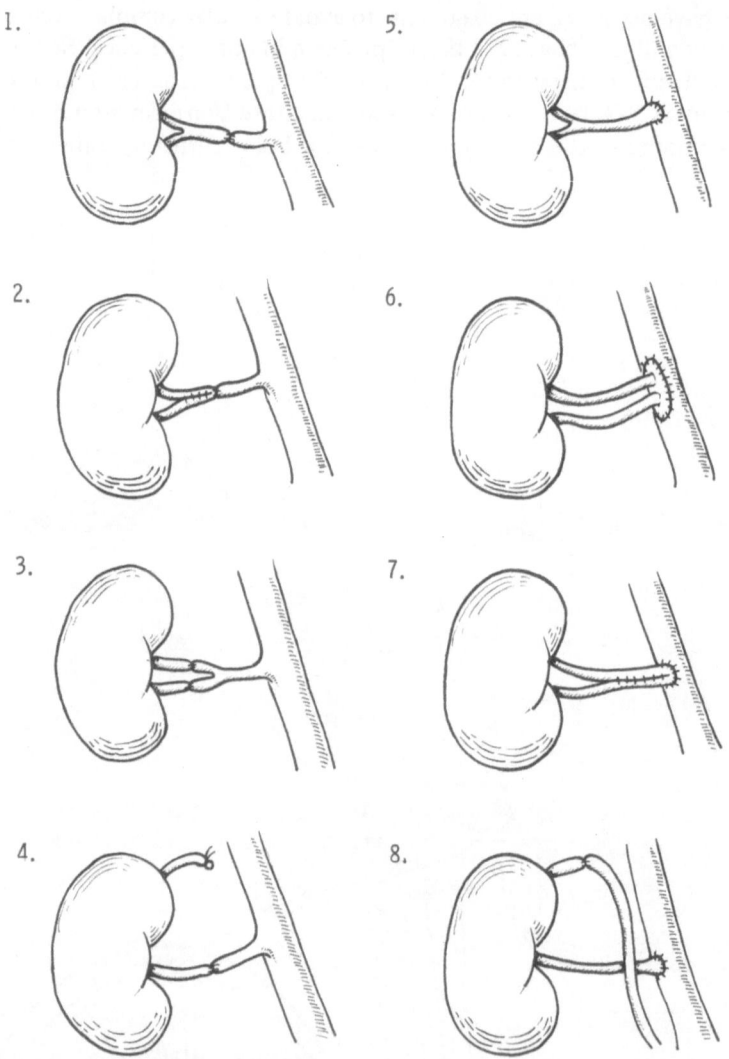

Figure 3   Methods for anastomosing multiple renal vessels. (1) Internal iliac end-to-end with renal artery. (2) Two renal arteries pantalooned. (3) Two renal arteries to branches of the internal iliac. (4) Ligation of *small* polar vessel. (5) External iliac and renal artery end-to-side. (6) Patch on external iliac. (7) Renal arteries pantalooned and joined to side external iliac. (8) Polar vessel to inferior epigastric artery

lower quadrant muscle-cutting incision; all lymphocyte vessels are diathermized or ligated to prevent lymphocoele. I usually ligate the inferior epigastric vessel (unless they are required for a polar anastomosis). In the male the spermatic cord is carefully preserved. We anastomose the artery first with 6/O Ethiflex and an everting suture. Out of choice, I usually anastomose the renal artery to the divided internal iliac artery. When a vascular patch is available, or the internal iliac artery is unsuitable, the end of the renal artery can be anastomosed to the side of the external iliac artery. A variety of techniques are available to deal with multiple vessels (Figure 3). Occasionally endarterectomy of the recipient arteries is necessary. I no longer undertake capsulotomy of the kidney. We then anastomose the renal vein with 5/O Ethiflex end-to-end to the external iliac vein.

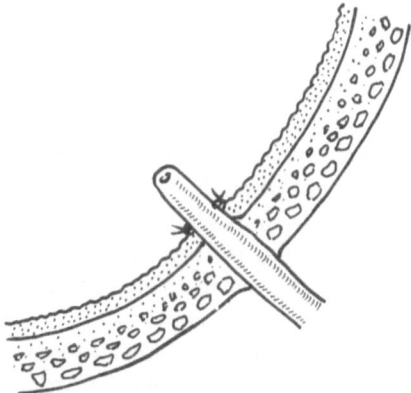

Figure 4   A simple method of ureteroneocystostomy. Tip of transplant ureter protruding into bladder lumen. Free segment should be 1 cm in length

Most centres connect the ureters by ureteroneocystotomy, passing the ureter behind the vas, and a variety of techniques are available for anastomosing ureter and bladder. We fill the bladder with saline containing antibiotic through the indwelling catheter and then use an anterior cystotomy and a simple 'drop-in' technique (Figure 4). The adventitia of ureter is fixed to the bladder mucosa with interrupted 4/O Dexon sutures. The cystotomy is closed in two layers. Some units use a Leadbetter-Politano technique, others a hooded cuff and others a bifurcated ureter. A few centres still prefer uretero-ureterostomy as a primary procedure. Splinting of the ureter is used by some. I usually drain the wound by vacuum drainage, but some surgeons prefer not to employ drainage. Topical antibiotics are also a matter of choice.

Postoperative management

Postoperative management is far simpler in patients having postoperative diuresis. The essence of fluid replacement is to regard blood loss and the replacement of other fluids as totally separate. Blood is replaced as necessary. Other fluids are balanced in the usual way, allowing for insensible loss. Replacement is judged hourly, dependent on the urinary output. Occasionally there is a massive diuresis, due both to the osmotic diuretic effects of urea and partial tubal damage. In this situation it is better to replace only 75% of the fluid loss or a continuing forced diuresis will occur.

Patients with anuria are more difficult to manage. Blood replacement, using a CVP line for assessment, should be complete, but electrolytic fluids should be restricted to the normal levels on dialysis. Dialysis may be required. If the peritoneum is intact, peritoneal dialysis may suffice, but if catabolism is great, haemodialysis may be preferred.

A sudden decline in urinary output or anuria in a kidney that was secreting at operation may result from catheter or ureteric obstruction due to a blood clot. Stenosis or twisting of the ureter are other causes. Vascular occlusion will also cause anuria. Renal scans, ultrasound, urography or arteriography may all help to make the diagnosis, but laparotomy may be indicated. If a cadaver kidney has failed to work in 2 weeks, we undertake open or closed renal biopsy to differentiate severe ATN rejection or infarction.

Drains, if present, are moved when they stop draining – usually by 48 h. Bladder catheters are left between 3 and 14 days. Catheter spasms may necessitate administration of antispasmodics or early removal of the catheter. If the ureter is splinted transvesically it is our policy to remove them at 7 days and the bladder catheter 4 days later.

The question of where and how long to intensively nurse the patient is a contentious one. Reverse barrier nursing, special wards, or cubicles on the open ward are variously used. Local facilities may govern the decision. Close observation and careful nursing is imperative. Oral fluids and food are given as soon as bowel sounds are heard. We encourage early ambulation and physiotherapy. Regular observations of blood pressure, pulse and CVP appropriate to any major operation is required. Any rise of temperature necessitates an extensive search for infection, including blood cultures. It is wise to measure the serum potassium 3–4 h after completion of the operation and then daily estimates of blood and urinary electrolytes are necessary. Throughout this period the existing vascular access sites must be protected for later dialysis may still be necessary. Particularly a limb with a functioning arteriovenous fistula should not be used for pressure measurements or for intravenous infusion.

Follow-up care

The frequency of post-transplant hospital visits varies greatly, dependent on hospital policy, the well-being of the patient and the duration of hospitalization. Certainly attendance three times weekly for the first 6–8 weeks, followed by weekly visits for a further 2 months, would seem to be necessary. Thereafter attendance depends upon the progress of the patient but even well patients should attend 3-monthly for the first 2 years. After 5 years an annual check is adequate. Each visit should include a history, a physical examination as well as measurements of blood pressure, full blood count and measurement of plasma creatinine, blood urea and electrolytes. Urine should be analysed, microscoped and cultured. Patients should be urged to attend the clinic at any time if a change in health occurs.

Prophylactic immunosuppression

The key to success in transplantation is an understanding of the application and correct use of immunosuppressive drugs. The mainstays of immunosuppressive therapy are steroids and corticosteroids. Despite the importance, practice varies widely: McGeowan[51] reviewed the method of immunosuppression used in 16 centres in the United Kingdom, carrying out a total of 957 grafts. The dose of azathioprine given at the time of transplantation varied from 1 to 5 mg/kg body weight, and the dosage did not appear to be a critical factor for graft survival. However, azathioprine should probably be given before the vascular anastomosis is completed. McGeowan found that a dose of 200 mg hydrocortisone given i.v. at operation seemed to be as effective as 1 g predisolone and a total dose of 800 mg hydrocortisone given over the first 24 h was as effective as higher doses. A maintenance dose of 3 mg/kg gave the best results. A dose of 15–20 mg prednisolone was adequate for maintenance of immunosuppression. Higher doses of prednisolone were no more beneficial and had various disadvantages. There is considerable debate as to the rate of decrease of steroids and one commonly employed scheme is shown in Table 2.

Table 2 One commonly employed scheme of immunosuppressive therapy

Period	Prednisone	Azathioprine	Others
Day of transplant	150 mg	5 mg/kg	± methylprednisolone 1 g
First 3–7 days	100 mg/day	2.5 mg/kg or 1 mg/kg*	± radiotherapy 150 r × 4 ± ALG
First 2–4 weeks	75 mg/day 40 mg/day	2.5 mg/kg or 1 mg/kg	± ALG
Second month onwards	30 mg/day 15 mg/day	2.5 mg/kg	

*Azathioprine reduced to 1 mg/kg if the patient develops postoperative oliguria

We now use smaller doses than these, giving 1 g methylprednisolone i.v. when the anastomoses are complete and then 30 mg prednisolone daily, reducing to a maintenance dose of 15 mg daily within 3 months.

Immunosuppressive drugs are usually necessary for the life of the graft. Steroids may often be stopped in the case of HLA identical sibling transplants but in general both azathioprine and steroids must be maintained, although there are reports of the drugs being stopped without rejection of the graft occurring[52].

In 1961 Reichlung and Kligman[53] proposed the use of alternate-day corticosteroid therapy in an effort to reduce the complication of steroid treatment whilst maintaining therapeutic efficiency. While the 48 h interval between doses was optimal in avoiding adrenal suppression, 72 h or longer was therapeutically ineffective[54]. This policy has been adopted more in the United States of America than in the United Kingdom. Diethelm et al.[55] gradually converted 45 patients with renal allografts from daily to alternate-day prednisolone therapy because of unacceptable side-effects. Eight of the patients developed acute or chronic rejection during or just after completion of the transfer to alternate-day steroid therapy. The use of alternate-day prednisolone therapy is of benefit in reducing the untoward side-effects of corticosteroids but the risk of precipitating allograft rejection is significant.

Corticosteroids exert anti-inflammatory effects; they can kill lymphocytes in vivo and there is good evidence to suggest redistribution of lymphocytes from the circulation of the bone marrow. Steroids are known to suppress antibody responses. The effects are better on the primary response than the secondary, and have maximal effect when given after antigens.

Corticosteroids are associated with significant morbidity arising from a multiplicity of actions relevant to immunosuppression (Table 3). Included amongst these are the development of features of Cushing's syndrome with salt and water retention, hypertension, diabetes and facial changes. More serious complications are the induction of severe osteoporosis and associated vascular necrosis, leading to the collapse of major weight-bearing joints. Facilitation of gastrointestinal ulceration, interference with wound healing through interference with collagen, and increased susceptibility to infection are manifestations of the anti-inflammatory effects of corticosteroids. In children the drugs inhibit skeletal growth.

Azathioprine is a most important drug for immunosuppression but is seldom given alone. It causes thrombocytopenia, and more rarely, liver dysfunction. A decrease of platelets or white cells is best diagnosed by the trend of measurements rather than absolute figures. At this stage we stop azathioprine and only when the white count has increased to 3500 do we recommence it, firstly at half the normal dosage, gradually increasing to the normal level if possible. More recently it has been shown that azathioprine can be stopped permanently if leukopenia occurs. The diagnosis of azathioprine-induced liver disease may be difficult and must be differentiated from infection with cytomegalovirus or other bilary pathology. Cyclophosphamide may be substituted if azathioprine is implicated in liver damage.

Because of these difficulties with azathioprine and steroids, other agents have recently been studied. In experimental studies heterologous anti-lymphocyte serum (ALS) is the most effective agent for the abrogation of cellular immunity. The remarkable ability of ALS to suppress allograft rejection in both small and large animals has generated much enthusiasm for its use in clinical transplantation. Unfortunately, despite its use for several years as an adjuvant immunosuppressive, its clinical effectiveness is still not established. In the United States, of 100 major centres, 67% use it, and half of these thought it to be beneficial[56]. The few controlled clinical trials of the agent have given equivocal results[57].

Table 3 Common side-effects of immunosuppressive drugs

1. Infections: new; latent
2. Bone disease: osteroporosis, avascular necrosis
3. Diabetes
4. Cataracts
5. Gastroduodenal ulceration
6. Pancreatitis
7. Liver dysfunction
8. Malignancy
9. Depression
10. Hypertension

Other agents have also been studied recently. The importance of vascular changes in graft rejection is well established and agents affecting platelet function have been investigated. In experimental allografts, sodium salicylate, acetylsalicylic acid, heparin and dicoumarol all prolong graft survival. In clinical studies, dipyrimadole improved vascular lesions, but did not improve results. Cyprohepadine is a safe antihistamine with antiserotonin activity and appears to be a useful drug when used in combination with convential treatment[58]. The antihelminth, niridazole, has been shown to prolong skin allograft survival in rodents and it is immunosuppressive in man. However, side-effects are common and current studies are directed at finding a non-toxic, immunosuppressive metabolite[59].

Calne[60] has recently emphasized the difficulties of finding suitable laboratory models of immunosuppression relevant to man. Asta 5122, which is a cyclophosphamide derivative, has only marginally superior immunosuppressive activity in dogs with renal allografts compared with cyclophosphamide and is much inferior to azathioprine. It does, however, appear to be useful in clinical practice for liver grafts. Lambda carrageenan, promethazine hydrochloride and azathioprine in combination are slightly immunosuppressive in dogs but disappointing in man. Particular interest has recently been expressed in Cyclosporin A, for in a series of *in vivo*[61,62] and *in vitro*[63] experiments it appears to be powerfully immunosuppressive. Limited experience with patients is very encouraging[12] but controlled clinical trials are now awaited.

There are, however, hazards inherent in immunosuppression itself. It has long been recognized that the humoral antibody response is part of the basic defence mechanism against bacterial invasion. It follows that any agent that depresses the ability of the organisms to respond in this fashion increases the risk of severe and opportunist infections. These include bacteria such as tubercle bacilli, fungi and viruses as well as a number of parasitic nematodes and helminths. Increased susceptibility to infection must be accepted as a direct consequence of non-specific immunosuppression and will manifest itself in proportion to the potency of the agents employed.

Another potential threat is the danger of potentiating malignancy. Recent experimental evidence suggests that immunosuppression alone may not be sufficient to induce the development of malignancy but in the presence of other factors immunosuppression considerably increases the risks of this complication.

Because of the difficulties of pharmacological immunosuppression, the search for a specific form of allogenic unresponsiveness that does not interfere with the remainder of the host's immunological defences is the central goal of transplantation research. The dividing lines between classical tolerance, enhancement and blocking have become increasingly tenuous. Although the classical experiments of Billingham et al.[64] on neonatal tolerance demonstrated the principles involved, approaches which may be now more clinically relevant utilize irradiation and bone-marrow transplantation. Other approaches to specific unresponsiveness involve the use of antisera against tissue incompatibility antigens, but more experimental work is needed before these techniques can be applied routinely to clinical practice.

Blood transfusion before transplantation

Originally most dialysis units restricted the use of blood transfusion in an attempt to reduce presensitization against HLA antigens, the occurrence of HLA antibodies seriously reducing the chance of finding a donor with a negative cross-match. However, in 1973 Opelz et al.[65] found that graft survival was better in those patients who had received blood transfusions when compared with those who had not. By 1977 Opelz and Terasaki[66] were able to compare 756 non-transfused patients with 2169 transfused patients and they found that the results of cadaver transplantation were 20% better in those given blood. The interpretation of these findings is difficult and three explanations exist:

(1) Blood transfusion preselects a group of high immunological responders who form antibodies and are unavailable for transplantation, thus transfusion eliminates immunologically high-risk patients.
(2) Blood transfusion may condition the recipient immunologically.

(3) Patients with chronic renal failure who do not require transfusion may have a more competent immune system because their uraemia is of recent onset or less severe, or for some other reason.

Until the importance of these three factors has been clarified, and until it has been established that transfusion improved the life-expectancy of the whole population with chronic renal failure it seems unwise to transfuse prospective recipients uncritically. Some units, however, have developed a policy of deliberate transfusion.

Diagnosis of rejection

From the clinical standpoint, three types of rejection can be identified: hyperacute, acute and chronic. The distinction is important as only acute rejection is amenable to treatment. Hyperacute rejection is usually evident at the time of transplantation, the kidney becoming blue and flaccid. Biopsy will confirm the diagnosis.

The conventional methods of detecting acute rejection rely on clinical signs and deterioration in standard biochemical estimations of renal function. Clinical features (Table 4) include graft enlargement and tenderness which occurs in 15–20% of cases, but it must be differentiated from abscesses, urine leakage and lymphocele; 60% of patients with rejection develop temperatures and it is frequently relapsing in type. It is essential to exclude local or systemic infection, for increased immunosuppression will exacerbate the infective process. Sodium retention may account for the increased weight gain which is sometimes seen in rejection episodes and it may partly be responsible (together with alterations in renin/angiotensin mechanism) for the hypertension which accompanies rejection in 50% of the patients.

Table 4 Clinical and biological features that signify a rejection episode

1. Enlargement and tenderness of the graft
2. Fever, hypertension and tachycardia
3. Decreased urine volume
4. Oedema and increased weight
5. Protein and lymphocytes in the urine
6. Decreased excretion of urea, creatinine and sodium
7. Rise in blood urea and creatinine, and fall in creatinine clearance

Urine output can be a useful indicator of rejection. Once dehydration has been excluded a persistent drop in urine output occurs in 20% of patients undergoing rejection. However, the most useful indicator of rejection is a rise or more than 20 SI units in the serum creatinine. It is our practice to accept such a rise as evidence for rejection until proven otherwise. However, it be remembered that dehydration, hypertension, urinary tract infection, some drugs (for example, Septrin and cimetidine), recurrence of original disease, ureteric obstruction, urinary leakage and vascular stenosis can all affect creatinine levels. Creatinine clearance is generally less accurate than serum creatinine because of the difficulties of accurate urine collection. Measurements of blood urea are less reliable than serum creatinine for they are affected by immunosuppression and large doses of corticosteroids. In the rare cases where a transplant has been connected to an ileal loop, or an ileal interposition used, urea will be reabsorbed and give an incorrect assessment of renal function[67]. Measurements of urinary urea concentration can be a particularly valuable monitor for a kidney recovering from ATN when the patient is being dialysed. Changes in 24 h urinary protein are neither early nor significant indicators of rejection[68].

A variety of immunological tests have been suggested for the diagnosis of rejection and they include:

(1) Lymphoblast activity in peripheral blood[69,70].
(2) Mixed lymphocyte culture[71].
(3) Leukocyte migration[72,73].
(4) Rosette inhibition[72,74].
(5) Leukocyte aggregation[75].
(6) Adenylcyclase response[76].
(7) Fibrinogen degradation products[77,78].
(8) Complement levels.

Other tests depend upon measurements in the peripheral blood and urine or direct investigation of the graft. Measurements of peripheral white cells or platelets are of no value for diagnosing rejection. Cytological examination of urine gives variable results[80]. A large number of enzymes have been measured in both serum and urine of transplant patients[81] and this approach merits further investigation. Other tests have concentrated on investigating the graft. Angiography[82], renography[83], ultrasound[84] and fibrinogen uptake[85], have all been used. There has been a suggestion that angiography may precipitate a rejection episode[86].

Most of these tests are difficult to perform, and expensive both in time and materials. With several of them, conflicting data have been obtained and with most of them rejection is diagnosed only a short while before the clinical diagnosis has been established. Furthermore, there is little evidence to show that earlier diagnosis of rejection affects the clinical outcome.

If a diagnosis of acute rejection is confirmed it is also important to search for a precipitating cause. It is now well established that cortisol metabolism can be influenced by anticonvulsant therapy[87] and so lead to an increased incidence of rejection[88]. There is also clear association between virus infections and biopsy-proven allograft rejection[89]. No simple explanation is available; it is possible that antigens that cross-react with histocompatibility antigens are expressed during the viral infection so that a response against virus may act against the graft. Some viruses have been shown to produce antigens in infected cells that cross-react with blood group substances. Another possibility is that virus infections induce a state of non-specific immunopotentiation.

The clinical picture of rejection can be mimicked by other events which require completely different treatments, and indeed that can be worsened by anti-rejection therapy. The most important of these is systemic infection. Another rare cause is thrombosis of the venous drainage of the kidney, but it is important because of its potential reversibility. Differential diagnosis from acute rejection is difficult, but a sudden decrease of renal function accompanied by proteinuria, a tender graft and frequency oedema of the upper thigh on the side of the transplant should point to the diagnosis. In renal artery thombosis urine output suddenly stops. Scanning or arteriography confirms the diagnosis. Obstruction of the ureter can simulate rejection. Failure to respond to anti-rejection therapy is an indication for further investigation with urography, ultrasound or retrograde catheterization. Urinary leakage or perirenal haematoma can occasionally simulate rejection. The most difficult time to diagnose acute rejection is during a postoperative period of acute tubular necrosis resulting from prolonged warm ischaemia. During this anuric phase the diagnosis of supervening rejection may be difficult. Scintiscanning and uptake of labelled fibrinogen may be useful. Tubular necrosis rarely occurs after renal function has been established, and any deterioration in this situation should be regarded as being due to rejection.

The value of renal biopsy in the diagnosis and prognosis of rejection is a contentious one. Some centres perform needle biopsies of transplants routinely and alter immunosupressive therapy according to their findings. Williams[90] biopsied all grafted kidneys at 1, 6 and 12 months, irrespective of the presence or absence of rejection. He found that even normally functioning grafts display many of the features of rejection and if anti-rejection treatment was given on the basis of histological findings it would require that the majority of patients are treated. In contrast the histological appearances of hyperacute rejection and chronic rejection are characteristic.

A different viewpoint is expressed by Frikelstein et al.[91] who partially quantified the histological appearances of the graft and predicted response to therapy. They concluded that renal biopsy is both helpful in diagnosing acute rejection and predicting response to therapy. It is our own usual practice to restrict biopsy to the kidneys that have failed to function 2 weeks after grafting, when the differential dignosis of ATN, rejection or mechanical problems may be difficult, or when rejection may have supervened on ATN. Then we either perform a closed-needle or an open biopsy. Renal biopsy is also useful in the later deterioration of renal function when chronic rejection or recurrent disease are possible. Specimens are examined by light, electron and immunofluorescence microscopy.

Treatment of rejection

Whilst occasional grafts may survive hyperacutè rejection if the patient is treated with heparin, we feel that allograft nephrectomy is the treatment of choice, once the diagnosis has been confirmed. Patients with this type of rejection are systemically ill and accompanying leukopenia and thrombocytopenia due to consumption coagulopathy can be fatal[92].

Acute rejection episodes are usually controlled by increased dosage of steroid, with or without the addition of actinomycin and/or local irradiation of the graft[51] (Table 5). An increase in steriod dose seemed to be more helpful in the treatment of rejection than an increase in azathioprine or the addition of other cytotoxic agents. Some centres advocate daily i.v. infusion of solu-Medrol for 3–5 days. Others employ increased amounts of oral prednisolone, giving as much as 200–400 mg on the first day and tapering this to maintenance levels. We believe these methods to be interchangeable. A comparative study of 50 rejection episodes treated by oral therapy and 49 by i.v. methylprednisolone showed both treatments achieved reversal of rejection in 60% of episodes[93]. Hypertension, oliguria, fluid retention and infection tended to be greater after oral treatment.

Table 5 Treatment of rejection

Treatment	Dose
Prednisone	200 mg/day for 3 days
Methylprednisolone	1 g 12-hourly for three doses
Actinomycin C	200 µg/day for 3 days
Local radiotherapy	150 r on alternate days × 4
ALG	
Heparin	
Plasmapheresis	

Drugs that can be used for treatment of rejection episodes. Usually large doses of steroids are given with or without one of the other agents

There was no evidence that i.v. methylprednisolone was nephrotoxic. However, there were no long-term studies, and our own impression was that avascular necrosis increased during a period when i.v. therapy was used. We do not use prophylactic antacids during high-dose steroid therapy but we do give oral Nystatin during this period. Irradiation of the graft with 150 R on three consecutive or alternate days is sometimes used. This may be employed to a total of three courses (3 × 450 R) if further rejection episodes occur. Occasionally actinomycin C and D, acetylsalicylic acid, heparin or antihistamines are used in the treatment of rejection.

Chronic rejection is difficult to treat. Occasionally the condition responds to steroid therapy and an increase may stabilize renal function. Some transplants may last several years with very slow deterioration, whereas others lose function in 1–2 months and the patients return to dialysis. The value of plasmapheresis in the treatment of allograft rejection has yet to be determined.

Allograft nephrectomy

The indication for removal of failed allografts is not clearly defined. In our own series 39 kidneys were removed within 6 months of transplantation mainly because of primary non-function or acute rejection. Nephrectomy at this time was associated with 7 deaths; 14 operations resulted in complications whereas 17 were trouble-free[94]. Wound infection is the most difficult problem. In addition to two deaths in which sepsis played a major role, 20% became infected after early nephrectomy. In other reported series, infection ranged from 17 to 56%[95,96]. Fifty per cent of our cases which developed postoperative sepsis had significant infection of the graft or urinary tract before nephrectomy. Contributory causes of infection may be early haemodialysis causing haematomas, difficulty in closing the dead space, and poor immunological resistance of the patient.

The definite indications for early graft removal include local and systemic signs and symptoms related to the graft, such as pain and pyrexia, graft infarction and severe uncontrollable hypertension. These symptoms are most likely to occur soon after non-function of the allograft and early nephrectomy is therefore encouraged in such cases. However, the operations are associated with a high incidence of mortality and morbidity. It is probable that this could be reduced by immediate nephrectomy of all kidneys which fail within 6 months of transplantation.

The indication for removal of kidneys which fail more than 6 months after transplantation is debatable[97]. In our series there were no deaths when nephrectomy was performed more than 6 months after transplantation. Haemorrhage at operation was the most critical complication.

We leave most chronically rejected kidneys *in situ*, as they frequently contribute to the excretion of fluids, and a similar policy is adopted by Gustagsson *et al.*[98] who found that only three out of 28 cases required removal. However, because of the complications of immunosuppression we discontinue this when the patient returns to haemodialysis. In contrast, Najarian maintains his patients on immunosuppressive therapy even after graft failure. It has recently been suggested that the non-functioning transplanted kidneys produce erythropoietin and that this reduces the need to transfuse patients when they are returned to haemodialysis[97].

When allograft nephrectomy is undertaken, I use an approach through the transplant incision and approach the kidney extraperitoneally. An extracapsular removal is desirable but intracapsular excision is sometimes necessary. Knowledge of the previous vascular anastomosis is important. Previous end-to-end arterial anastomoses are more easily ligated and secondary haemorrhage can be dealt with by simple ligation proximal to the anastomosis. When the kidney has been grafted using end-to-side arterial anastomosis, nephrectomy is more difficult and secondary haemorrhage may necessitate ligation of iliac vessels.

COMPLICATIONS AFTER TRANSPLANTATION

Complications may occur in the early postoperative phase or much later. They can be related to the graft operation or to the immunosuppressive therapy that is required.

Infection

Infection is the most serious and most frequent complication, and it is the commonest cause of death in transplant recipients[99,100]. It is more common in patients with frequent rejection episodes where larger doses of immunosuppression have been required. Prevention is important; infected donors should not be used; recipients with recent infection should not be transplanted and sources of chronic infection should be sought and treated in the potential recipient before patients are considered for grafting. Prophylaxis against infection must begin as soon as a patient is accepted on to a dialysis/transplant programme, particular care being taken of blood access sites and peritoneal catheters.

In the peroperative period there is a particularly high incidence of infection. The graft itself may be the source of Gram-negative enterococci[101], *Histoplasma*[102], *Cryptococcus*[103], *E. coli*, *Staph. aureus*[104], cytomegalovirus[105], and *Candida albicans*[106]. Postoperative renal failure augments the effects of azathioprine and results in hypogammaglobulinaemia or granulocytopenia[107,108]. The difficulty of differentiating infection and rejection has already been described. Bacterial infections often persist despite drainage and appropriate antibiotics. Primary transplant wounds, when otherwise uncomplicated, had an infection rate of 1·7%, but with secondary major operations this increased to 9%[95]. Prevention depends upon measures to reduce the incidence of wound haematomas with particular emphasis on carefully managed regional haemodialysis if this is required. Some workers[95] avoid wound drainage; we prefer a closed vacuum system. Wound infection may be associated with mycotic aneurysm and deep perinephric infections. Perinephric infection requires allograft nephrectomy in 75% of cases.

Diagnosis depends upon careful examination including pelvic and rectal examination. Ultrasound and gallium scanning may contribute to making the diagnosis, but they are not always useful.

Use of prophylactic topical antibiotics such as neomycin has been advocated. Appropriate systemic antibiotics are indicated if there are known foci of infection or if urine cultures are positive. Short courses of peroperative prophylactic antibiotics have recently been used and results are encouraging. Culture of swabs taken from the surface of cadaver kidneys or from the transport medium can be useful for anticipating future infection.

Treatment of wound infection is by early incision and drainage. When generalized infection is suspected, rapid isolation of the infecting agents by aggressive diagnostic tests may be required. Blood cultures should be undertaken repeatedly. In pulmonary infections, sputum cultures are often inadequate as superinfections may cause confusion. Bronchial washings, pleural aspiration or biopsy and lung biopsy give more information[109]. Myerowitz et al.[110] has stressed the importance of the urinary tract as a source of infection and in 15 patients in whom infection developed post-transplant, 19 separate urinary infections occurred within 6 weeks. In six, the organism was also detected in the blood[111]. Pretransplant recipient nephrectomy may be required to eliminate these sources of infection[112,113]. Urinary tract infections occurring more than 3 months after transplantation are less serious. There was no evidence that these infections affected the function of the transplanted kidney and a conservative approach to management is recommended[114]. Serious systemic infections should be treated as soon as bacteraemia is suspected, without waiting for bacteriological confirmation. We used triple therapy with tobramycin, flucloxacillin and metronidazole. With lower doses of corticosteroids, it is to be hoped that infection will be less of a problem[115].

In recent years increasing numbers of cases of Legionnaire's disease have been diagnosed, and some have occurred in transplanted patients with a compromised immune response. The illness usually starts with malaise, muscle aches, headaches and a rapidly rising fever with rigors. During the initial phase there may be chest pain and a productive cough. Flu-like symptoms occur for 2–6 days and may be associated with increasing mental confusion. In several cases, pneumonia develops and is unresponsive to antibiotics except tetracycline or erythromycin.

Listeria monocytogenes is a macroaerobic Gram-positive diphtheroid. Since 1967, when reporting of the disease started in the USA, 15 cases have been reported in transplant patients[116]. Occasional infections also occur in patients on dialysis. Infection after transplantation is usually associated with high cortisone dosage but occurs any time after the operation. Most patients have myalgia, fever and meningitis, but other presentations with septicaemia, conjunctivitis, pericarditis and pneumonia do occur. The majority of patients can be successfully treated with penicillin, but penicillin resistance can occur.

Tuberculosis is one of the more serious complications of renal transplantation. The aetiology of tuberculosis in chronically immunosuppressed patients is believed to be a recrudescence of an old, possibly asymptomatic, disease. Pretransplantation tuberculosis testing is of little help in predicting patients at risk because of anergy. Prophylaxis with isoniazid precipitates liver disease in an unacceptable number of patients[117]. We have found tuberculosis to present as a pyrexia, haematuria, miliary disease and in one case it was diagnosed incidentally when tissue was examined microscopically during parathyroidectomy. Early treatment with modern antituberculous therapy insures good results and immunosuppression can be continued during this time.

Fungal infections, particularly with *Candida albicans* and *Aspergillus fumigatus*, have become less of a problem recently[111,118] probably because of the shorter duration of high-dose corticosteroids. The predisposing causes of these infections are neutropenia, poor graft function and hyperglycaemia[119].

Pneumocystis carinii infection is also associated with high-dose steroid therapy[120]. General fungal and parasitic infections tend to occur several weeks after transplantation, particularly in patients on prolonged or frequent high-dose steroids. Indiscriminate use of broad-spectrum antibiotics predisposes to fungal infections, although modern antibiotics have less tendency to this[121]. Many of the therapeutic agents used against these infections are potentially noxious and unsatisfactory—for example, pentamidine for *Pneumocystis carnii*[122] and amphotericin B for aspergillosis and candidiasis[123]. The majority of renal allograft recipients have evidence of viral infections, usually with cytomegalovirus (CMV) during the 6 months after transplantation. These infections have been associated with various clinical manifestations, such as 'transplantation pneumonia', hepatitis, heterophile-negative infectious hepatitis, retinitis and encephalitis. Frequently the onset of viral infections is accompanied by a clinical illness characterized by fever, leukopenia and renal allograft malfunction[124].

Cytosine arabinoside has been used in treatment for CMV by Fiala *et al.*[125]. They used a continuous intravenous infusion at a mean dose of 35 mg/m² daily for 3–4 days and found side-effects were few and minor in nature. The response of patients with both CMV and herpes infection was satisfactory.

During the past 2 years, improved tissue matching, integrated dialysis and transplantation, and the use of more powerful antibiotics, have improved survival of patients; however, 30–40% of patients still die from infections. The balance between treatment of rejection and the occurrence of infection is precarious and until the ideal immunosuppressive agent or technique is found, it will remain so.

Vascular complications

Arterial thrombosis is usually a postmortem or post-nephrectomy finding with an incidence of 1–2%[126,127]. Predisposing factors are the formation of an intimal flap, multiple vessels, hypercoagulable state, pre-existent renal artery stenosis, complications of arteriography and damage by perfusion canula. Treatment depends primarily on prevention by minimizing predisposing factors. Attempts at thromboembolectomy are probably worthwhile, if the occlusion is less than 24 h.

Venous thrombosis is unusual, ranging from 0·5 to 4%[127,128]. Predisposing causes are angulation of the iliac vein, thrombotic extension from the iliac veins or venous compression by haematoma, lymphocoele, urinary extravasation or oedema of the transplanted kidney. The diagnosis is suggested clinically by oliguria, sudden anuria, graft swelling, proteinuria, haematuria and ipsilateral groin swelling. The diagnosis can be confirmed by exploration or venography. Thrombectomy may restore function. Conservative treatment with heparinization and use of other anticoagulants may stabilize function and reduce proteinuria. The prophylactic use of heparin is a matter for debate, for reduced thrombosis may be countered by increased haematuria and bleeding[128].

Haemorrhage

A massive secondary haemorrhage due to leakage at the anastomosis or rupture of a mycotic aneurysm occurs between 1·9 and 4·4%[129]. Early postoperative bleeding is due to faulty technique or a missed polar vessel. Delayed haemorrhage is usually due to infection. Reconstructive surgery is usually possible with early bleeding, but with delayed haemorrhage nephrectomy is usually necessary. Careful ligation or oversewing is essential to prevent recurrence of the bleeding. We have found it necessary in life-threatening situations to ligate the iliac vessels. Only very rarely does this result in serious ischaemia of the involved limb.

Kidney rupture

This complication occurs in 3·6–6·0%, the majority occurring in the first 4 weeks after transplantation. Severe rejection is probably the major aetiological factor, although ischaemic damage, renal biopsy or preservation damage may contribute. Rupture usually occurs on the convex border of the kidney. The preventive role of capsulotomy at the time of transplant is not clear and it is not fully protective as rupture has been reported in kidneys treated in this way. The clinical presentation is of pain, swelling and vascular collapse. Nephrectomy is the usual treatment.

Lymphocoele

The incidence of lymphocoele varies between 2 and 18% and is probably dependent on the diagnostic techniques used to look for it. It has been reported 1 week to 17 months after transplantation. The most likely cause is leakage from the external iliac chain during vessel mobilization. Presentation is usually as a mass in the region of the transplant and this must be differentiated from a rejecting, obstructed or extravasating kidney. The presentation can be significantly different if the lymphocoele causes secondary obstruction to the ureter, or if it becomes infected or induces hypertension because of the vascular compression. Diagnosis is helped by intravenous pyelography, cystography or ultrasound examination of the pelvis which may delineate a cystic mass. Analysis of the fluid will differentiate a lymphocoele from a urinary leak. Prevention by careful ligation or diathermy of lymph vessels is important. Expectant treatment of lymphocoele is usually successful but active treatment is indicated if complications occur. In such cases, intra-abdominal marsupialization or aspiration may be indicated.

Renal artery stenosis

This occurs in 3–12% of cases. Diagnosis is made angiographically during investigation of hypertension. Sometimes there is erythraemia and in advanced cases deterioration of renal function may occur. Three-quarters of the cases have renal bruit. Aetiological factors include faulty technique, atherosclerosis, angulation of the artery, intimal tears during perfusion or harvesting, and vascular rejection.

We investigate by transplant angiography when hypertension is difficult to control by medication or if deterioration or transplant function occurs despite control of blood pressure. Such cases are the ones which may benefit from surgical correction. Intraluminal dilatation of the stenosis has been reported to be successful in some instances. Surgical correction is best approached transabdominally and involves either excision and reanastomosis, a vein patch, or bypass grafting with vein or synthetic material.

Urological complications

At present urological complications occur in 3–8% of transplanted patients. This represents a steady improvement that can be attributed to improved technique both in kidney harvesting and the transplantation operation.

Vesicocutaneous fistula

The identification of urine in persistent wound leakage can be made by measurement of the creatinine, urea, potassium or sodium concentrations of the discharge. Localization of the leakage is made radiologically, first by cystography. An alternative presentation is with diffuse lower abdominal pain, abdominal distension and a decrease in urinary output. Differentiation from graft rejection, wound infection, lymphocoele, ureteric obstruction and vascular obstruction is important.

In most uraemic, immunosuppressed patients, spontaneous closure rarely occurs and early operative treatment is needed. This complication is best avoided by careful cystotomy closure and adequate catheter drainage.

Ureterocutaneous fistula

The incidence of this complication depends on the method used to establish continuity of the urinary system. Kiser[130] reported 17% leakage following ureteroureteral anastomosis and a 33% incidence following 12 pyeloureteric anastomoses. The complication occurred in only four of 220 allografts when ureteroneocystostomy was used, and this usually results from the ureteric ischaemia following faulty harvesting. Radiological diagnosis is usually made by excluding a bladder leakage during cystography. Pyelography is not particularly helpful unless coexistent obstruction is present. Treatment is by early operation. The continuity of the urinary tract can be re-established by reimplantation of the ureter, a psoas hitch, Boari flap, ureteroureterostomy or ureteropyelostomy. In the latter case I use the extended loin incision and after recipient nephrectomy anastomose the recipient ureter to the transplanted kidney in similar fashion to an Anderson–Hynes operation. Ureteric intubation for 7–10 days is advisable.

Calyceal–cutaneous fistulae

These occur most frequently when multiple arteries are present in the transplanted kidney. They are best avoided by microvascular anastomosis of polar vessels. Diagnosis can be made by pyelography or an area of underperfusion on scanning. Drainage using a rat-tailed nephrostomy tube or other drainage tube for 2–3 weeks may allow closure. Occasionally, polar nephrectomy or omentapexy will be necessary. As with all cases of urinary leakage, it is important to exclude distal obstruction.

Urinary obstruction

Transplanted patients are subject to the common causes of urinary obstruction that occur in the non-transplanted population. In some, urological obstruction may have been the cause of the patient's renal failure, but this would have been diagnosed during dialysis or in the pretransplant assessment.

Ureteric obstruction

This was reported in 8 of 220 patients undergoing ureteroneocystostomy[130]. In the immediate postoperative phase this may be due to ureteric oedema and will resolve spontaneously or by ureteric catheterization. Other early causes of obstruction are due to twisting of the ureter, blood clots or compression. Ureteric necrosis may initially present as stenosis followed by fistula if left untreated.

Later obstruction can be exogenous due to compression by abscess, lymphocoele or periureteric fibrosis. Intrinsic fibrosis may be due to ischaemia or rejection. They are best treated by ureteropyeloplasty or ureteroureterostomy.

Stones in transplanted kidneys

Development of calculi in successful renal allografts is extremely uncommon. We reported three patients who developed calculi. Hypercalcaemia and secondary hyperparathyroidism were present in two cases, urinary stagnation and infection resulting from ureteric stenosis was the cause in the third[131]. Treatment is by usual urological principles.

Urinary tract infection

Urinary tract infection occurs in approximately 75% of patients. It is more common in females than males. Twenty-five per cent of patients will have a urinary infection by the 5th postoperative day[114,132]. A single course of antibiotics will cure more than 40% of patients. Krieger[132] found that unsuccessful transplants were associated with a higher incidence of urinary infections and the organism was usually S. faecalis, whereas successful transplants had a lower incidence of infection, which was usually due to E. coli.

Vesicoureteric reflux

Hamshere[114] found vesicoureteric reflux occurred in 10% of transplanted patients with urinary infection. It has also been shown that graft failure occurred in 14 of 29 refluxing grafts compared with 14% of 90 non-refluxing grafts[133]. Treatment of the reflux is usually conservative with long-term antibiotics and in the absence of infection radiological investigation is not necessary[134].

Hypercalcaemia

In renal failure and after renal transplantation increased serum calcium is common[135]. Elevation may occur immediately after transplantation or be delayed for 6 months[136]. It may be transient or last for several years.

The cause of hypercalcaemia after renal transplantation is a matter for debate. Most attention has been given to secondary hyperparathyroidism for this is a frequent complication of chronic uraemia which lasts for variable periods after grafting[137,138]. In such cases of secondary hyperparathyroidism, the characteristic radiological changes in bone may be absent and the biochemical changes may remain masked until revealed by low serum phosphate levels after transplantation. Phosphate chelating agents, such as aluminium hydroxide, which have been used for prophylaxis against steroid-induced gastrointestinal ulceration, can initiate such hypophosphataemia.

Other factors may contribute to hypercalcaemia. Dominguez et al.[139] have suggested that it is related to improved renal function occurring after transplantation. Certainly, hypercalcaemia is more common in transplanted patients with creatinine clearance greater than 60 ml/min. Others believe that steroids used for immunosuppression may be important, whilst renal tubular acidosis and alteration of vitamin D metabolism in the graft are other possible aetiological factors. Steroids can cause skeletal decalcification and increased urinary clearance of phosphorus with hypophosphataemia. In renal tubular acidosis the urine is alkaline and this facilitates precipitation of calcium phosphate. An increase in hydroxylated metabolites of vitamin D has been reported in renal allograft recipients and this may cause hypercalcaemia by enhancing absorption of calcium from the bowel[140].

Proponents of conservative treatment for hypercalcaemia following transplantation argue for administration of phosphate supplements, at least in the early stages. They believe that low serum calcium levels initiate hyperparathyroidism and hypercalcaemia. If this is true, parathyroidectomy should be reserved for resistant cases and those with evidence of metastatic calcification or secondary bone disease[141].

Established secondary hyperparathyroidism demands parathyroidectomy. Indeed, Leapman[140] advocates early surgery when secondary hyperparathyroidism and recurrent transplant calculi occur.

Bone disease

With improvements in the management of patients undergoing renal transplantation the number of long-term survivors has increased and therefore the number of complications involving the musculoskeletal system has also increased. These complications, may be the most serious long-term problem of patients with successful renal allografts. In our own experience, 22 patients (14·9%) developed orthopaedic complications. The incidence and type of complications are shown in Table 6. Some patients developed more than one complication, the commonest being avascular necrosis of bone which occurred in 14 patients (7·5%) at an average age of 37 years (range 20–61). Nine patients developed avascular necrosis of the femoral head; this was bilateral in six, giving a total of 15 avascular hip joints. One patient was asymptomatic and the condition was discovered on a routine intravenous urogram. In three patients the condition affected the femoral condyle; in one this was bilateral. One patient developed avascular necrosis of one humeral head and another had the condition in the second metatarsal head.

Table 6 Orthopaedic complications of renal transplantation (225 patients)

Complication	Number of patients
Renal osteodystrophy	4
Avascular necrosis of femoral head	9
Avascular necrosis of femoral condyle	3
Avascular necrosis of humeral head	1
Avascular necrosis of metatarsal head	1
Joint effusion	1
Spontaneous rupture of tendo-achilles	1
Spontaneous fracture of thoracic spine and ribs	1
Web space infection	1

Patients usually presented with severe pain and limitation of movement. When a weight-bearing joint was affected pain was often sufficient to make walking – even short distances – difficult. Symptoms usually progressed rapidly. The average interval between transplantation and the development of avascular necrosis was 30 months (range 12/67).

Early radiographic changes were a linear subchondral fracture, often best seen on the lateral view with patchy porosis and sclerosis followed in the later stages by collapse of the femoral head, loss of joint space and a tendency for protrusion acetabulare to occur. A stress fracture of the neck preceded avascular necrosis of the head in one patient. [99Tc]MDP bone scans demonstrated increased activity before radiological changes became apparent, suggesting an increased blood supply and isotope uptake in the femoral head.

Five patients with avascular necrosis of the femoral head responded to 6 months of conservative treatment consisting of regular analgesics, periods of bed-rest and traction. They improved symptomatically and radiographic changes failed to progress. Four patients failed to respond symptomatically to conservative management and progressive joint destruction occurred. These patients were treated surgically by total joint replacement. The bone was found to be unusually soft and bled profusely, and in one patient the femoral component of a prosthesis went through the shaft.

In a single instance the prosthesis loosened due to infection although no organism was isolated, and 2 months after insertion the joint was removed and a Girdlestone excision athroplasty performed – the patient remains pain-free and mobile.

In patients with progressive hip joint destruction despite conservative treatment, we believe that total joint replacement is justifiable when performed early, and although bone appears softer and more vascular than normal there were no particular surgical difficulties in our small group of patients.

Tumours in transplanted recipients

Transplanted cancer

Penn[142] reported 63 patients who received kidneys from donors with cancer; 22 (35%) subsequently developed malignancy. In some, but not all, tumour regression occurred when immunosuppression was stopped[143]. With regard to tumour-bearing donors, it is now considered ethical to use only kidneys from patients with primary intracerebral tumours and low-grade skin cancers. In all cadaver donors it is imperative that a search be made for unsuspected malignancy at the time of donor nephrectomy.

De novo tumours

In patients taking immunosuppressive drugs after renal transplantation there is an increased incidence of tumours. Penn[144] reported an overall corrected incidence of 5·6%; 100 times greater than a normal age-matched population. Tumours appear within a few months up to 13 years after transplantation (average 3 years) at an average patient age of 39·6 years. The distribution of the histological types of these tumours is markedly different from that found in the normal population, for nearly 50% of the tumours were mesenchymal in origin and many were reticulum cell sarcomas and these may be multicentric in origin.

There is also high incidence of skin cancers, particularly in Australia, and these are more aggressive than normal[145]. As well as malignant tumours there is a high incidence of warts. Spencer and Anderson[146] reported an incidence of 42% on transplant recipients. Occasionally these lesions become widespread.

Early diagnosis and treatment is imperative. Cervical dysplasia has been reported to occur more frequently in female transplant patients. The incidence of pre-existing dysplasia is unknown. In our own prospective study[147] of urinary and cervical cytological screenings of 50 transplant patients, two of 38 patients before transplantation had pre-existing dysplasia. No new cases of dysplasia were found during the study (mean surveillance of 3 years). A high incidence of urinary viral infection was found, but a relation to cervical dysplasia was not noted. The increased frequency of cervical abnormalities previously reported might have been due to different immunosuppressive regimes or to failure to exclude pre-existing disease. Despite the low incidence of abnormalities the use of cytological screening provided valuable reassurance to our patients, and its use is recommended.

With skin lesions induced by sunlight, prevention by the use of barrier cream is important. Any persistent skin lesion should be biopsied. Basal cell carcinomas are probably best treated by cryotherapy, radiotherapy or excision. Squamous cell carcinomas are probably best treated by wide local excision (sometimes with skin grafting) and if lymph nodes are involved block dissection is indicated. In general, most localized malignancies have been treated by standard excisional or radiotherapeutic methods. Immunosuppression has been maintained in most patients with localized tumours. When metastases have developed immunosuppressive drugs have been stopped but unfortunately regression has not been reported and kidney rejection invariably occurs.

Hypertension

Although a successful renal allograft may relieve hypertension[148], hypertension after transplantation occurs in 18–83% of patients[149,150]. The maximal incidence occurred 3 months after grafting and remained stable for the next 5 years when it decreased slightly. Patients whose original renal failure was due to hypertensive disease were particularly at risk. Cadaver kidney recipients and those with their own kidneys *in situ* also have a high incidence. Measurement of renal vein renin activity may, or may not, be useful for assessing the contribution of the retained diseased kidney to the high blood pressure[151]. Other causes of hypertension include acute and chronic rejection, expansion of the ECV, prednisone administration, renal artery stenosis or the inadvertent transplantation of a diseased kidney.

The management of hypertension depends upon defining the cause and instituting specific treatment. In other cases combination of a beta-adrenergic blocking agent with a vasodilator and/or a diuretic is usually most effective and best tolerated by the patient.

Hypertension in transplanted patients is probably the main factor leading to the higher incidence of coronory heart disease, cerebrovascular disease, congestive heart failure and occlusive arterial disease.

Alimentary tract complications

A range of complications affecting all parts of the alimentary tract have been reported. They are frequently lethal and are the third major cause of death in transplant recipients. We found that it was not possible to predict those patients who later develop these complications[18].

Upper gastrointestinal tract

Incidence varies from 1 to 22·3% with an average of 10–15%[152,153]. There is 65% mortality for bleeding or perforated ulcers[153]. Diagnosis is usually straightforward and gastroscopy during bleeding is frequently useful. The place of visceral angiography with embolization in these cases is yet to be established. Resuscitation with nasogastric suction and i.v. fluids should be started. Parenteral steroids should be given and azathioprine discontinued if infection or thrombocytopenia is suspected. Early operation is indicated; local lesions should be dealt with, but severe haemorrhage may require gastrectomy, with or without vagotomy and for perforation vagotomy and antrectomy or vagotomy and pyloroplasty. Cimetidine, a histamine H_2-receptor antagonist, is of increasing interest in the treatment of peptic ulcer[154,155]. Rapid symptomatic relief with healing of the ulcer and avoidance of operation has considerable advantages, especially in uraemic or immunosuppressed patients. However, there is some doubt concerning the use of cimetidine in patients with renal transplants. Significant increases in mean plasma creatinine have been reported after administration of the drug[156,157] and this could be confused with graft rejection, though Jones et al.[158] showed no alteration in biochemistry in their patients. Furthermore, agranulocytosis after cimetidine has been described[159] and combination with azathioprine may result in severe bone-marrow toxicity causing azathioprine to be stopped. In mice, H_2-receptor antagonists inhibit histamine-mediated T-lymphocyte cytolysis. Cimetidine also prevents histamine-mediated migration inhibition of immune guinea-pig peritoneal exudate cells[161]. A limited study in humans showed that cimetidine had no effect on mean lymphocyte migration inhibition by BCG and antibody production, but it did cause lower serum concentrations of IgA and IgM in some patients, and increased response to BCG in others[162]. No immunological abnormalities were detected during 2 years of cimetidine treatment of patients with Zollinger-Ellison syndrome[163]. In our own preliminary study[164] we found cimetidine to be of some value in the management of patients who develop peptic ulceration following renal transplantation. The previously reported immunological effects of H_2-receptor antagonists did not appear to provoke allograft rejection. Agranulocytosis was not seen in our patients.

Colonic complications

Diverticulitis, bleeding, ulceration, perforation, acute colitis, gangrenous acute appendicitis, necrotizing enterocolitis and faecal impaction all occur. Incidence ranges from 1·5 to 12% with the average approximating to 6%[165,166]. Mortality is high and for perforation of the colon 75% mortality is common. Diagnosis and resuscitation follow general principles, but early operative treatment is indicated. We have tended to exteriorize the affected loop in the acute phase with a double-barrelled colostomy. However, some centres practise primary treatment with colostomy. Bleeding from the colon requires angiography, conservative treatment initially, and surgery only if this fails.

Pancreatitis

At post-mortem significant pancreatic disease was found in 56% of patients with chronic renal failure requiring haemodialysis[167], although none had a clinical history of the disease.

Pancreatitis was first recognized as a complication of renal transplantation in 1964[168]. Subsequent reports describe an incidence of 2–3%. It has been shown that 53% of these patients with pancreatitis die and a higher mortality for patients who developed pancreatitis later than 3 months after transplantation has been described[169].

The aetiology of pancreatitis in patients with chronic renal failure and those who have undergone transplantation is not clear, but many factors have been suggested. Pancreatic vascular lesions have been noted in animal models of experimental renal diseases. Hyperparathyroidism is another factor, for pancreatitis occurs in 7–12% of patients with primary hyperparathyroidism, and the incidence of hyperparathyroidism following renal transplantation approaches 20%. The association between these two diseases may be explained by an excess ionic calcium ion concentration which accelerates the conversion of trypsinogen or trypsin which promotes pancreatic autodigestion.

Alternatively, calcium may precipitate in pancreatitic juice causing ductal obstruction by calculi. Thirdly local areas of thromboendarteritis and necrosis of pancreatic tissue have been demonstrated after high doses of parathyroid hormone[170]. These include changes due to the hormone itself or high calcium levels that result. It has been suggested that immunosuppressive therapy may cause pancreatitis: azathioprine-induced pancreatitis has been reported[171]. Steroids have been shown to cause the disease in man and animals. In reported autopsies on 108 patients with collagen and haematological disorders, half of whom received steroids, 16 of 44 had pancreatitis in the steroid-treated group but only two in those not receiving the drug[172]. Forty per cent of children with nephrosis treated by steroids had pancreatitis compared with 15% in those who did not receive this treatment. The mechanism by which corticosteroids produce pancreatitis is unknown. Relationship between dosage or duration of therapy and the incidence of pancreatitis has been found[173]. It has also been suggested that pancreatitis may result from 'rejection pancreatitis' in which the host forms antibodies reactive to pancreatic cell surfaces. Two reported cases of haemorrhagic pancreatitis showed severe vascular rejection of the graft and vasculitis in the pancreas[174].

Patients undergoing haemodialysis with renal transplantation have an increased incidence of virus infection. Viral hepatitis, a well-recognized complication in these patients, may in itself cause pancreatitis and the presence of cytomegalovirus in the pancreas has been found but its pathogenic significance is uncertain. Alcohol and hyperlipaemia are other factors which may be important aetiological factors.

Treatment is difficult but we have used supportive therapy including nasogastric suction and intravenous fluids as well as Trasylol 400 000 units 8-hourly for 5 days and glucagon 2 mg 6-hourly for 5 days. Recrudescence of the disease demands further treatment.

Ocular complications

Ocular disorders are unusual but well-recognized complications of chronic renal failure. Those occurring in patients on maintenance haemodialysis have usually been related to disorders of calcium homeostasis and those after renal transplantation to corticosteroids used for immunosuppression. In our experience (Williams and Castro, unpublished) of 215 patients treated by haemodialysis and transplantation, 19 patients had a total of 26 ocular conditions. Seven had conjunctival irritation, nine cataracts and three retinal vein disorders. Specific ocular infections occurred in three, and two had neurological disorders involving the eye; a further two had glaucoma. Astle and Ellis[175] found 39% of their patients developed ocular symptoms requiring ophthalmic consultation. Indeed the incidence of corneal or conjunctival calcification in patients on dialysis has been reported to be as high as 89%[176], so the majority of these must be symptom-free.

The occurrence of cataracts in patients on regular dialysis is now recognized more frequently. Only incidental mention of bilateral posterior subcapsular cataracts occurring in patients on haemodialysis was made in 1966[177] and 1975[178] but it was suggested as a definitive association in 1970[179,180], the latter paper suggesting that calcium phosphate disturbance during dialysis was the aetiological factor. Chronic persistent hypocalcaemia has also been implicated as a cause of cataracts[181]. Cataracts produced by systemic steroid therapy are well documented[182] and most reports describe patients who have been receiving moderate steroid doses for many years. In such reports the earliest cataract was 2 years after beginning steroids but most occurred after 4.

It has been suggested that age is an important factor in the development of posterior subcapsular cataracts. In one series 47% of the patients who developed cataracts were less than 25 years old[183]. In ours, the nine patients ranged from 25 to 53 years (mean of 40). Although steroid-induced cataracts have been reported to be almost always bilateral they were unilateral in three of our patients.

The association between chronic renal failure and retinal vein thrombosis is increasingly recognized. Hypertension is a feature common to both conditions and the concept that venous occlusion is secondary to retinal artery disease has been suggested. Infections are common in immunosuppressed patients and herpetic keratitis or tuberculous choroiditis occur in these patients.

Rehabilitation

The eventual degree of rehabilitation after transplantation depends upon numerous factors, such as the primary disease, the patient's age and general state before transplantation, his employability and his desire to return to a normal life. In considering a candidate for renal transplantation, possible rehabilitation should be a concern. Whilst full activity and a normal life without dietary restriction are the ultimate aims, in high-risk patients a more realistic approach is to achieve a state of health and activity acceptable to the patient.

Both haemodialysis and transplantation cause psychological stress to patients, relatives and medical and nursing staff. Renal transplantation is usually regarded as less stressful than maintenance haemodialysis because there should be less dependency on machines and on nursing, technical and medical staff and family. Nevertheless, patients who have had transplants have to cope with changes of body image due to steroid treatment and the risks and implication of graft rejection. Many of them still have varying degrees of chronic renal failure and associated complications such as hypotension requiring continuous drug treatment. Posnanski et al.[184] examined the quality of life in 18 children and adolescents after renal transplantation. They compared nine patients with good renal function on low doses of steroids with nine who were undergoing intermittent short-term or long-term rejection and were receiving high doses of steroids. Those with a good, functioning renal transplant fared very much better; seven of the nine were at school or work full-time. De Nour and Shanan[185] compared the quality of life in 20 patients having dialysis and in 11 patients with transplants. Vocational rehabilitation was only slightly better in the transplanted patients with no differences in the social activities of the two groups. Nevertheless, two-thirds of the transplanted patients, but only one-third of those on dialysis, were free of psychiatric complications such as anxiety, depression, suicidal tendencies or psychotic symptoms.

Table 7 Assessment of work patterns after treatment of renal failure

Treatment	Number	Percentage of all patients	Medically fit for work				Unable to work	
			Full-time work	Part-time work	Unable to find work	Social benefits exceed salary	Home	Hospital-ized
Hospital dialysis	7606	43.3	36.4	23.0	13.9	13.2	12.2	1.2
Home dialysis	2655	61.8	64.6	12.8	8.6	8.4	5.1	0.5
Living donor transplant	444	57.7	77.9	6.8	4.5	8.6	2.0	0.2
Cadaver donor transplant	2008	55.6	64.7	11.4	7.6	8.0	7.5	0.9

A more objective assessment of rehabilitation is an assessment of employment prospects. Figures analysed by Jacobs et al.[186] are shown in Table 7. It is clear that the best rehabilitation occurs after living-donor transplantation. Almost identical results for full-time employment are obtained after cadaver transplantation and home dialysis. After a successful transplant a patient is restored virtually to a normal life with the proviso that immunosuppressive drugs remain necessary usually during the life of the graft. Steroids may often be stopped in the case of HLA-identical sibling transplants, but in general both azathioprine and steroids must be maintained.

Fertility

Chronic renal failure requiring dialysis or renal transplant therapy is usually preceded by a period of relative infertility in the male and female patient. This is the result of a combination of toxic, endocrine and general ill-health which accompanies the onset of severe renal failure resulting in anaemia, hyperprolactinaemia and loss of libido[187]. After treatment libido is increased in the male and comparative sexual activity is shown in Figure 5. In the female successful transplantation is followed by the restoration of normal renal and endocrine function. This can occur quite rapidly, the hormonal abnormalities can be corrected within a matter of weeks and conception is possible within the first 3 months of a successful transplant. However, there is no doubt that a pregnancy in the first year following transplantation – with its more frequent rejection episodes, higher steroid dose and more frequent complications within the transplanted kidneys – should be avoided.

The first live birth to a transplanted recipient was recorded in the *Montreal Star* on 4 April 1967. Since then there have been many reported. Table 8 shows the number of pregnancies recorded in the *European Dialysis and Transplant Registry* from 1967 to 1977. There is a high incidence of surgical abortion, probably due to the early restoration of normal ovulation and conception, coupled with the anxiety of the transplant surgeons and physicians that a pregnancy might complicate their management in the early months of a successful transplant. It stresses the need for contraceptive advice to be readily available. Management of the pregnancy has been summarized by Parson et al.[188]. Their patients were seen in obstetric and transplant clinics, and immunosuppression with oral prednisone and azathioprine was continued throughout pregnancy. Supplements of folic acid, iron and vitamins were given, and one patient with hypoparathyroidism received vitamin D 1α-hydroxycholecalciferol throughout pregnancy. Patients were seen monthly in the first two trimesters but as often as weekly in the last few weeks. Weight, blood pressure, urinary protein and oestriol were estimated regularly with the usual blood counts and electrolytes. Ultrasound in the last trimester monitored fetal growth. Vaginal delivery is now considered to be the norm.

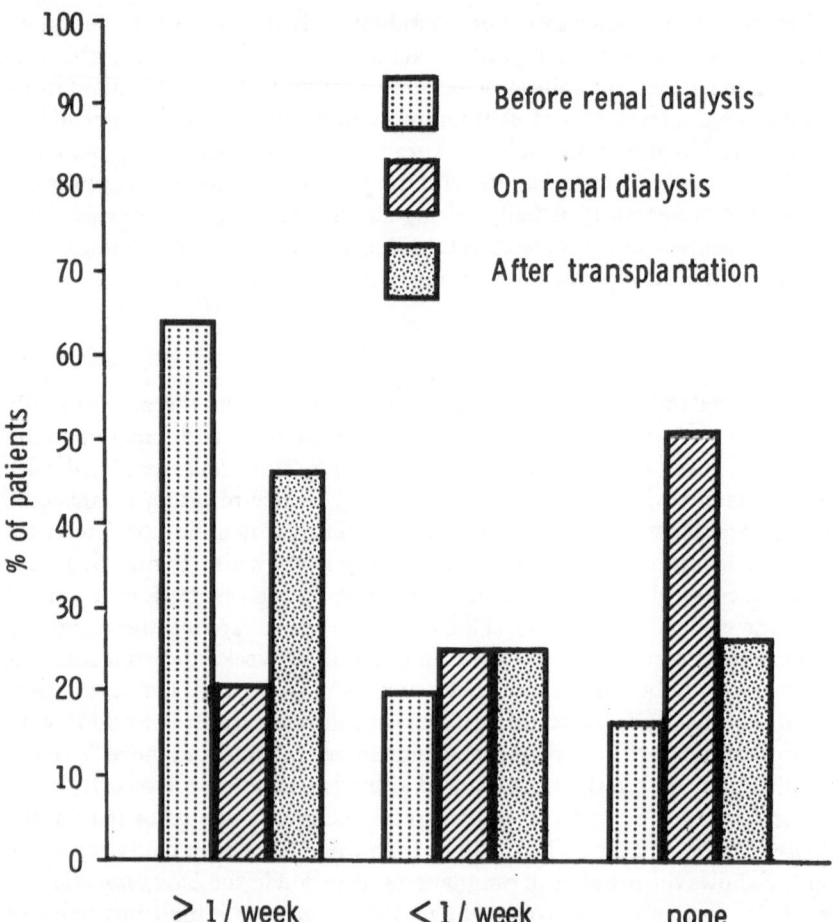

Figure 5   Male sexual function: frequency of coitus (after Salvatierra, Fortmann and Belzer (1975), *Urology*, **1**, 64)

Results

The number of truly high-risk patients who undergo renal transplantation greatly influences the results of any centre. Many factors will influence the successful outcome for a particular individual. The underlying cause of renal failure, age of recipient, age of donor, tissue matching and the centre performing the transplant operation are all relevant factors.

These are clearly documented in detail in the reports of the *ACS/NIH Transplant Registry*, the *Proceedings of the European Dialysis and Transplant Association* and the publication of the NOMS, Bristol. Some indication of graft and patient survival is given in Table 9. Individual units have reported

Table 8 Pregnancies in transplanted and dialysed women documented by the EDTA in 1967–77

Mode of treatment	Live births		Abortions		Pregnant on 31 December 1977
	Normal child	Abnormal child	Surgical	Spontaneous	
Transplanted	75*	4	57	16	18
Dialysed	15	1	45	54	1

*Includes two pairs of normal twins and two patients with two separate pregnancies

significantly better results[189,190]. It is to be hoped that with the introduction of new immunosuppressive agents and improved tissue matching, results will improve still further. Perhaps the real key to future success will be the ability to selectively manipulate the immune response so that the body will accept foreign tissue grafts, yet maintain its own protective barriers. The possibility of transplanting almost every organ could then be considered.

Table 9 Actuarial graft and patient survival related to donor source

Donors	Year of transplant	Sample size	Percentage graft survival			Percentage patient survival		
			1 year	3 years	5 years	1 year	3 years	5 years
Sibling	1968	203	80	71	62	88	80	73
Parent	1968	208	73	60	51	80	72	66
Cadaver	1968	649	48	35	30	59	47	43

Adapted from 12th report of the ACS/NIH Transplant Registry, 1975.

Economics

It is generally accepted that successful renal transplantation as a routine therapy for end-stage renal failure has various medical advantages over chronic haemodialysis. The economic problems faced by government require optimal allocation of funds in different public-spending areas. Comparisons of costs of different methods of treatment for chronic renal failure show considerable differences in favour of transplantation.

Although cost factors vary considerably in different centres and in different countries, there is no doubt that a successful kidney graft is the least expensive. In the United States an uncomplicated case can be undertaken for between £8000 and £11 000 (including donor and short-term dialysis expenses). The initial year's cost of in-centre dialysis may run from £8000 to £16 000, excluding multiple hospitalizations if complications occur. These high costs continue through the ensuing years, whilst follow-up costs for a transplanted patient are minimal. Home dialysis is considerably less expensive than hospital dialysis after the initial purchase and installation of equipment and training. However, the continuing costs exceed those for transplantation. For both dialysis and transplant patients, costs can become astronomical when complications develop[191].

In Holland[192] renal transplantation, including 12 months of postoperative care, requires £10 000 whereas 1 year of chronic in-centre haemodialysis costs £15 000. The cost of a patient with a well-functioning graft does not exceed £1500 per year. There have been few comparative studies in the United Kingdom, but unpublished data (Parsons and Glass, 1970) estimate a successful transplant operation to cost £1750 with monthly maintenance costs of £100. In home dialysis, capital costs average from £5000 to £6000 with additional monthly maintenance of £500. The monthly cost of hospital dialysis is £900.

However, dialysis and transplantation are complementary to each other and the best usage of resources and the best clinical results can be obtained by an integrated programme of dialysis and transplantation. The major objective is to achieve a successful transplant, using dialysis to maintain patients who are awaiting transplantation and those who are, at present, unable to undergo transplantation for medical and immunological reasons.

The central question is whether these relatively high costs to treat end-stage renal failure are justified. The patients are usually young, with dependents. Treatment offers a real chance of re-establishing a fully productive member of society. The results of patient survival are now excellent, and improving. It has frequently been pointed out that treating patients who have terminal renal failure by means of dialysis and transplantation is far better than can be achieved for many cancers.

Paediatric renal transplantation

The incidence of end-stage renal failure in children is unknown and depends upon the criteria used to define children – be it age alone, or assessment of physical and psychological maturity which may be retarded in children with renal failure. Estimation of incidence may vary between one and five children per million population per year[193,194]. There is a higher incidence of congenital malformations of the urogenital tract, renal hyperplasia and hereditary neuropathies than found in adults. The factors which determine the acceptance of a child on to a transplant programme are similar to those for adults, although careful assessment of multisystem disease and psychological assessment will be necessary. The lowest age for transplantation is unclear. Some clinicians only accept patients over the age of 5. However, encouraging results for the age group 1–5 by Mauer et al.[195] and Fine[196] have been reported. Few attempts have been made to transplant infants below 1 year of age, and a conservative approach should be generally accepted.

Choice of donor

Either live or cadaver grafts can be used, and similar factors to those applicable to adults are relevant to paediatric transplantation. Kidneys from adults may be used in recipients aged 2 and above and weighing more than 10 kg[197]. In younger children a kidney from a paediatric donor is preferred. The operative technique is similar to that used in adults for most cases, but Starzl et al.[198] recommended a transperitoneal approach in young children, anastomosing the renal vein and artery to the vena cava and aorta.

Immunosuppression

Corticosteroids and azathioprine are the usual drugs used for immuno-suppression. Dosage schedules used by Fine[199] are shown in Table 10. If the graft is functioning adequately 1 year after transplantation then alternate-day corticosteroid can be used. Two and a quarter times the normal daily dose is given on alternate days in order to minimize side-effects and maxi-mize growth. Such treatment does not adversely affect graft function and survival.

Acute rejection episodes can be treated with pulse doses of i.v. methyl-prednisolone. Each treatment consists of three daily infusions of 30 mg/kg.

Table 10 Immunosuppression used in paediatric recipients

AZATHIOPRINE AND PREDNISONE DOSAGES AFTER RENAL TRANSPLANTATION

Time	Azathioprine ($mg\ kg^{-1}\ day^{-1}$)	Prednisone ($mg\ kg^{-1}\ day^{-1}$)
Preoperative (3 days)	2–3	3
Postoperative	2–3	3
with oligo-anuria	0·5–1	3
Rejection		
acute	2–3	30×3 days (i.v.)
chronic	0·5–2	–

PREDNISONE DOSAGES ($mg\ kg^{-1}\ day^{-1}$) AFTER
RENAL TRANSPLANTATION

Time post-transplant	Patient weight (kg)			
	<20	20–35	35–50	>50
3 weeks	2	2	2	2
6 weeks	1	1	1	1
9 weeks	0·5	0·5	0·5	0·5
6 months	10	12·5	15	20
1 year	7·5	10	12·5	15

Details from Ref. 193, p. 362.

The serum creatinine may continue to rise during therapy, only reducing 4–5 days after treatment. Severe rejection episodes may require two or three treatment courses over a 2-week period. Chronic rejection is not amenable to treatment.

Growth

Failure of children to grow after transplantation is a serious problem. Failure to grow accompanies chronic renal failure and this fails to respond to adequate haemodialysis. The factors inhibiting normal growth after successful transplantation are not clear; corticosteroids and decreased allograft function certainly contribute. No growth should be expected in a patient whose bone age is > 12 years at the time of transplantation. In recipients with a bone age of < 12 years, alternate-day steroid therapy may be associated with normal growth in 40–60%. The status of the allograft also influences growth after transplantation. Significant reduction of growth accompanies only slight to moderate reduction in graft function.

Results

The results of paediatric transplants are not dissimilar to those for adults and, indeed, may be better. Live-donor parent grafts give better results at all ages – approximately 60% functioning at 3 years – but more surprising is good functional survival in children aged 0–5 years, where 53% of grafts were functioning at 3 years. Results of cadaver grafts in this particular group are not satisfactory, only 15% functioning at 3 years. Half of the children receiving cadaver transplants are dead by 3 years. However, the results of units more experienced in treating children are significantly better[199], and if the success is measured by survival of the patient, children above the age of 5 years undergoing all forms of transplantation achieve greater success than any adult age group. The long-term survival of a child with a transplant remains in doubt, but despite this, approximately 1700 transplants have been undertaken in children below the age of 16 years.

The quality of life achieved is difficult to quantify and it is this aspect that is used to question the value of transplantation in children. However, 80% of transplanted children return to full school activity. Severe problems remain, particularly regarding bone disease, sexual motivation and psychological adjustment[200]. Most children adapt psychologically within 1 year of transplantation if the transplant is successful. The specific attributes of the child that correlate with poor psychological adaptation, especially non-compliance, are poor school performance, pre-existing emotional problems and low self-esteem. Factors in the family associated with poor adaptation are low income, single-parent families and poor communication among family members.

The problems associated with paediatric renal transplantation can only be resolved by the passage of time and a great deal of careful investigation. Many of the children currently being treated should be alive to benefit from the technical and immunological advances which are currently being developed in the laboratory. At the present time, results for treating paediatric renal failure are superior to the treatment of childhood malignancies including leukaemia.

References

1 Hume, D. M., Merrill, J. P., Miller, B. F. and Thorn, G. W. (1955). Experiences with renal homotransplantation in human: report of nine cases. *J. Clin. Invest.*, **34**, 327

2 Dempster, W. J. (1953). Kidney homotransplantation. *Br. J. Surg.*, **40**, 447

3 Hamburger, J., Vaysse, J., Crosnier, J., Tubiana, M., Lalanne, C. M., Antoine, B., Auvert, J., Soulier, J. P., Dormont, J., Salmon, C., Maisonnet, M. and Amiel, J. L. (1959). Transplantation of a kidney between non-monozygotic twins after irradiation of the recipient. *Lyon Med.*, **92**, 297

4 Branch, R. A., Clark, G. W., Cochrane, A. L. *et al.* (1971). Incidence of uraemia and requirements for maintenance haemodialysis. *Br. Med. J.*, **1**, 249

5 Pendreigh, D. M., Heasman, M. A., Howitt, L. F., Kennedy, A. C., MacDougal, A. I., MacLeod, M., Robson, J. S. and Stewart, W. K. (1972). Survey of chronic renal failure in Scotland. *Lancet*, **1**, 304

6 Najarian, J. S., Sutherland, D. E. R. and Simmons, R. L. (1978). In Friedman, E. A. (ed.). *Strategy in Renal Failure.* (New York)

7 Joint Scandinavian Report (1978). Renal transplantation in insulin-dependent diabetics. A joint Scandinavian report. *Lancet*, **2**, 915

8 Triger, D. R., Joekes, A. M. (1973). Renal amyloidosis: a 14-year follow-up. *Q. J. Med.*, **42**, 15

9 Kennedy, C. L. and Castro, J. E. (1977). Transplantation for renal amyloidosis. *Transplantation*, **24**, 382

10 Richardson, J. A. (1973). Haemodialysis and kidney transplantation for renal failure from scleroderma. *Arthritis Rheum.*, **16**, 265

11 Penn, I. (1976). Second malignant neoplasms associated with immunosuppressive medications. *Cancer*, **37**, 1024

12 Calne, R. Y. (1980). Transplant surgery: current status. *Br. J. Surg.*, **67**, 765

13 Peterson, G. J., Danielson, B. and Raij, L. (1976). Renal transplantation in Lindau von Hippel disease. *Ann. Intern. Med.*, **85**, 99

14 Matthews, T. H., Matthews, D. C., Hobbs, J. B. *et. al.* (1975). Glomerular lesions after renal transplantation. *Am. J. Med.*, **59**, 177

15 Cameron, J. S. and Turner, D. R. (1977). Recurrent glomerulonephritis in allografted kidneys. *Clin. Nephrol.*, **7**, 47

16 Chatterjee, S. N., Payne, J. E., Bischel, M. D. *et al.* (1974). Successful renal transplantation in hepatitis B antigen positive patients. *N. Engl. J. Med.*, **291**, 54

17 Castro, J. E., Mustapha, N., Mee, D. and Shackman, R. (1975). Ileal urinary diversion in patients with renal transplants. *Br. J. Urol.*, **47**, 603

18 Chisholm, G. D., Mee, A. D., Williams, G. and Castro, J. E. (1977). Peptic ulceration, gastric secretion and renal transplantation. *Br. Med. J.*, **1**, 1660

19 Vertes, V., Cangiano, J. L., Berman, L. B. *et al.* (1969). Hypertension in end-stage renal disease. *N. Engl. J. Med.*, **280**, 978

20 Weidmann, P., Maxwell, M. H., Lupu, A. N., Lewin, A. J. and Massry, S. G. (1971). Plasma renin activity and blood pressure in terminal renal failure. *N. Engl. J. Med.*, **285**, 757

21 Lee, C., Neff, M. S., Slifkin, R. F. and Leiter, E. (1978). Bilateral nephrectomy for hypertension in patients with chronic renal failure on a dialysis programme. *J. Urol.*, **119**, 28

22 Aronian, J. M., Stubenbord, W. T., Stensel, K. H., Whitsell, J. and Rubin, A. N. (1973). Bilateral nephrectomy in chronic haemodialysis and renal transplant patients. *Am. J. Surg.*, **126**, 635

23 Mendez, R., Mendez, R. G., Payne, J. E. and Berne, T. V. (1975). Renal transplantation in adult patients with end stage polycystic kidney disease. *Urology*, **5**, 26

24 Mitcheson, H. D., Williams, G. and Castro, J. E. (1977). Clinical aspects of polycystic disease of the kidneys. *Br. Med. J.*, **1**, 1196

25 Salaman, J. R. (1976). In Castro, J. E. (ed.). *Immunology for Surgeons*, p. 315. (Lancaster: MTP Press)

26 Boczko, S., Tellis, V. and Veith, F. J. (1978). Transplantation of children's kidneys into adult recipients. *Surg. Gynacol. Obstet.*, **146**, 387

27 Morling, N., Ladefoged, J., Lange, P., Nerstrom, B., Nielson, B., Staub Nielson, L. and Sorensen, B. L. (1975). Kidney transplantation and donorage. *Tiss. Ant.*, **6**, 163

28 Filoso, A. M. and Cho, S. I. (1976). Analysis of 75 discarded cadaver kidneys. *Arch. Surg.*, **111**, 1129

29 Nelson, S. D. and Tovey, G. H. (1964). National organ matching and distribution service. *Br. Med. J.*, **1**, 622

30 Medawar, P. B. and Medwar, J. S. (1977). *The Life Science. Current Ideas of Biology*, p. 8. (London: Wildwood House)

31 Forrester, A. C. (1976). *Health Bulletin (Edinburgh)*, **34**, 199

32 Editorial (1977). *Ann. R. Coll. Surg.*, **59**, 170

33 Morres, B., Clarke, G., Lewis, B. R. and Mallick, N. P. (1976). Public attitudes towards kidney transplantation. *Br. Med. J.*, **1**, 629

34 Jeddolph, N, P. and Chatterjee, S. N. (1978). Legal problems in organ donation. In Chatterjee, S. N. (ed.). *Surg. Clin. N. Am.*, **58** (No. 2)

35 Skegg, P. D. G. (1974). *Medicine, Science and the Law*, **14**, 53

36 Stuart, F. P. (1977). Progress of legal definition of brain death and consent to remove cadaver organs. *Surgery*, **81**, 68

37 Guttmann, R. D., Morehouse, D. D., Meakins, J. L. *et al.* (1978). Donor pre-treatment in an unselected series of cadaver renal allografts. *Kidney Int.*, **13** (Suppl.), 99

38 Zincke, H., Woods, J. E., Khan, A. U. *et al.* (1978). Immunological donor pretreatment in combination with pubatile preservation in cadaveric renal transplantation. *Transplantation*, **26**, 207

39 Dienst, S. G. (1977). Statewide donor pre-treatment study. *Transplant. Proc.*, **9**, 1597

40 Collins, G. M., Bravo Shugarman, M., Terasaki, P. I. *et al.* (1969). Kidney preservation for transplantation initial perfusion and 30 hours in storage. *Lancet*, **2**, 1219

41 Sacks, S. A., Petrisch, P. H. and Kaufman, J. (1973). Canine kidney preservation using a new perfusate. *Lancet*, **1**, 1024

42 Clarke, E. A., Terasaki, P. I., Opelz, G. *et al.* (1974). Cadaver kidney transplant failure at 1 month. *N. Engl. J. Med.*, **291**, 1099

43 Sheil, A. G. R., Boulas, J., Drummond, J. M. *et al.* (1975). A controlled clinical trial of machine perfusion of cadaveric donor renal allografts. *Lancet*, **2**, 287

44 Dvorak, K. J., Braun, W. E., Magnusson, M. O. *et al.* (1976). Effect of high dose methylprednisolone on the isolated perfused canine kidney. *Transplantation*, **21**, 149

45 Cross, D. E., Whittier, F. C., Cuppage, F. E. *et al.* (1974). Hyperacute rejection of renal allografts following pulsatile perfusion with a perfusate containing specific antibody. *Transplantation*, 17, 626

46 Boijsen, E. (1959). Angiographic studies of the anatomy of single and multiple renal arteries. *Acta Radiologica*, Suppl. 183

47 Sherwood, T., Ruutu, M. and Chisholm, G. D. (1978). Renal angiography problems in live kidney donors. *Br. J. Radiol.*, 51, 99

48 McLoughlin, M. G. (1976). Related living donor nephrectomy. *J. Urol.*, 116, 304

49 Smith, M. J. V., (1973). Living kidney donors. *J. Urol.*, 110, 158

50 Edgren, J., Laasonen, L., Kock, B., Brotherus, J. W., Pasternack, A. and Kuhlback, B. (1976). Kidney function and compensatory growth of the kidney in living kidney donors. *Scand. J. Urol. Nephrol.*, 10, 134

51 McGeowan, M. G. (1973). Immunosuppression for kidney transplantation. *Lancet*, 2, 310

52 Sherif, M. H., Yayha, T. and Lee, H. A. (1978). Is azathioprine necessary in renal transplantation? *Lancet*, 1, 118

53 Reichling, G. H. and Kligman, A. M. (1961). Alternate day corticosteroid therapy. *Arch. Dermatol.*, 83, 980

54 Harter, J. G., Reddy, W. J. and Thorn, G. W. (1963). Studies on an intermittent corticosteroid dosage regimen. *N. Engl. J. Med.*, 269, 591

55 Diethelm, A. G., Sterling, W. A., Hartley, M. W. and Morgan, J. M. (1976). Alternate day prednisolone therapy in recipients of renal allografts. *Arch. Surg.*, 3, 867

56 Monaco, A. P., Campion, J.-P. and Kaprick, S. J. (1977). Clinical use of antilymphocyte globulin. *Transplant. Proc.*, 9, 1007

57 Launois, B., Campion, J.-P., Kerbaol, M. and Cartier, F. (1977). Prospective randomized clinical trial in patients with cadaver kidney transplants. *Transplant. Proc.*, 9, 1027

58 Rattiazzi, L. C., Simmons, R. L., Markland, C., Casali, R., Kjellstrand, C. M. and Najarian, J. S. (1977). Use of cyproheptadine in human cadaver transplantation. A controlled randomized prospective study. *Transplant. Proc.*, 9, 985

59 Salaman, J. R., Bird, M., Godfrey, A. M., Jones, B., Millar, D. and Miller, J. (1977). Niridazole as an immunosuppressive agent. *Transplant. Proc.*, 9, 989

60 Calne, R. Y. (1979). Pharmacological immunosuppression in clinical organ grafting. *Clin. Exp. Immunol.*, 35, 1

61 Kostakis, A. J., White, D. J. G. and Calne, R. Y. (1977). Prolongation of the rat heart allograft survival by Cytosporin A. *IRCS Med. Sci.*, 5, 595

62 Calne, R. Y. and White, D. J. G. (1977). Cyclosporin A.—a powerful immunosuppressant in dogs with renal allografts. *IRCS Med. Sci.*, 5, 595

63 Borel, J. F., Feurer, C., Gubler, H. U. *et al.* (1976). Biological effects of Cyclosporin A: a new antilymphocytic agent. *Agents Actions*, 6, 468

64 Billingham, R. E., Brent, L. E. and Medawar, P. B. (1956). Quantitative studies on tissue transplantation immunity. III. Actively acquired tolerance. *Phil. Trans. R. Soc.*, (London), B, 239, 357

65 Opelz, G., Sengar, D. P., Mickey, M. R. *et al.* (1973). Effect of blood transfusion on subsequent kidney transplants. *Transplant. Proc.*, 5, 253

66 Opelz, G. and Terasaki, P. I. (1977). Factors influencing effect of HLA matching on cadaver kidney transplants. *Transplant. Proc.*, 9, 1795

67 Castro, J. E. and Ram, M. (1970). Electrolyte imbalance following ileal urinary diversion. *Br. J. Urol.*, 42, 29

68 Chisholm, G. D., Papadimitriou, M., Kulatilake, A. E. and Shackman, R. (1969). The diagnosis of rejection of renal allotransplants in man. *Lancet*, 1, 904

69 Hersh, E. M., Butler, W. T., Rossen, R. D., Morgan, R. O. and Suki, W. (1977). *In vitro* studies of the human response to organ allografts: appearance and detection of circulating activated lymphocytes. *J. Immunol.*, 107, 571

70 Pauly, J. L., Han, T., Varkarakis, M. J., Sokal, J. E., Sampson, D. and Murphy, G. P. (1973). Leukocyte [^{3}H] thymidine uptake in short-term whole-blood cultures of human and canine renal allograft recipients. *J. Surg. Res.*, 15, 301

71 Hattler, B. G., Rocklin, R. E., Ward, P. A. and Rickles, F. R. (1973). Functional features of lymphocytes recovered from a human renal allograft. *Cell. Immunol.*, 9, 289

72 Wood, R. F. M. and Gray, A. C. (1973). Evaluation of rosette inhibition test in renal transplantation. *Br. Med. J.*, 4, 649

73 Dunningham, T. and Castro, J. E. (1976). Assessment of the leukocyte migration test for predicting renal allograft rejection. *Transplantation*, 22, 18

74 Munro, A., Berwick, M., Manuel, L., Cameron, J. S., Ellis, F. G., Boulton-Jones, M. and Ogg, C. S. (1971). Clinical evaluation of a rosette inhibition test in renal allotransplantation. *Br. Med., J.*, 3, 271

75 Kahan, B. D., Tom, B. H., Mittal, K. K. and Bergan, J. J. (1974). Immunodiagnostic test for transplant rejection. *Lancet*, 1, 37

76 Wood, R. F. M., Alston, W. C., Goudie, R. and Gray, A. C. (1975). Lymphocyte adenylcyclose activity in canine renal transplant rejection. *Transplantation*, 19, 188

77 Naish, P., Peters, D. K. and Shackman, R. (1973). Increased urinary fibrinogen derivatives after renal allotransplantation. *Lancet*, 1, 1280

78 Hall, C. L. Pejhan, N., Thomson, R. W., Dawson-Edwards, P., Barnes, A. D., Robinson, B. H. B., Meynell, M. J. and Blainey, J. D. (1973). Serial estimations of urinary fibrin/fibrinogen degradation products in kidney transplantation. *Br. Med. J.*, 3, 204

79 Yokoyama, T., Torisu, M., Durst, A. L., Schroter, G., Groth, C. G. and Starzl, T. E. (1972). The complement system in renal homograft recipients. *Surgery*, 72, 611

80 Murphy, G. P., Williams, P. D. and Merrin, C. E. (1973). Diagnostic value of lymphocyturia in renal allograft rejection in man. *Urology*, 2, 227

81 Wellwood, J. M., Ellis, B. G., Hall, J. H., Robinson, D. R. and Thompson, A. E. (1973). Early warning of rejection? *Br. Med. J.*, 2, 261

82 Pastershank, S. P., Chow, K. C., Baltzan, M. A. *et al.* (1973). Renal homotransplantation. Angiographic features in first 180 days following surgery. *J. Can. Assoc. Radiol.*, 24, 104

83 Hayes, M. and Moore, T. C. (1972). Early detection of canine renal allograft rejection by reduction in the scan bladder/kidney isotope intensity ratio. *Surgery*, 71, 60

84 Sampson, D., Abramczyk, J. and Murphy, G. P. (1972). Ultrasonic measurement of blood flow changes in canine renal allografts. *J. Surg. Res.*, 12, 388

85 Yeboah, E. D. Chisholm, G. D. Short, M. D. and Petrie, A. (1973). The detection and prediction of acute rejection episodes in human renal transplants using radioactive fibrinogen. *Br. J. Urol.*, 45, 273

86 Heiderman, M., Claes, G. and Nilson, A. E. (1975). The risk of renal allograft rejection following angiography. *Scand. J. Urol. Nephrol.* Suppl. 29, 91

87 Werk, E. E., MacGee, J. and Shohton, L. J. (1964). Effect of diphenylhydantoin on cortisol metabolism in man. *J. Clin. Invest.*, 43, 1824

88 Wassner, S. J., Pennisi, A. J., Malekzaden, M. H. and Fine, R. N. (1976). The adverse effect of anticonvulsant therapy on renal allograft survival. *J. Pediatr.*, 88, 134

89 Lopez, C., Simmons, R. L., Mauer, S. M. *et al.* (1974). Association of renal allograft rejection with virus infections. *Am. J. Med.*, 56, 280

90 Williams, G. M. (1978). Status of renal transplantation today. *Surg. Clin. N. Am.*, 58, 273

91 Finkelstein, F. O., Siegal, N. J., Bastl, N. J., Forrest, J. N. and Kashgarian, M. (1976). Kidney transplant biopsies in the diagnosis and management of acute rejection reaction. *Kidney Int.*, 10, 171

92 Starzl, T. E., Boehmig, H. J., Amemiya, H. *et al.* (1970). Clotting changes including disseminated intravascular coagulation during rapid renal homograft rejection. *N. Engl. J. Med.*, 283, 383

93 Gray, D., Daar, A., Shepherd, H., Oliver, D. O. and Morris, P. J. (1978). Oral versus i.v. high dose steroid treatment of renal allograft rejection. *Lancet*, **1**, 117

94 Sinha, S. N. and Castro, J. E. (1976). Allograft nephrectomy. *Br. J. Urol.*, **48**, 413

95 Schweizer, R. T., Kountz, S. L. and Belzer, F. O. (1973). Wound complications in recipients of renal transplants. *Ann. Surg.*, **117**, 58

96 Moore, T. C. and Hume, D. M. (1969). The period and nature of hazard in clinical renal transplantation: the hazard to patient survival. *Ann. Surg.*, **170**, 1

97 Shapiro, D. J., Blumenkrantz, M. J., Shinaberger, J. H. and Coburn, J. W. (1975). Useful function of 'non-functioning' renal homograft. *Br. Med. J.*, **3**, 140

98 Gustafsson, A., Groth, C. G., Halgrimson, C. G., Penn, I. and Starzl, T. E. (1973). The fate of failed renal homografts retained after transplantation. *Surg. Gynaecol. Obstet.*, **137**, 40

99 Rifkind, D., Marchioro, T. L., Schneck, S. A. and Hill, R. B. (1967). Systemic fungal infections complicating renal transplantation and immunosuppressive therapy. *Am. J. Med.*, **43**, 23

100 Chandler, C., Donckerwoecke, R. A., Brunner, F. P. *et al.* (1977). Combined report on regular dialysis and transplantation of children in Europe, 1976. *Proc. Eur. Dial. Transplant. Assoc.*, **14**, 70

101 McCoy, G. G., Leoning, S., Braun, W. E., Magnusson, M. O., Banowsky, L. H. and McHenry, M. C. (1975). The fate of cadaver renal allografts contaminated before transplantation. *Transplantation*, **20**, 467

102 MacLean, L. D., Dassetor, J. B., Gault, M. H., Oliver, J. A., Inglis, F. G. and MacKinnon, K. J. (1965), Renal homotransplantation using cadaver donors. *Arch. Surg.*, **91**, 228

103 Ooi, B. S., Chen, B. T. M., Lim, C. H., Khoo, O. T. and Chan, K. T. (1971), Survival of a patient transplanted with a kidney infected with *Cryptococcus neoformans*. *Transplantation*, **11**, 428

104 Leigh, D. A. (1969). The outcome of urinary tract infections in patients after human cadaveric renal transplantation. *Br. J. Urol.*, **41**, 406

105 Doig, R. L., Boyd, P. J. and Eykyn, S. (1975). *Staphylococcus aureus* transmitted in transplanted kidneys. *Lancet*, **2**, 243

106 McLeish, K. R., McMurray, S. D., Smith, E. J. and Filo, R. S. (1977). The transmission of *Candida albicans* by cadaveric allografts. *J. Urol.*, **118**, 513

107 Ku, G., Varghese, Z., Fernando, O. N. *et al.* (1973). Serum IgG and renal transplantation. *Br. Med. J.*, **4**, 702

108 Starzl, T. E., Porter, K. A., Husbeg, B. S. *et al.* (1974). Renal homotransplantation. I. *Curr. Probl. Surg.*, **3**, 59

109 Vereerstraeten, P., De Koster, J. P., Vereerstraeten, J. *et al.* (1975). Pulmonary infections after kidney transplantation. *Proc. Eur. Dial. Transplant. Assoc.*, **11**, 300

110 Myerowitz, R. L., Medeiros, A. A. and O'Brien, T. F. (1972). Bacterial infection in renal homotransplant recipients. A study of 53 bacteremic episodes. *Am. J. Med.*, **53**, 308

111 Walker, P. R. and Moorhead, J. F. (1978). Infection in the renal transplant patient. *J. R. Soc. Med.*, **71**, 84

112 Hricko, M., Birtch, A. G., Bennett, A. H. *et al.* (1973). Factors responsible for urinary fistulae in the renal transplant recipient. *Ann. Surg.*, **178**, 609

113 Love, W. B. (1969). Infection complicating organ transplantation. *Southern.Med. J.*, **62**, 1259

114 Hamshere, R. J., Chisholm, G. D. and Shackman, R. (1974). Late urinary tract infection after renal transplantation. *Lancet*, **2**, 793

115 McGeown, M. G., Kennedy, J. A., Laughridge, W. G. *et al.* (1977). One hundred kidney transplants in the Belfast City Hospital. *Lancet*, **2**, 648

116 Ascher, N. L., Simmons, R. L., Marker, S. and Najarian, J. S. (1978). Listeria infection in transplant patients. *Arch. Surg.*, 113, 427

117 Bell, T. J. and Williams, G. B. (1978). Successful treatment of T.B. in renal transplant recipients. *J. R. Soc. Med.*, 71, 265

118 Hall, C. L., Sansom, J. R., Obeid, M. *et al.* (1976). Results of 250 consecutive cadaver kidney transplants. *Br. Med. J.*, 1, 547

119 Anderson, O. S., Tissot, R. G., Cohen, C. and Jonasson, O. (1973). Platelet survival test. An accurate prediction of hyperacute rejection of renal allografts in rabbits. *Transplantation*, 15, 105

120 Rifkind, D. (1976). *Pneumocystis carinii* pneumonia in renal transplant recipients. *Natl. Cancer Inst. Monogr.*, 43, 49

121 Noone, P., Pattison, J. R. and Davies, D. G. (1974). *Postgrad. Med. J.*, 50, Suppl. 7, 9

122 Western, K. A., Perera, D. R. and Schultz, M. G. (1970). Pentamidine isethionate in the treatment of *Pneumocystis carinii*

123 Ultz, J. P. (1963). Chemotherapeutic agents for the systemic mycoses. *N. Eng. J. Med.*, 268, 938

124 Balfour, H. H., Slade, M. S., Kalis, J. M. *et al.* (1977). Viral infections in renal transplant donors and their recipients: a prospective study. *Surgery*, 81, 487

125 Fiala, M., Chow, A. W., Miyasaki, K. *et al.* (1974). Susceptibility of herpes viruses to three nucleoside analogues and their combinations and enhancement of the antiviral effect of acid pH. *J. Infect. Dis.*, 129, 82

126 Goldman, M. H., Vineyard, G. C., Lakes, H. *et al.* (1975). A twenty-year survey of arterial complication of renal transplantation. *Surg. Gynaecol. Obstet.*, 141, 758

127 Vidne, B. A., Leapman, S. B., Butt, K. M. *et al.* (1976). Vascular complications in human renal transplantation. *Surgery*, 79, 77

128 Butt, K. M., Rao, T. K. S., Friedman, E. A. *et al.* (1975). Venous complications of enal transplantation. *Proc. Dial. Transplant. For.*, 5, 77

129 Leapman, A. B. Vidne, B. A., Butt, K. M. *et al.* (1976). Elective and emergency surgery in renal transplant patients. *Ann. Surg.*, 183, 266

130 Kiser, W. S., Hewitt, C. B. and Moutie, J. E. (1971). The surgical complication of renal transplantation. *Surg. Clin. N. Am.*, 51, 1133

131 Lucas, B. St. C. and Castro, J. E. (1978). Calculi in renal transplants. *Br. J. Urol.*, 50, 302

132 Kreiger, J. N., Tapia, L., Stubenbord, W. T. *et al.* (1977). Urinary infection in kidney transplantation. *Urology*, 9, 130

133 Matthews, T. H., Kincaid Smith, P. and Vikraman, P. (1977). Risks of vesicoureteric reflux in the transplanted kidney. *N. Engl. J. Med.*, 297, 414

134 Mitterdorfer, A. J., Williams, G. and Castro, J. E. (1981). Vesicoureteric reflux following renal transplantation; a simple method of ureteric implantation. *Br. J. Urol.*, 53, 111

135 McPhaul, J. J., McIntosh, D. A., Hammond, W. S. and Park, O. K. (1964). Autonomous secondary (renal) parathyroid hyperplasia. *N. Engl. J. Med.*, 271, 1342

136 Wilson, R. E., Bernstein, D. S., Murray, J. E. and Moore, F. D. (1965). Effects of parathyroidectomy and kidney transplantation on renal osteodystrophy. *Am. J. Surg.*, 110, 384

137 Latimer, R. G., Renning, J., Stevens, L. E., Northway, J. D. and Reetsma, K. (1970). Tertiary hyperthyroidism following successful renal allografting. *Ann. Surg.*, 172, 137

138 Johnson, J. W., Hattner, R. S., Hampers, C. L., Bernstein, D. S., Merrill, J. P. and Sherwood, L. M. (1971). Secondary hyperparathyroidism in chronic renal failure. *J. Am. Med. Assoc.*, 215, 478

139 Dominguez, J. M., Mautalen, C. A., Rodo, J. E., Barcat, J. A. and Molins, M. E. C. (1970). Tertiary hyperparathyroidism diagnosed after renal homotransplantation. *Am. J. Med.*, 49, 423

140 Leapman, S. B., Vidne, B. A., Butt, K., Waterhouse, K. and Kountz, S. L. (1976). Nephrolithiasis and nephrocalcinosis after renal transplantation. A case report and review of the literature. *J. Urol.*, **115**, 129

141 Geis, W. P., Poportzer, M. M., Corman, J. L., Halgrimson, C. G., Groth, C. G. and Starzl, T. E. (1973). The diagnosis and treatment of hyperthyroidism after renal homotransplantation. *Surg. Gynaecol. Obstet.*, **137**, 997

142 Penn, I., (1977). Development of cancer as a complication of renal transplantation. *Transplant. Proc.*, **9**, 1121

143 Wilson, R. E., Hager, E. B., Hampers, C. L., Corson, J. M., Merrill, J. P. and Murray, J. E. (1968). *N. Engl. J. Med.*, **278**, 479

144 Penn, I. (1975). The incidence of malignancies in transplant recipients. *Transplant. Proc.*, **7**, 323

145 Marshall, V. C. (1974). Premalignant and malignant skin tumours in immunosuppressed patients. *Transplantation*, **17**, 272

146 Spencer, E. S. and Anderson, H. K. (1970). Clinically evident non-terminal infections with herpes virus and the wart virus in immunosuppressed renal allograft recipients. *Br. Med. J.*, **3**, 251

147 Ingoldby, C. J. H., McWhinney, N. A., Wachtel, E. and Castro, J. E. (1980). Serial urinary and cervical cystological studies in women undergoing renal transplantation. *J. Clin. Pathol.*, **33**, 990

148 Kolff, W. J., Nakamoto, S., Poutasse, E. F., Stratton, R. A. and Figneroa, J. E. (1964). Effect of bilateral nephrectomy and kidney transplantation on hypertension in man. *Circulation*, **29, 30**, Suppl. 1123–7

149 Papadimitriou, M., Chisholm, G. D. and Shackman, R. (1969). Hypertension in patients on regular haemodialysis and after renal allotransplantation. *Lancet*, **1**, 902

150 Bachy, C., Alexandres, G. P. J. and Ypersele de Strihou, C. Van (1976). Hypertension after renal transplantation. *Br. Med. J.*, **2**, 1287

151 Grunfeld, J. P. and Bankir, L. (1976). Méthodes d'étude de la circulation intrarénale. *J. Urol. Nephrol. (Paris)*, **82**, 727

152 Kuhlback, B. and Lilius, P. (1976). Late complications after primary successful transplantation. *Acta Med. Scand.*, **200**, 21

153 Hadjiyannakis, E. J., Smellie, W. A. B., Evans, D. B. *et al.* (1971). Gastrointestinal complication after renal transplantation. *Lancet*, **2**, 781

154 Domschke, W., Domschke, S. and Demling, L. (1977). A double blind study of cimetidine in patients with duodenal ulceration: clinical, kinetic and gastric and pancreatic secretory data. In Barland, W. L. and Simpkins, M. A., (eds.). *Proceedings of the 2nd International Symposium on Histamine H_2—Receptor Antagonists*, pp. 217–33. (Amsterdam: Excerpta Medica)

155 Gillespie, G., Gary, G. R., Smith, I. S. *et al.* (1977). Short term and maintenance cimetidine treatment in severe duodenal ulceration. In Barland, W. L. and Simpkins, M. A. (eds.). *Proceedings of the 2nd International Symposium on Histamine H_2—Receptor Antagonists*, pp. 217–33. (Amsterdam: Excerpta Medica)

156 Blackwood, W. S., Maudgal, D. P., Pickard, R. G. *et al.* (1976). Cimetidine in duodenal ulcer—controlled trial. *Lancet*, **1**, 174

157 Haggie, S. J., Fermont, D. C. and Wyllie, J. H. (1976). Treatment of duodenal ulcer with cimetidine. *Lancet*, **2**, 983

158 Jones, R. H., Rudge, C. J., Bewick, M. *et al.* (1978). Cimetidine: prophylaxis against upper gastrointestinal haemorrhage after renal transplantation. *Br. Med. J.*, **1**, 398

159 Craven, E. R. and Whittington, J. M. (1977). Agranulocytosis four months after cimetidine therapy. *Lancet*, **2**, 294

160 Plaut, M., Lichenstein, L. M., Gillespie, E. *et al.* (1973). Studies on the mechanisms

of lymphocyte mediated cytolysis III. The role of microfilaments and microtubules. *J. Immunol.*, **3**, 89

161 Rocklin, R. E. (1975). Regulation of migration inhibitory factor (MIF) production by histamine receptor-bearing lymphocytes. *Fed. Proc.*, **34**, 977 (abstr. 4296)

162 McGregor, C. G. A., Cochrane, A. J., Ogg, L. J. *et al.* (1977). Immunological and other laboratory studies of patients receiving short term Cimetidine therapy. *Lancet*, **1**, 122

163 De Pauw, B. E., Lamers, C. B. H. E., Wagener, F. J. T. *et al.* (1977). Immunological studies after long term H₂ receptor antagonist therapy. *Lancet*, **2**, 616

164 Williams, G. and Castro, J. E. (1979). Cimetidine in the treatment of peptic ulceration following renal transplantation. *Br. J. Surg.*, **66**, 510

165 Aldrete, J. S., Sterling, W. A., Hathaway, B. M. *et al.* (1975). Gastrointestinal and hepatic complications affecting patients with renal allografts. *Am. J. Surg.*, **29**, 115

166 Powis, S. J. A., Barnes, A. D., Dawson-Edwards, P. *et al.* (1972). Ileocolonic problems after cadaveric renal transplantation. *Br. Med. J.*, **1**, 99

167 Avram, M. M. (1977). High prevalence of pancreatic disease in chronic renal failure. *Nephron.*, **18**, 68

168 Starzl, T. E. (1964). *Experience in Renal Transplantation.* (Philadelphia: W. B. Saunders)

169 Johnson, W. C. and Nabseth, D. C. (1970). Pancreatitis in renal transplantation. *Ann. Surg.*, **171**, 309

170 Heuper, W. (1927). *Arch. Pathol.*, **3**, 14

171 Kawanishi, H., Rudolph, E. and Bull, F. E. (1973). Azathioprine-induced acute pancreatitis. *N. Engl. J. Med.*, **289**, 357

172 Carone, F. A. and Liebow, A. A. (1957). Acute pancreatic lesions in patients treated with ACTH and adrenal corticoids. *N. Engl. J. Med.*, **257**, 690

173 Riemenschneider, T. A., Wilson, J. F. and Vernier, R. L. (1968). Glucocorticoid-induced pancreatitis in children. *Paediatrics*, **41**, 428

174 Tilney, N. L., Collins, J. J. and Wilson, R. E. (1966). Haemorrhagic pancreatitis. A fatal complication of renal transplantation. *N. Engl. J. Med.*, **274**, 1051

175 Astle, J. N. and Ellis, P. P. (1974). Ocular complications in renal transplant patients. *Ann. Ophthalmol.*, **6**, 1269

176 Demco, T. A., McCormick, A. Q. and Richards, J. S. F. (1974). Conjunctival and corneal changes in chronic renal failure. *Can. J. Ophthalmol.*, **57**, 339

177 Abrams, J. D. (1966). Corneal and other ocular findings in patients on intermittent dialysis for renal failure. *Proc. R. Soc. Med.*, **59**, 533

178 Thomson, G. E., Waterhouse, K., McDonald, H. P. and Friedman, E. A. (1967). Haemodialysis for chronic renal failure. *Arch. Intern. Med.*, **120**, 153

179 Straub, W. and Freund, J. (1970). Katarakt Nach extra Rorporaler dialyse behandlung. *Klin. Manatsbl. Augenheilkd.*, **157**, 50

180 Perrini, S., Burschi, E. and Muolo, A. (1970). Cataratta sotto capsulare posteriore come complicanza della terapia emodialitica periodica. *Annali Ottal Clin. Ocul.*, **96**, 111

181 Berlyne, G. M., Benari, J., Danovitch, G. M. and Blumenthal, M. (1972). Cataracts of chronic renal failure. *Lancet*, **1**, 509

182 Giles, C. L., Mason, F. L., Duff, I. F. and McLean, J. A. (1962). The association of cataract formation and systemic corticosteroid therapy. *J. Am. Med. Assoc.*, **182**, 719

183 Berkowitz, J. S., David, D. S., Sakai, S., Shoji, H., Cheigh, J. S., Riggio, R. R., Stenzel, K. H. and Rubin, A. L. (1973). Ocular complications of renal transplant recipients. *Am. J. Med.*, **55**, 492

184 Posnanski, E. O., Miller, E., Salgnero, C. and Kelsh, R. C. (1978). Quality of life for long-term survivors of end stage renal disease. *J. Am. Med. Assoc.*, **239**, 2343

185 De Nour, A. K. and Shanan, J. (1980). Quality of life of dialysis and transplanted patients. *Nephron.*, **25**, 117

186 Jacobs, *et al.*

187 Wills, M. R. (1978). *Metabolic Consequences of Chronic Renal Failure.* (Aylesbury)

188 Parson, V., Bewick, M., Elias, J., Snowden, S. A., Weston, M. J. and Rooleck, C. H. (1979). Pregnancy following renal transplantation. *J. R. Soc. Med.*, **72**, 815

189 McGeown, M., Kennedy, J. A., Loughridge, W. G. G. *et al.* (1977). One hundred kidney transplants in the Belfast City Hospital. *Lancet*, **2**, 648

190 Morris, P. J., Oliver, D. O., Bishop, M. *et al.* (1979). Results from a new renal transplant unit. *Lancet*, **2**, 1353

191 Woods, J. E. (1976). In Munster, A. M. (ed.). *Surgical Immunology*, p. 93. (New York: Grune & Stratton)

192 Schippers, H. M. A. and Kalff, M. W. (1976). Cost comparison haemodialysis and renal transplantation. *Tiss. Ant.*, **7**, 86

193 Potter, D. E. (1976). In Lieberman, E. (ed.). *Clinical Paediatric Nephrology*, p. 442. (Philadelpha: Lippincott)

194 Scharer, (1971). Incidence and causes of chronic renal failure in childhood. *Proc. Eur. Dial. Transplant. Assoc.*, **8**, 211

195 Mauer, S. M., Kjellstrand, C. M., Buselmeier, T. J. *et al.* (1974). Renal transplantation in the very young child. *Proc. Eur. Dial. Transplant. Assoc.*, **2**, 247

196 Fine, R. M. (1979). Transplantation in children. In Morris, P. J. (ed.). *Kidney Transplantation*, p. 353. (London: Academic Press)

197 Fine, R. M. (1975). In Hamburger, J., Crosnier, J. and Maxwell, M. (eds.). *Advances in Nephrology.* Vol. 5, pp. 201–228. (Chicago: Year Book Medical Publishers)

198 Starzl, T. E., Marchioro, T. L., Porter, K. A. *et al.* (1966). The role of organ transplantation in pediatrics. *Pediatr. Clin. N. Am.*, **13**, 381

199 Belzer, F. O., Schweitzer, R. T., Holliday, M. *et al.* (1972). Renal transplantation in children. *Am. J. Surg.*, **12**,

200 Francis, V. R., Fine, R. M. and Korsch, B. M. (1970). Psychologic and social adjustment to extended haemodialysis and renal homotransplantation in 42 children. *Proc. Eur. Dial. Transplant. Soc.*

Index